A synopsis of

Infectious and Tropical Diseases

A synopsis of

Infectious and Tropical Diseases

A. W. Woodruff CMG MD PhD FRCP FRCPE DTM&H

Professor of Medicine, University of Juba, Sudan
Honorary Consulting Physician, Hospital for Tropical Diseases, London
Emeritus Wellcome Professor of Clinical Tropical Medicine (University of London)
London School of Hygiene and Tropical Medicine

S. G. Wright MB MRCP(UK)

Associate Professor, Department of Medicine,
College of Medicine, King Saud University, Riyadh
and Senior Lecturer, Department of Clinical Tropical Medicine
London School of Hygiene and Tropical Medicine

Third edition

WRIGHT
1987 Bristol

Published under the Wright imprint by
IOP Publishing Limited, Techno House, Redcliffe Way, Bristol BS1 6NX, England.

First edition, 1968
Second edition, 1978
Third edition, 1987

British Library Cataloguing in Publication Data
Woodruff, A. W.
  A synopsis of infectious and tropical
  diseases. —— 3rd ed.
  1. Communicable diseases   2. Tropical medicine
  I. Title   II. Wright, S. G.
  616.9   RC111

ISBN 0 7236 0826 1

Typeset by
Activity Limited, Salisbury, Wiltshire

Printed in Great Britain by
Billing and Sons Ltd, Worcester

Preface to the Third Edition

Since the second edition of this work was published international travel has increased enormously. In 1980 the number of travellers worldwide on scheduled air services topped 800 millions for the first time and included an estimated 270 millions of holiday visitors, many of them to tropical and subtropical regions. In Great Britain approximately 1 in 10 of the population have, during the preceding year, visited the tropics or subtropics. All practitioners therefore now need to have at their elbow a synopsis giving up-to-date information on the diagnosis and management of diseases with which they may be confronted by these travellers. It is the aim of this synopsis to fulfil this need.

It contains, in short compass, the essential information required by general practitioners, specialists, medical students and graduates preparing for higher examinations, the nursing profession and health workers in order that they may handle properly infective and tropical diseases.

The subject matter has been extensively and carefully revised and brought up to date. Therapy in particular has made many important strides forward in recent years. There are new sections on toxocariasis and several viral infections. The chapters on staphylococcal and streptococcal diseases has been almost entirely rewritten.

Dr S. Bell has now retired from practice and his place as co-author has been taken by Dr Stephen Wright. Dr Wright's experience as Senior Lecturer in the Department of Clinical Tropical Medicine, London School of Hygiene and Tropical Medicine; Consultant Physician, Hospital for Tropical Diseases, London, and currently Associate Professor at King Saud University, Saudi Arabia, makes him particularly well-equipped to have taken on the task and I am very grateful to him for the thorough work he has done.

I am also grateful to Dr P. W. R. Woodruff, MRCP, Lecturer in Medicine, King's College Medical School, London, for reading much of the manuscript and giving valuable advice and comments. Mr Roy Baker, Staff Editor to John Wright & Sons Ltd, has been most helpful at all stages in the production of this edition and my special thanks are expressed to him.

AWW

Preface to the First Edition

The increase in knowledge of tropical diseases in the past two decades has been matched by an increase in the number of doctors practising in the tropics, by the number of persons going from temperate to tropical regions and coming from tropical to temperate regions. These events are of course closely interrelated and their many results include an increasing difficulty in maintaining familiarity with the range of material in this field, and an increasing need for practitioners both in tropical and temperate regions to have available a small volume in which the essential knowledge is condensed. The aim of this book is to present that essential knowledge in a form in which it is readily accessible to the busy practitioner, to postgraduate students and senior undergraduates engaged in a study of the subject. For this purpose, Sir Henry Tidy was in former years able to include in his synopsis general medicine and special subjects in a single volume, but expansion of all these fields has rendered this no longer possible and infective and tropical disease have been placed together in a volume of their own. Extensive revision of Sir Henry Tidy's original synopsis has been necessary and much new material has been included in new sections, and many chapters are entirely new, but the original aim of presenting condensed readily available material has been adhered to. It is hoped that the volume may be found useful to practitioners in the English-speaking tropics and non-tropics.

We wish to thank Mr L. G. Owens for his invaluable help and inexhaustible patience.

AWW SB

Contents

Chapter 1

HERPESVIRUS INFECTIONS

Herpes Simplex

Commonly exhibited by bunch of vesicles on skin, most often of lips, nostrils or genitalia. Due to infection with *herpes simplex virus* (HSV).

Virus
DNA-containing herpesvirus.
   1. Infectious (contagious). Probably many people are life-long carriers.
   2. Transmissible to animals by conjunctival inoculation: results in encephalitis, transmissible in series. Thus is neurotrophic in animals. May be grown on chorio-allantoic membrane of chick embryo.
   3. Present probably in normal saliva. Acute infections lower resistance and allow it to act.
   Two distinct serotypes recognized: HSV1 causes lesions above the waist and HSV2 causes genital herpes. HSV1 transmitted by infected saliva, HSV2 by sexual contact or from mother to baby during childbirth.

Clinical Forms
1. HSV type 1
Common. Grouped vesicular eruption preceded by itching or burning sensation ('cold spots'). Also herpetic gingivostomatitis, and herpetic whitlow. *Usual site*: Nasolabial area. Any area may be affected. Tends to be fixed for a patient. *Associations*: Febrile episodes especially common cold, pneumonia, influenza, malaria. *Less common.* Recurrent herpetic keratitis. Eczema herpeticum. *Rare.* Disseminated HSV infection: pneumonitis; carditis; nephritis; encephalitis. Thought that HSV1 reaches CNS via sensory fibres of trigeminal nerve. Encephalitis severe but rare. 70% mortality. May be associated with impaired immune responsiveness. Neonatal herpes simplex encephalitis associated with HSV2 (q.v.). Diagnosis of encephalitis difficult: clinical — febrile patient with encephalopathy plus focal signs: CSF findings: raised protein and cells (lymphocytes), normal sugar. Demonstrate HSV in brain biopsy material.
2. HSV2
Common. 1. Primary genital herpes has an incubation period of 2–7 days. Initial symptom is burning pain at the site where the vesicular eruption will appear. Lesions appear on cervix, vaginal mucosa, labia etc. Vesicles rupture leaving painful, small ulcers. Lymphadenopathy occurs. Healing is slow but complete by 5 weeks. In the male lesions appear most often on the penis but the scrotum and skin around genitalia can also be involved. 2. Recurrent genital herpes vesicles appear after initial local burning discomfort in males and females. Inguinal

adenopathy occurs in recurrences. *Less common*. HSV2 viral meningitis. Young, sexually active and otherwise healthy adults. Usual symptoms and signs associated with meningitis. Raised protein and lymphocyte count in CSF. HSV2 usually grown from CSF.

Treatment

Acyclovir effective in HSV infections.

1. Initial and recurrent labial or genital infections. 5% cream applied topically 5 times daily (4-hourly) for 5 days. Start at the first symptom of recurrence. Tablets (200 mg each) may be given orally, 5 times daily (4-hourly) for 5 days.

2. Herpes simplex keratitis. 3% ophthalmic ointment. 1 cm ribbon of ointment put into lower conjunctival sac 5 times daily (4-hourly). Commence as soon as possible during initial infection and at first hint of recurrence. Continue for 3 days after healing complete.

3. Severe and disseminated HSV infections. Acyclovir 5 mg/kg 8-hourly by slow i.v. infusion over 1 hour. Modify dosage according to age and renal function (acyclovir excreted by kidneys).

Varicella-zoster Infections

Infectious Agent

Varicella-zoster virus, a DNA-containing virus of the *Herpes virus* group, causing either varicella (chickenpox) or herpes zoster (HZ).

Transmission

Person to person by direct contact, droplet or airborne spread of respiratory tract secretion in varicella. Also vesicle fluid from a patient with HZ. Scabs not infective. Varicella much more readily communicable than HZ. Patients with varicella are infective for others from usually 2 days (up to 5 days possible) before the appearance of the rash, up to 6 days after the appearance of the first crop of vesicles. Patients with HZ are infective for a week after the appearance of vesicopustular skin lesions. One attack of varicella usually prevents a subsequent attack but virus latency causes later herpes zoster.

Morbid Anatomy

Initial infection of vascular endothelium and then epithelial cells of skin. These swell and later are destroyed to form vesicle. Giant cells seen. Virus can be seen as intranuclear inclusions.

Quarantine Period of Contacts

Usually not required except for children in hospital. Contacts must be kept away from immunocompromised persons for 21 days.

Chickenpox (*Varicella*)

Symptoms

Incubation period. Ten to twenty days, usually 14–16 days. Limit 24 days. No infectivity under 10 days from exposure.

Stage of invasion. In *children*, usually slight fretfulness and anorexia. In *adults*, pyrexia, slight chill, vomiting, pains in back, usually slight, rarely severe and suggestive of smallpox. *Prodromal rash*, a general erythema, occasionally occurs. Initial symptoms often overlooked until eruption attracts attention.

Eruption. On first or second day. Fever does not disappear with eruption, but symptoms are slight throughout.

Order of appearance of eruption. Earliest on trunk, either back or chest. Rarely on forehead or limbs. Few spots in mouth at same time. No constant sequence subsequently.

Distribution of full eruption. Usually characteristic: (*a*) Trunk and scalp most affected; spots in axilla almost constant; (*b*) Face and limbs less so, and *proximal* portions more affected than distal. Few spots on palms and soles, often none. May occur on palate and other mucosal surfaces including respiratory tract, gastrointestinal tract and vagina. On scalp, hands and feet the vesicles are small and may be 'shotty'.

Character of eruption. Rose-coloured *papules*, changing in few hours into superficial *vesicles*, size of match-head. Contain clear serum No umbilication. Unilocular, and collapse on pricking. Firm, but more superficial than, and without shotty feel of, smallpox. Always discrete. Skin around normal, or slight red areolae. Oval spots present in groins and folds of skin. *Pustules* form in 48 h: later shrivel and form crusts.

> *Successive crops.* On subsequent days. Usually three in all.
> *All stages of eruption simultaneously present*, even among those of similar date in any area.
> *Number of spots.* Ten to several hundreds. Specially numerous in hollows and on protected surfaces.
> *Progress of eruption.* The progress of different spots usually varies; some vesicles may not become pustular:
> 1. Pustule remains unruptured, falls off in 5 days to 2 or, rarely, 3 weeks, leaving dry surface, no scar.
> 2. Pustule ruptures from scratching or injury. Thin crust forms, dries rapidly, scab falls in 1–3 weeks.
> 3. Pustule ruptures, skin around becomes inflamed, crust forms with suppuration below, falls off in 1–2 weeks. Surface ulcerated but heals rapidly. *Scar* often results. More common in children, especially on face.

Severity. Mildest cases in infants and most severe cases in adults. Inapparent infections rare. Immunosuppressed patients may get severe, disseminated infections.

Constitutional Symptoms

General disturbance depends on number of spots, amount of pustulation and ulceration. *Itching* may be severe and cause insomnia. *Temperature* 37·2–38·3 °C (99–101 °F); occasionally 39·4 °C (103 °F), as long as new lesions are produced. Falls rapidly. May rise again in second week with suppuration under crust. *Constitutional symptoms* rarely severe, even with the higher temperatures, except in debilitated subjects. In adults both eruption and constitutional symptoms often severer.

Primary varicella pneumonia major complication in adults (16% of young males with varicella). May be cough, dyspnoea, pleuritic pain in some patients. Signs usually minimal. X-ray shows diffuse nodular densities through both lung fields. X-ray changes clear shortly and may leave residual calcification.

Encephalomyelitis (encephalitis) is a rare sequel (1 per 1000 cases). Most commonly acute cerebellar ataxia beginning a few days after rash. Also meningoencephalitis, transverse myelitis, peripheral neuritis, Reye's syndrome.

Pyrexia, headache, vomiting and various nervous symptoms. Mortality very low.

Diagnosis
Usually simple. Characteristics are: (*a*) Order of onset of rash; (*b*) Distribution; (*c*) Successive crops; (*d*) Various stages of eruption simultaneously present—papules, vesicles and pustules; (*e*) Symptoms slight, but temperature does not fall with appearance of rash.

Where available electron microscopy of material from vesicles provides rapid and definite identification of varicella virus.
Variola. See Smallpox: Diagnosis, p. 61.
Impetigo contagiosa. Mostly on face. Mucous membranes not affected.
Herpes zoster. Definite distribution corresponding to nerve roots.

Treatment
For mild cases, no special treatment. *Itching*: sponge with warm boracic lotion, or dust with starch and zinc oxide powder. Prevent scratching. Warm bath hastens separation of scabs, but these re-form if separated too early. Treat secondary bacterial infections of skin or lungs with antibiotics. Acyclovir as for herpes zoster.

Herpes Zoster (*Zona; Shingles*)
An acute infection due to reactivation of latent infection with varicella-zoster virus (q.v.) in sensory root ganglia, characterized clinically by erythema, vesicles and pain in the cutaneous area corresponding to one, or rarely two, dorsal roots, and pathologically by inflammation of dorsal root ganglia. Factors precipitating reactivation are poorly understood: they include immunosuppression either due to disease such as Hodgkin's or drugs, irradiation of tumours of the spinal cord, heavy metal poisoning or treatment.

Those areas where varicella lesions are most numerous are most often affected by zoster.

Epidemiology
All races and both sexes affected with equal frequency. Incidence rises from childhood when it is uncommon to 2·5 per 1000, age 20–50. Peak incidence 10 per 1000 in those 80 and over. Incidence in immunosuppressed patients increased up to × 100.

Morbid Anatomy
Dorsal root ganglion: Necrotic, swollen and hyperaemic, with minute haemorrhages, and intense lymphocytic infiltration. Anterior horn and meninges may also show changes. In old cases, secondary glial reaction.

Symptoms
Onset. Pain and paraesthesiae in involved dermatome preceding eruption by several days. Fever, headache and malaise in 5% of cases.
Eruption. Commences with erythema about third day, then formation of vesicles. Commonest on trunk and unilateral. Distribution: area supplied from a dorsal root (partial or complete); appears first where cutaneous branch reached surface, and spreads to its termination. Vesicles commence to dry and scab from fifth to tenth day, leaving scars.
Occasionally. Lymph nodes enlarged, especially in axilla. Sensory changes, slight and variable. Paresis rare, e.g. abdominal muscles with corresponding segments: usually transient.

Herpes of geniculate ganglion. Vesicles in external auditory meatus; may also be on fauces. *Pain* in same sites as mastoid. *Facial palsy.* Loss of taste over anterior two-thirds of tongue.

Ophthalmic division of Vth nerve. Common in old age. Corneal vesicles may ulcerate: scarring results which impairs vision. May be IIIrd nerve palsy with ptosis and squint.

CSF. Increased lymphocytic and globulin content.

Sequelae
Postherpetic neuralgia, occasionally very severe in old people. Second attacks very rare. *Disseminated infections* in immunosuppressed individuals.

Treatment
Acyclovir, topically for corneal involvement and oral, 400 mg ×5/day for 5 days, reduces appearance of new lesions and virus shedding if given early. Intravenous infusions of acyclovir in immunocompromised patients with varicella-zoster infections. Does not affect occurrence of post-herpetic neuralgia. Analgesia used as necessary. May be intractable severe pain.

Epstein–Barr Virus

Glandular Fever (*Infectious Mononucleosis*)
An acute infectious disease caused by infection with the Epstein–Barr virus (EBV) in which EBV infects B-lymphocytes.

Aetiology
The EBV is a herpesvirus (DNA-containing). Infection with EBV is world-wide but glandular fever (GF) is only seen in populations where infection occurs in older children, teenagers or adults.

Epidemiology
GF occurs in areas of the world where housing, personal hygiene and socio-economic conditions generally are good. Peak incidence at 15 years in girls and 17–18 in boys. Kissing is the most common route of infection. This epidemiological situation has to be compared to that in the tropics where GF is not seen and infection with EBV is universal by the age of 10 years, probably the result of poor socio-economic conditions and the high frequency of oropharyngeal shedding of virus.

Pathology and Pathogenesis
Enlargement of lymph nodes, spleen and liver caused by infiltration with atypical lymphocytes which are cytotoxic T-cells and their local proliferation. The systemic illness in GF results from the destruction of EBV-infected B-lymphocytes by these cytotoxic T-lymphocytes sensitized to viral antigens on the B-lymphocyte surface membrane.

Incubation Period
4–7 weeks.

Duration of Communicability
A year or more after infection, 15–20% of young adults in N. America shed EBV from the oropharynx.

Clinical Features

50% of cases in young adults have typical features, 30% are asymptomatic, 20% have a range of symptoms e.g. upper respiratory tract symptoms, that do not suggest GF.

1. Pharyngitis: Common. Sore throat, fever, malaise and lethargy. Examination shows pharyngitis with cervical adenopathy. Greyish exudate on tonsils. Often petechiae at junction of hard and soft palate. Adenopathy at other sites and splenomegaly may be present. Self-limiting illness, resolves within 1–3 weeks. GF is commonest cause of pharyngitis in 15–20 year olds in USA.

2. Systemic upset with adenopathy. Common. Malaise, fever, sweats, headache. Diffuse tender adenopathy which may affect all groups of glands. Liver and spleen enlarged. Jaundice uncommon. Illness more marked and more prolonged with increasing age among adults.

3. Hepatitis. Fever, hepatosplenomegaly, adenopathy and biochemical abnormalities of liver function.

4. Miscellaneous features. Periorbital oedema, arthropathy, maculopapular rash (present in 80% of GF patients given ampicillin).

Complications

Neurological involvement (meningism, aseptic meningitis, encephalitis, Guillain–Barré syndrome). Splenic rupture. Haemolytic anaemia. Persisting post-GF lethargy syndromes (effort syndrome).

Laboratory Studies

Elevated WBC count with relative and absolute lymphocytosis. Atypical lymphocytes in blood films (>20% of lymphocytes). Heterophile antibody test (Paul–Bunnell–Davidsohn test) positive. Heterophile antibodies are IgM antibodies produced by polyclonal activation of EBV infected B-lymphocytes. They agglutinate cells of other species, e.g. rabbit erythrocytes. Specifically in GF this agglutination is abolished by absorption of test serum with ox red cells but not with guinea-pig kidney. Monospot test positive, this is a slide test for heterophile antibody. Note that heterophile antibody is associated only with GF. Specific EBV serology shows positive anti-EBV IgM or a rising titre to EBV in paired sera. Elevated transaminases common but elevated bilirubin uncommon.

Diagnosis

Cytomegalovirus infection causes a very similar illness with negative monospot and Paul–Bunnell–Davidsohn tests. Toxoplasmosis causes fever, adenopathy and sometimes hepatosplenomegaly. Toxoplasma dye test strongly positive. Tuberculosis, brucellosis, secondary syphilis, leishmaniasis, deep mycoses and lymphoma can all cause fever, adenopathy and hepatosplenomeagly and may come into the differential diagnosis.

Management

Symptomatic treatment. Analgesics and antipyretics. Steroids for severe neurological complications or haemolytic anaemia.

EBV and Malignant Disease

Burkitt's lymphoma: described by Denis Burkitt in 1958. A non-Hodgkin's malignant lymphoma occurring most often in children aged 5–7 years. Affects the jaw commonly but other sites including nervous system and ovary as well.

Distribution
Predominantly in holoendemic falciparum malaria areas, especially Africa and Papua-New Guinea. Occasional cases outside the tropics.

Aetiology
EBV was first isolated from Burkitt's lymphoma cell lines in culture. EBV genome is incorporated into host B-lymphocyte genome. High EBV titres in serum samples from affected children and in serum samples taken over the year before disease is apparent. It seems likely that there are additional promoting factors such as the immunosuppression caused by falciparum malaria and genetic susceptibility that act with EBV in oncogenesis.

Pathology
Tissue shows sheets of immature B-lymphocytes with large pale macrophages scattered through the tumour.

Clinical Features
Tumours of the upper and lower jaws. Abdominal lymph node masses, ovarian tumours, spinal cord compression and other neurological deficits including multiple cranial nerve palsies with deposits in the neuraxis.

Treatment
Combinations of cytotoxic drugs, e.g. cyclophosphamide, vincristine and methotrexate, are effective and cure a proportion of cases.

Nasopharyngeal Carcinoma
Common in Chinese populations in the Far East. Also in the Sudan, Tunisia and highland areas of Kenya. EBV isolated from tumour cells and high titres of anti-EBV antibody in patients. Cases usually present with cervical adenopathy and not because of the primary tumour. Diagnosis made histologically. Treatment with radiotherapy and cytytotoxic drugs.

Cytomegalovirus Infection (CMV)

A viral infection causing a characteristic syndrome due to intrauterine infection and features like those of glandular fever in later infections.

Aetiology
Cytomegalovirus (CMV) is a herpesvirus (DNA-containing) 150–200 nm in diameter. It is indistinguishable from other herpesviruses on electron microscopy. Infected cells develop typical, large intranuclear inclusions.

Epidemiology
Worldwide distribution. Infection is more common in those areas where accommodation is overcrowded and living condition are poor. About 50% of women of childbearing age are seropositive. Up to 7% of newborn infants excrete the virus making it a very common intrauterine infection.

Clinical Features

Congenital infection. Hepatosplenomegaly, jaundice, purpura, microcephaly, cerebral calcifications and choroidoretinitis are common features. Neurological damage is the most severe outcome of intrauterine infection with a considerable range in severity of the effects from, at one extreme, a vegetative state to impaired coordination, behaviour or speech at the other. Congenital abnormalities such as club foot, inguinal hernia, and squint are more common with intrauterine CMV.

Acquired infection. Can be very much like glandular fever with sore throat and generalized lymphadenopathy with hepatosplenomegaly. Petechial rash may occur. Pneumonic symptoms and signs can occur. Reactivation of latent infections can occur in immunosuppressed patients. CMV infection is common in patients with AIDS, p. 58.

Diagnosis

Congenital infection. Toxoplasmosis and rubella infection are causes of congenital infections which may produce a similar clinical picture. Microphthalmia, choroidoretinitis and hydrocephalus are often associated with congenital toxoplasmosis. Positive serological tests for toxoplasmosis with IgM antibody to the parasite suggest this infection. Cataract and the presence of congenital cardiac lesions suggest rubella on clinical grounds and serological tests confirm this infection.

Acquired infection. Glandular fever and toxoplasmosis are causes of a similar clinical picture. CMV causes most of the glandular fever-like illnesses that have a negative monospot test. Specific serological tests will distinguish between these three infections. CMV can often be isolated from urine.

Treatment

Most infections are self-limiting and the patient makes a full recovery after a convalescent period of variable duration. Steroids and antiviral drugs have been used in treatment but no firm recommendation for their use can yet be made.

Chapter 2　　　　# INFLUENZA

An acute infectious disease due to strains of virus characterized by sudden onset, headache, pains in back and limbs and pyrexia often complicated by involvement of the respiratory tract.

Widespread epidemics and pandemics occur irrespective of season, climate and race.

Epidemiology

A pandemic occurred in 1889–90. It commenced probably in Turkestan, and spread from East to West, becoming world-wide within 12 months. Epidemics recurred in 1891 and 1892, in the latter year being almost pandemic. In subsequent years, local epidemics occurred, but on a smaller scale. Epidemics are independent of personal, seasonal, and usual epidemiological factors. Often severer in young and healthy adults than in infants and aged.

Epidemic of 1918. Healthy young adults attacked. Cyanosis early and marked; pneumonia frequent. Mortality very high. Little variability in symptoms, and complications rare other than pulmonary.

Epidemic of 1957 was described as Asian 'flu.

Mode of Infection

Direct by droplet. Infectivity very high. Spread very rapid. One attack in no way protects, but the progress and cessation of epidemics suggest that a nation may acquire some immunity. The rapidity of spread depends on the shortness of the incubation period, universal susceptibility and the frequency of mild neglected cases.

Aetiology

Caused by viruses, the presence of which has been established in certain epidemics. Search for such viruses in other epidemics *clinically identical* have failed. Research is advancing rapidly. *H. influenzae* now known to be secondary invader, and with streptococci and other organisms to be cause of respiratory and other complications and fatal terminations.

Influenza virus. Belongs to the RNA viruses in the group known as orthomyxoviruses. Laidlaw and others, 1933, established existence of a virus, now known as Influenza Virus A. Ferrets inoculated nasally with filtrate of human influenzal garglings develop influenzal symptoms, transmissible back to man by nasal inoculation. This, like virus B is recognized to be a group of related viruses. These have been called 'A prime' viruses, and the type recovered in the 1957 epidemic (Asian 'flu) was distinct and is called A2. Type A tends to cause pandemics. Virus B, found in USA, has similar features but differs serologically and in pathogenicity to animals. Virus C has been found much less frequently and is medically insignificant. The influenza viruses have a considerable capacity for antigenic variation in the H and N surface glycoproteins which appear to be concerned with adhesion to cells and the release of virions respectively. Minor variations do not alter reactivity with antisera to the parent strain but the antigenic drift continues until cross-reactions are lost and then a new subtype designation is given.

Identification of virus

1. *Culture*: Nasal washings are inoculated into embryonated hens' eggs. Types A and B can also be grown in primary kidney cell culture. Virus is detected in allantoic or tissue culture fluid by haemagglutinating activity.

2. Virus antigen may also be detected in exfoliated nasopharyngeal cells or in sputum by fluorescent antibody methods.

3. Antibodies to virus can be detected using a range of techniques but the 4-fold rise in titre usually signifying recent infection may not occur in proven infections. Haemagglutination inhibition is the preferred serological technique in influenza diagnosis.

Virus vaccine: Animals can be immunized. Vaccines containing inactivated A and B virus used in humans give some protection for about 6 months.

Haemophilus influenzae (*B. influenzae*). Discovered by Pfeiffer in 1892: long held to be causal organism of influenza. Now recognized to be a secondary invader. Together with streptococci, pneumococci and staphylococci is cause of bronchopneumonia; essential factor in mortality from influenza. (*See also* p. 10.)

Morbid Anatomy

In fatal cases, inflammatory changes in the lungs are invariably present, most commonly bronchopneumonia: no specific lesions. In 1918 lungs were often slate-blue and haemorrhagic.

Quarantine Period
Five days is sufficient.

Symptoms
Incubation period. Uncertain. Probably 24–48 h. The symptoms are extraordinarily complex and variable, but certain types can be recognized: (1) Simple influenza, general febrile type; (2) Respiratory; (3) Malignant type.
1. General febrile type. Under this heading are described the general features commonly seen in an attack of influenza.
Onset abrupt. May be sudden vertigo.
Characteristic features: Chill (may be rigor). *Headache* severe, frontal or *back of eyes*: photophobia. *Aching pains* in back and limbs, of great severity when lying in bed. *Cough*: dry and distressing; *Temperature*: rises rapidly, but may be normal. *Prostration rapid*. Mouth, throat and larynx dry and irritable. *Drenching sweats* develop.
Physical signs: Few râles at bases: or nothing.
Acute symptoms usually last about 1 week.
The general febrile form may develop into any of following types, or these may dominate the symptoms from onset.
2. Respiratory type. May commence as simple form. After few days catarrh of respiratory tract increases and cough becomes severe. Infection progresses from larynx to trachea to bronchi, bronchioles, and to alveoli; may be localized to bases, If all lung affected, condition is very serious and mortality high.
Tracheobronchitis: this was a feature of the 1957 epidemic.
Bronchitis, Bronchopneumonia: Signs slight and atypical at onset: faintness of breath sounds and few moist sounds. Sputum may be frothy, pink, and very copious, or thick and viscid. Cyanosis early. *Radiographs*: may show numerous scattered shadow areas.
Pneumonia: Always serious; may be purely viral, bacterial or a mixture of the two. *Staphylococcus aureus*, *Streptococcus pneumoniae* and *Haemophilus influenzae* are usual pathogens.
3. Malignant type. Especially in large epidemics. Fulminating onset and course. Especially in the very young and elderly.
Toxaemia: Rapid and intense.
Cyanosis: 'Heliotrope' tint.
Fever: Varies, may be none.
Progress: Other symptoms slight. Rapid heart failure. Mortality high within few days.
THE HEART. May be especially affected. Myocarditis.
FEVER. Variable, no typical course, usual duration about 5 days; may last 3 weeks.
BLOOD. Leucopenia (4000–2000/mm^3) with relative lymphocytosis. Polynuclear leucocytosis occurs with complications, especially pulmonary.

Complications and Sequelae
There is almost invariably temporary depression of physical and, more especially, mental powers.

Patients may be left weak with marked lethargy after relatively minor exertion. Tachycardia and postural hypotension may occur. Purulent mucus may accumulate in paranasal air sinuses. Rarely among children after influenza B, or less commonly A, Reye's syndrome may occur in which encephalopathy is accompanied by hepatic failure. Epidemiological evidence of recent aspirin ingestion among some of these cases.

Diagnosis
During an epidemic, diagnosis is usually easy. In sporadic cases and small outbreaks, diagnosis frequently made solely by the extreme prostration in the postfebrile stage: often very uncertain. Culture of nasal washings or serological studies confirms clinical impression. Community surveillance warns of epidemics with new strains.

Prognosis
Mortality very low in absence of complications. With respiratory infections may be very high.

Treatment
General treatment. Confine to bed until temperature has been normal several days and *no râles are present in lungs*.
Drugs. There is no specific. Aspirin (0·6–1·0 g, t.d.s.) of most value and partly relieves pains. Paracetamol may be used instead of aspirin.
Chemotherapy. No evidence of effect on virus. Antibiotics are valuable in secondary bacterial pneumonias, flucloxacillin for *Staph. aureus*, penicillin for *Strep. pneumoniae* and amoxycillin for *H. influenzae*.
Oxygen. In all cases with cyanosis.
  Headache: Aspirin in 0·6 g q.d.s. or paracetamol 1·0 g q.d.s.
  Severe General Pains: Aspirin.
  Cough: For dry cough, steam inhalations (tinct. benz. 3 ml/l).

Chapter 3   *COMMON COLD (Acute Coryza; Acute Rhinitis)*

Acute inflammation of mucous membrane of upper air passages associated with the presence of rhinoviruses which contain RNA and belong to the large group of picornaviruses.

Aetiology
Distribution. Widespread in temperate and cold regions.
Seasons. Especially at changes of temperature, as in early winter and early spring.
Age. No age immune: children very susceptible.
Causal organism. Rhinoviruses are 25 nm in size, probably consist of several serotypes, and are readily spread by droplets from the oronasal cavities.
Infectivity. Varies greatly with: (1) Individual: marked idiosyncrasies; (2) Outbreak: schools and households often affected.

Symptoms and Signs

Initial stage. Chill, sneezing, head feels heavy, skin dry.

Nasal mucous membrane. *First Stage*: congested; unable to breathe through nose; duration 1–3 days. *Second Stage*: watery discharge; duration 2–7 days. *Third Stage*: mucopurulent discharge; gradually subsides. Chronic rhinitis may persist.

Inflammation often spreads to: (*a*) *Tonsils*: Sore throat, common initial symptom. (*b*) *Pharynx*: Swallowing painful. (*c*) *Larynx*: Voice husky. (*d*) *Ears*: Deafness from blocked Eustachian tubes, also otitis media. (*e*) *Conjunctivae and tear ducts*: Eyes 'run'. (*f*) *Oesophagus*.

Temperature and pulse moderately raised.

Smell, taste and appetite affected.

Extension to trachea or bronchi produces 'cold on the chest' (acute bronchitis). Herpes labialis occasional.

Treatment

No treatment is reliable to abort attack. Inhalation of steam from hot water to which menthol or Friar's balsam (tinct. benz. co.) has been added will relieve upper respiratory congestion.

Antibiotics are only indicated when a complication due to secondary bacterial invaders has occured.

Vaccine treatment. Not practicable because of the large number of serotypes.

Diagnosis

Measles commences with typical coryza.

Chapter 4   *MEASLES (Rubeola; Morbilli)*

Acute infectious disease caused by a paramyxovirus (RNA virus). Highly infectious; characterized by coryza, a skin eruption and catarrh of upper portion of respiratory tract.

Aetiology

Geographical distribution. Endemic and epidemic in temperate and tropical regions, but no zone exempt.

Epidemics. In Britain usually recur every 2 years. Periodicity was interrupted by World War II, but is now becoming re-established.

Season. In British Isles, mainly winter and spring.

Susceptibility. Universal. *Most contagious* of all fevers.

Age. No age immune. Infants under 3 months possess immunity transmitted from mother: rare under 6 months.

One attack protects. Exceptions extremely rare.

Morbid Anatomy

Nothing characteristic. *Bronchopneumonia* almost invariable in fatal cases. *Tuberculosis* may be a sequel.

Mode of Infection

Specific virus present in secretion of nose, mouth and respiratory tract. *Transmitted* by droplet infection via respiratory tract. 90% of susceptible contacts in close proximity to patient shedding virus will develop disease.

Duration of Infectivity

Contagiousness is especially marked in catarrhal pre-eruptive stage, probably greatest on first day of prodromal symptoms until 4 days after the appearance of the rash.

Quarantine

Ineffective in most cases.

Symptoms

Incubation period (to onset of prodromal symptoms). Usually 8–14 days; most commonly 10 days, viz. 14 days to rash. Limits, 7–21 days. No infectivity under 7 days from exposure to infection.

Prodromal stage. Period of invasion and catarrhal symptoms. Duration usually 4 days. Extremes 3–6 days.

  Onset of Symptoms: Usually abrupt, but may be insidious. (1) Coryza with sneezing and thin nasal discharge; (2) Redness of the conjunctiva and lids, lacrimation, often photophobia. (3) Pyrexia moderate, commonly 38·9 °C (102 °F). Diarrhoea in young children (especially in poorly nourished children in the tropics). Cough and voice hoarse, tongue furred. Patient thirsty, restless, and irritable. May be nausea or vomiting and headache. Occasionally epistaxis. Convulsions in severe cases.

  On Second and Third Day: *Face becomes puffy*: coryza, bronchitis and conjunctivitis increase, and appearance becomes suggestive.

  Koplik's spots now appear.

  Temperature commonly falls. A distinct remission of symptoms may occur and be deceptive.

  Mucous membrane of mouth and throat hyperaemic and dry.

  Laryngitis is common.

  Glands behind jaw frequently palpable.

  Prodromal Rashes: Occasionally seen. May simulate scarlet fever.

Koplik's spots. Minute white specks surrounded by red areolae on buccal mucous membrane, most commonly at level of lower second molar or milk molars. Numbers very variable; and distribution may be extensive. Areolae frequently absent, when distribution extensive. Appear usually on second day. Disappear rapidly after eruption comes out. Strongly suggestive but not pathognomonic (difficult to see by artificial light).

Stage of Eruption. Symptoms increase until fourth day, when the eruption appears.

  Order of Onset of Eruption: Earliest on temples, on forehead at margin of hair, and behind ears. Spreads rapidly in a few hours over face, trunk and finally limbs. Feet and hands are last affected. Maximum in 1–3 days. Amount of eruption varies, but some normal skin is always present.

  Character of Rash: Early stage: small brownish macules, disappearing on pressure; become papular and fuse. *Typical eruption* develops a few hours later: irregular blotchy, crescentic patches of erythema, dusky red; edges feel raised to the finger; do not disappear entirely on pressure. The rash fades with cold, and becomes more marked with warmth.

Progress: *Catarrhal symptoms do not subside* with eruption, but continue until fifth or sixth day. *Bronchitis* develops, scattered rhonchi and râles in lungs. *Laryngitis* common. Diarrhoea occasionally. *Fever* raises to maximum (40 °C, 104 °F) with appearance of rash. Pulse and respiration rapid. Dry cough. Restlesness and insomnia: may be delirium.

Duration of Eruptive Stage: Three or four days; rarely six. *Commences to fade in 24 h*, in order of appearance: may fade on face before appearing on limbs; last on hands, wrists, and feet. Brownish stain lingers. Desquamation of fine branny scales, varying with profuseness of rash: duration up to 10 days.

Temperature curve. In typical cases, moderate pyrexia on first day (38·9 °C, 102 °F); fall on second day (37·8–38·3 °C, 100–101 °F) rises to maximum at onset of rash (40–40·5 °C, 104–105 °F). Falls rapidly as rash commences to fade, and normal about seventh day from onset. Delayed by pulmonary or other complications.

Variations in rash. *Petechiae* occur with lice or cachexia: usually near joints. The typical rash, in areas where confluent, may resemble scarlet fever.

Convalescence. Rapid, *in absence of complications*. Usually no symptoms in 10 days from onset. Cough persists longest.

The Blood
Leucopenia with reduction in lymphocytes: some plasma cells but not constant.

Variations in Clinical Type
All are rare.

Mild forms. Catarrhal symptoms absent: convalescence by fifth day. Common in Europe and N. America.

Morbilli sine morbillis. Clinical symptoms without an eruption. Occurs in mild cases (rash may be transient).

Haemorrhagic measles (*'Black Measles'*). Rare, but occasionally in epidemics in tropics. Widespread haemorrhages of skin and mucous membranes, marked toxaemia. Death second to sixth day. Many epidemics of 'black measles' formerly described were probably erroneous diagnoses, e.g. smallpox.

Mortality
1 : 1000 patients in developed countries; in tropics up to 25%, though 1–5% usually.

Relapses
Very rare. Once in several thousand cases.

Complications
Severe complications are:

1. Bronchitis and Bronchopneumonia. *Bronchitis* is practically constant. Usually first evident during eruption. *Bronchopneumonia* serious and not uncommon, is cause of most deaths; convalescence slow. Pleurisy and empyema may follow. Rarely a giant-cell primary interstitial pneumonia in immunocompromised persons. Other respiratory complications: *Laryngitis*, mild form almost constant; severe form followed rarely be oedema glottidis, pseudomembranous laryngitis, or perichondritis (may be diphtheria). *Lobar pneumonia* rare.

2. *Stomatitis*. Mucous membrane of mouth constantly affected in some degree. May be severe ulceration: serious. Cancrum oris in malnourished children.

3. *Otitis media*. Not uncommon. Mastoid abscess, meningitis, etc., may follow.

4. *Diarrhoea*. Serious in debilitated subjects. Protein loss into the gut. May be chronic.

5. *Kwashiorkor*. In children likely to suffer from protein-calorie malnutrition severe kwashiorkor may be precipitated by an attack of measles.

6. *Xerophthalmia and keratomalacia* due to vitamin A deficiency in measles-induced malnutrition leading to blindness.

7. *Encephalomyelitis (Encephalitis)*. Rare complication. Sudden onset during or few days after attack. Fever, headache, drowsiness, or irritability: occasionally vomiting, hyperaesthesia, paralyses. CSF under pressure: cells increased. *Mortality* about 10%; complete recovery 25%; residual symptoms common. *Treatment*: Management of the comatose or excited patient, care of electrolyte and fluid balance, early appropriate antibiotic therapy of respiratory infection, and in serious cases possibly corticosteroid therapy.

Sequelae

Pulmonary tuberculosis not uncommon: high mortality. *Chronic bronchitis, bronchiectasis* and recurrent bronchitis. *Enlarged tonsils and adenoids*. Occasionally pustular eruptions. Subacute sclerosing panencephalitis (SSPE) is an ill-understood late sequela of measles. Behavioural changes, intellectual deterioration and motor inco-ordination. Death follows in 6 months. High titres of measles antibody in serum and antibody to measles in CSF. Measles-like antigen detected in brain.

Association with other Disease

Common with other specific fevers, especially diphtheria (serious), scarlet fever and whooping cough. Owing to these conditions being common at same age as measles, exact relations of their association are still in dispute.

Diagnosis

Koplik spots are earliest sign. Difficulty may arise with:

Scarlet fever. In measles: (1) Longer prodromal period; (2) Affects mouth rather than throat; (3) Marked catarrhal symptoms and conjunctivitis; (4) Rash: blotchy, crescentic, commences on forehead, and affects face; no circumoral pallor; (5) No leucocytosis; (6) Koplik spots strongly suggestive. Vomiting less common. Desquamation branny only. In anginose scarlet fever, rash on extremities is often macular.

Rubella. In rubella: (1) Shorter prodromal period; (2) Slight symptoms, eyes clear; (3) Occipital glands enlarged; (4) Rash discrete rose-pink spots.

Drug allergy. May suggest the rash of measles, but conjunctivitis absent.

Smallpox. Prodromal rash and early symptoms may resemble measles, and vice versa.

Prognosis

Immediate prognosis. Very low mortality now in Western World but still high in less privileged communities. *Bronchopneumonia* causes most fatalities. Highest in young children: deaths 20–50% (with antibiotics). *Otitis media*, diphtheria and diarrhoea may be fatal. Mortality varies with age, being higher in infancy and in old age, with poor social conditions and environment, and also in different epidemics. Epidemics among unaccustomed adult populations have caused enormous mortalities.

Remote prognosis. Pulmonary complications may result in chronic bronchitis, bronchiectasis. *Tuberculosis* not uncommon. Deafness from otitis media. Conjunctivitis, if untreated, may cause keratitis and leave opacities.

Prophylaxis
Prevention of spread difficult, owing to long prodromal period and contagiousness in early stages. Cessation of infectivity rapid: disinfection of room apparently unnecessary after patient's discharge.

Specific prophylaxis. Gammaglobulins: Passive immunization may be given (0·25 mg/kg) to protect certain at-risk groups, e.g. pregnant women, immunosuppressed patients (prevents measles if given within 48 h of contact and modifies measles if given within 5 days), but this is not practicable in the tropics where measles is most important.

Vaccines. Measles vaccines are safe and effective, giving protection that is probably lifelong. Maternal antibody may persist through most of the first year of life and so measles vaccine is given at about 9 months in the tropics and at 15 months in developed countries.

Treatment
Danger arises from the respiratory complications. Treatment aims at: (1) Avoiding complications; (2) Treating symptoms; (3) Preventing spread of infection.

Bronchopneumonia. On onset of pulmonary symptoms commence antibiotics, e.g. amoxycillin or co-trimoxazole.

Otitis media. Penicillin.

Mouth and stomatitis. Oral toilet.

Skin and rash. For itching: carbolized petroleum jelly. During desquamation, rub with oil.

Chapter 5   *RUBELLA (German Measles; Röteln)*

Mild, acute, specific infection due to an RNA virus in togavirus group, characterized by rose-pink papular or macular eruption, appearing early, by enlarged glands in neck and slight constitutional disturbance. Congenital defects in child may follow maternal rubella during pregnancy.

Mode of Infection
By direct contact (droplets). Moderately infectious. Adults often attacked. Second attacks extremely rare.

Duration of Infectivity
One week before and 4 days after the appearance of the rash.

Quarantine Period for Contacts
None.

Symptoms

Incubation period. Fourteen to twenty-one days: rarely up to 21 days; usually 17 or 18.

Onset. Slight malaise, headache, conjunctivitis and pyrexia.

Distribution: Commences on face, or face, trunk and arms simultaneously. Spreads to lower extremities in 24 h; often fading from face. Rarely, face free.

Character: Discrete numerous rose-pink spots; on trunk and limbs often coalesce rapidly, becoming indistinguishable here from scarlet fever. Occasionally macules form, but smaller than measles.

Duration: One to two days, rarely 3: disappears from feet last. Leaves slight stain: desquamation rare and slight.

Occipital glands. Enlarged and tender: less constantly, also posterior cervical and mastoid and elsewhere. Never suppurate.

Constitutional symptoms. Mild. (1) *Fauces*: dryness and slight redness. May be rash on soft palate. (2) *Temperature*: often normal: may rise to 40 °C (104 °F) for 1 or 2 days.

Polyarthritis has been a feature of some epidemics, unassociated with later joint sequelae.

Blood. Often many varieties of mononuclear cells, especially type known as Türk cells.

Complications

Arthralgia and arthritis self-limiting.

Diagnosis

(1) History and rash with cervical adenopathy. (2) Leucopenia often with many Türk cells. (3) Rubella virus may be identified early by a haemagglutination inhibition test, where laboratory facilities available. Differentiate from:

Scarlet fever. Rash may simulate scarlet fever on second day when faded from face and coalescent on trunk, but remains discrete on feet; constitutional symptoms slight; no circumoral pallor; no typical changes on tongue; no peeling.

Measles. No coryza, prodromal symptoms, or bronchitis: conjunctivitis slight; rash is brighter tint.

Glandular fever. Rash may be indistinguishable. Monospot test and Paul–Bunnell test may be of help.

Treatment

No special treatment necessary.

Congenital Defects due to Maternal Rubella

Congenital defects in babies may follow rubella in pregnant mothers (Gregg, Swan). Ascribed to virus damaging rapidly developing embryonic tissue. About 50% of women affected in the first four months of pregnancy will produce infants having congenital defects, falling to 20% and 4% in the 2nd and 3rd trimesters respectively.

Provisional conclusions

1. Incidence of defects is highest when rubella occurs in first three months of pregnancy and very rare after the fourth.

2. Defects vary. May be: *Cataract* (of unusual type)—apparently from rubella in second month; *Deaf-mutism* (rarely absolute); *Cardiac defects* particularly

persistent patent ductus and septal defects; *Mental deficiency*. Other defects recorded. Are usually small, poorly developed children.

  3. Acute self-limiting lesions such as thrombocytopenia, hepatitis, pneumonitis, myocarditis, encephalitis.

  4. Spontaneous abortion and stillbirths more common in rubella-infected pregnant women than in non-infected pregnancies.

Prophylaxis
Passive immunity. Gammaglobulin given in large dose (1500 mg) causes rise in rubella antibody in blood, but usual dose does not necessarily cause detectable rise. Nevertheless there may be some protective effect for fetus of mother exposed to rubella.

Active immunity. Natural infection in childhood protects, and damage to fetus in those growing up and becoming pregnant is prevented. Attempts have been made to produce attenuated rubella virus vaccine and antibodies develop in those vaccinated giving 95% protection. Spread of virus in the community from those vaccinated does not occur. Obviously the group who should receive such a vaccine are girls at about puberty. Very important to avoid giving vaccine to woman in pregnancy and pregnancy should be avoided for 2 months after vaccination.

| *Chapter 6* | **MUMPS** *(Epidemic Parotitis)* |

Acute specific infection due to RNA virus of the group of myxoviruses, characterized by swelling of salivary glands, especially parotids.

Aetiology
Widespread. Endemic in most towns. Large epidemics common.

Age. Mainly 5–15 years: infants rare: adults not immune. Probably many subclinical infections.

Season. Prevalent in winter and spring.

Morbid Anatomy
Degeneration of parenchyma; repair takes place without scar formation.

Mode of Infection
By direct contact, spread by droplets of saliva: exposure often very short but infectivity not very great. One attack protects.

Virus. Present in blood from fourth to ninth day after onset of parotid swelling. Grows in a range of cell lines from saliva of patient. Initial distribution probably systemic or neurotrophic before localization in certain secretory glands.

Duration of Infectivity
Virus isolated from saliva from 6 days before salivary gland enlargement to 9 days thereafter. Viruria for up to 14 days after onset of illness.

Symptoms
Incubation period. Twelve to twenty-five days, rarely 30. Usually 18–22 days.

Prodromal. Malaise for 1–2 days: often absent.

Parotid gland. Swelling and tenderness, commences *behind jaw and behind ear*, lifting the lobe of the ear: *spread forward over jaw and down neck* beneath sternomastoid; doughy: skin may be red; pain on opening mouth, varies with degree of swelling and tension. Papillitis visible at orifice of Stensen's duct. Saliva becomes scanty, and mouth dry. When severe, oedema of neck and enlarged cervical glands. *Unilateral at onset*; other side usually follows in 1–5 days. Facial nerve is never affected.

Submaxillary glands. Usually enlarged: occasionally without parotid enlargement. *Lingual glands* less often.

Temperature. About 38·3 °C (101 °F).

Blood. Initial leucopenia; returns to normal in few days. Lymphocytosis and monocytosis develop to moderate degree; may be marked in children.

Lymphatic glands. Rarely enlarged.

Duration. Glands attain maximum in 3–4 days: subside in 7–10 days. Relapses rare.

Complications
Rare, except orchitis, but sometimes severe.

1. Orchitis. Rare before puberty. In 20–40%, especially young adults. Onset about eighth day, with fever and malaise, swelling of one or both testes: occasionally urethral discharge. Duration 3–5 days. *Atrophy may follow*. In epidemics, cases of orchitis occasionally occur without parotitis. *Ovaritis* may occur: suggested by pain and tenderness in lower abdomen, and pyrexia.

2. Encephalomyelitis (encephalitis). Onset during or even previous to parotitis. Pyrexia, headache, vomiting and various nervous symptoms. CSF under pressure, clear, lymphocytes normal, glucose present. Mortality low. Very rarely, optic atrophy or nerve deafness.

3. Acute pancreatitis. Pyrexia, epigastric pain and abdominal discomfort. Rarely serious but may be obstinate. Diabetes recorded.

4. Parotid glands. Chronic hypertrophy. (Possibly connected with carious teeth or oral sepsis.)

5. Inner ear disease. Rare. Serious. May cause deafness, vertigo, tinnitus, vomiting.

6. Suppuration of glands. Extremely rare.

7. Mastitis occasionally occurs.

Various Rare Sequelae
Peripheral neuritis, paralyses, affections of special senses, nephritis.

Diagnosis
Simple. 'Bull-neck' of diphtheria gravis must not be confused. A septic parotitis may occur in conditions when mouth becomes dry. In glandular fever the salivary glands are not affected.

Where adequate laboratory help available virus can be isolated and haemagglutination–inhibition by mumps antiserum demonstrated. Antibodies in the patient's blood can be demonstrated,

Treatment
Rest in bed for 10 days at least. Mouth washes. *Diet*: jellies, custards and

semi-solids swallowed more easily than fluids. *Local to gland*: if very tender, hot or cold compresses as desired. *Orchitis*: rest in bed; support testes. Pain may be controlled with aspirin but sometimes morphine is necessary.

Prevention

Active immunity has been produced by live attenuated vaccine (freeze-dried). Immunity appears solid and long lasting.

Chapter 7   ROTAVIRUS INFECTION

Acute viral infection causing watery diarrhoea that is rarely fatal but may cause dehydration.

Aetiology

Virus is a 70 nm RNA-containing spherical particle.

Epidemiology

Worldwide distribution. Probably the most common pathogen causing dirrhoea in children < 2 years old, and second most common pathogen in older children. Can infect adults to produce acute watery diarrhoea. Occurs most often in colder months of the year in temperate parts of the world. Less seasonal variation in incidence in tropics.

Transmission by faecal-oral route from asymptomatic virus excreters to susceptible children. Infection is common in hospital nurseries and special care baby units where staff infect babies. Infected children may infect adults in the home.

Pathology

Jejunum mainly affected. Mucosa shows shortened villi with deeper crypts. Increased lamina propria cellularity. Patchy changes in the gut. Diarrhoea results from net secretion of fluid into the gut lumen. Stools contain 30–40 mEq/L of sodium and about the same amount of potassium. Diarrhoea does not result from accumulation of cyclic adenosine monophosphate (c'AMP) in epithelial cells (cf. cholera and enterotoxinogenic *Escherichia coli* infection). Damage to the brush border causes disaccharidase deficiency and disaccharide intolerance may contribute to diarrhoea.

Clinical Features

Incubation period about 48 hours. Mild fever and upper respiratory tract symptoms are common at onset, followed by watery diarrhoea. Vomiting is common and may precede diarrhoea. Anorexia is usual. Illness is self-limiting in most cases within 3–8 days. Dehydration more common and more severe than in diarrhoea due to other causes. Mortality is very low but fatalities occur, particularly in developing countries. Main findings on examination relate to degree of dehydration present.

Diagnosis

Fever, upper respiratory tract symptoms and vomiting at onset, together with watery diarrhoea, are suggestive of rotavirus infection. Diagnosis confirmed by detecting virus antigen in stools using enzyme-linked immunosorbent assay techniques (ELISA).

Management
Rehydration giving estimated volume of fluid lost over first six hours and additional fluids to replace continuing faecal losses and insensible and urinary losses. Oral rehydration solution with the standard WHO/UNICEF formula can be used (*see* p. 190) for all but the most severely affected who will require initial intravenous fluids. Fluids to replace insensible and urinary losses can be water, breast milk, tea, etc. but not oral rehydration solution so as to avoid the risk of sodium overload. Early attempts to replace fluid losses with oral rehydration solutions in the home prevent more severe dehydration developing.

Prevention
Attention to personal hygiene with careful hand washing before handling infants and food preparation. Boiling of water for drinking and storage of this water in clean, covered vessels in tropics . No vaccine available.

Chapter 8   ***ENTEROVIRUSES***

RNA viruses first isolated from the human intestinal tract in the course of epidemiological investigations of poliomyelitis. The family of viruses are called picornaviruses. They include:
1. Poliomyelitis viruses (*see* p. 23).
2. Coxsackie viruses.
3. ECHO viruses.

Coxsackie Viruses
First isolated (Dalldorf and Sickles, 1948) from two children living in the town of Coxsackie, New York.

Clinical Features
About 30 viruses are now included, classified as Group A with 24 subtypes and Group B with 6 subtypes.
1. Aseptic meningitis: Relatively mild illness of 1–2 weeks' duration. The CSF shows a plecoytosis of up to 100 cells/mm^3; and the protein content is normal or only slightly increased.
    Virus has been isolated from the pharynx and from the faeces of patients with this condition. May be either Group A or Group B virus.
2. Epidemic myalgia, pleurodynia, or Bornholm disease (epidemic myalgia, epidemic dry pleurisy): An infectious disease due to a virus, characterized by spasmodic attacks of pain affecting the intercostal muscles particularly. Abdominal pain when anterior abdominal wall muscles affected. Tends to occur in epidemics, usually in summer or autumn. Can be of any degree of severity.
           Virus: Coxsackie Group B viruses. Group A viruses and echoviruses will cause this as well. Mode of transmission virus probably enters through the gut.

Incubation period: Probably 2–8 days.

Symptoms:

Onset. Pain often initial presenting symptom. First spasm may be sudden and severe. *Prodromal symptoms*: Before severe attacks, short period of malaise and headache.

Constitutional Symptoms. Slight. Does not appear to be ill. No cough: moderate laryngeal congestion. *Temperature*: Usually raised for few days in severe attacks: in milder forms may be normal throughout. No enlargement of glands. Blood count within normal limits.

Pain. In spasms: extreme on movement, no pain on complete rest. Not affected by ordinary respiration. *Area*: centred on diaphragm; extends to muscles above and below costal margin and round to back. May be felt in shoulder. Muscles rigid, especially in abdomen: tenderness severe on pressure. Muscles may be swollen.

Rub. 25% of patients. May be very loud and coarse and unlike pleural rub: in other instances may be indistinguishable. No relation to pain, may first appear after spasms subside or on opposite side. Origin doubtful: probably in muscles and not pleural. Incidence varies greatly in different epidemics.

Lungs. No pulmonary symptoms, physical signs, or sequelae.

Note: Pleural effusion has followed in a few cases.

Course: Spasms subside after a few days, muscles may subsequently ache. Spasms may be absent for a few hours or a day, patient feeling well, and then return. Recurrences frequent. Milder forms may be ambulatory throughout and last several weeks.

Complications: Benign lymphocytic meningitis may develop: encephalitis less often. Further observations required.

Prognosis: Recovery complete, though pain may persist for several months.

Diagnosis: Mild forms often mistaken for muscular strain or fibrositis. With rub, diagnosed as acute dry pleurisy. Complement-fixation test with Coxsackie virus may be still positive after several months.

3. *Herpangina*: There is sudden onset of fever often with anorexia and dysphagia associated with sore throat. Some patients suffer from vomiting and abdominal pain.

The pharynx shows hyperaemia and, most commonly on the fauces, vesicles each with a surrounding red areola or small punched-out ulcers if vesicles have ruptured. These persist from 4 to 6 days after the onset of the fever. The illness is self-limiting but in some patients leucocytosis is probably attributable to secondary bacterial infection. Usually associated with Group A, B and ECHO viruses.

4. *Myocarditis in the newborn*: When the mother suffers from Coxsackie Type B virus infection there is the possibility of her newborn infant suffering from

myocarditis, of which the mortality rate in reported cases is high. There is some evidence to incriminate these viruses in causing myocarditis and pericarditis in older children.

5. *Hand, foot and mouth disease*: A febrile infection with blisters in the mouth and a maculopapular rash on the hands and feet, of short duration, usually ascribed to Group A 16 particularly.

Diagnosis
Clinical features are suggestive, and with special laboratory help viruses may be isolated from oropharyngeal washings, faeces, or specimens obtained at post-mortem in the case of myocarditis. In addition, neutralizing antibodies against the virus may appear in serum taken at intervals during the patient's illness.

Treatment
No specific treatment is known. Symptomatic treatments are used.

Echoviruses (*E*nteric *c*ytopathogenic *h*uman *o*rphan viruses)
These viruses have been isolated from respiratory tract in some patients, as well as from faeces. There are 26 strains in this group and these are known by Type numbers. Correlation of virus with clinical state is not yet complete, but following clinical conditions have been associated with echovirus infection:

Aseptic meningitis. Many possible causes for this but in some outbreaks echoviruses have been isolated, and in some due to ECHO Type 9 and Type 4 there has been a maculopapular eruption in patients suffering from meningitic signs and symptoms.

It is to be expected that much more information will become available about epidemiology and clinical illnesses associated with these viruses.

Chapter 9   *POLIOMYELITIS* (*Heine–Medin Disease; Polioencephalitis; Infantile Paralysis*)

Acute infection due to neurotropic virus with special affinity for anterior horn cells of spinal cord and corresponding cells of brain stem, and characterized by fever and paralyses. Many more inapparent or mild cases than paralytic cases, especially in childhood.

Distribution
Widespread in tropical climates. Sporadic cases in temperate regions. Epidemics may be extensive.

Season. Late summer and autumn, greatest prevalence. Epidemics diminish with cool weather.

Age. Great majority *under 5 years*. In environments of good hygiene and sanitation a greater proportion of sufferers are young adults.

Sex. Both sexes.

Virus
Poliovirus contains RNA molecule and is included in enteroviruses of picorna-
virus group. Virus of 28 nm in size now recognized to be widely distributed in
humans. Has been obtained from nasopharyngeal washings as well as from faeces
of patients and contacts. Types I to III may cause paralytic poliomyelitis in
humans; Type I most likely to produce paralysis. There are group antigens
common to Types I and II. While the virus is rapidly killed by drying it is resistant
to cooling and to many chemical agents though oxidizing agents act best against it.
Several studies have shown that a proportion of cases diagnosed as poliomyelitis
clinically are not caused by poliovirus but by other enteroviruses.

Mode of Entry of Virus
(1) Nasopharynx; (2) Alimentary canal. Virus isolated from pharynx of patients
5 days before and up to 7 days after onset of illness. Virus has been isolated from
faeces up to 3 weeks before onset of illness. Faecal excretion of virus continues in
most patients for 10–14 days from onset of illness, but after sixth week only 25%
of patients are still carriers, and very few at twelfth week. Transmission occurs by
the faecal-oral route.
Distribution in tissues. (1) Nasopharynx; (2) Intestinal wall; (3) Nervous
system—especially in anterior horn, grey matter of brainstem and cerebral motor
cortex. CNS involvement is believed to occur only in a minority of those infected,
and probably this is consequent upon viraemia.
 Transmission to animals: Monkey infected experimentally by inoculation of
virus into: (1) Nasal mucosa, also by insufflation; (2) Large nerve trunks
(paralysis commences locally); (3) Intracerebral and intradural. Rodents have
been infected by intracerebral inoculation of the Lansing strain.

Mode of Spread of Infection
1. Nasopharynx. Virus present in secretions for short period before and after
prodromal symptoms commence. The infection is most common in summer
months when opportunity for spread by the droplet route is least.
2. Alimentary canal. Virus in faeces: may be present several weeks before and
after acute attack. Virus present in numerous unaffected healthy contacts.
Spreads by close contact; person to person. Faecal contamination of milk and
food rarely involved.
Accelerating factors
1. Removal of tonsils and adenoids liable, during epidemics, to be followed by
   brainstem poliomyelitis.
2. Injection of irritants, e.g. DPT vaccine or arsenicals predisposes to paralysis
   localized in the inoculated limb.
3. Heavy physical exercise liable, during epidemics, to predispose to paralytic
   polio.
4. Transportation by air over long distances during acute phase has trebled
   mortality.

Development of Epidemics
Virus present in faeces of 2–10% of non-contacts in an area where polio is
occurring. Human adult serum contains antibodies in 80%: suggests previous
infection without symptoms and may explain comparative immunity of adults.
Estimated that only few per cent of infected persons develop symptoms (50% of

these developing paralysis), remainder constituting healthy carriers spreading infection.

An attack gives immunity against the infecting strain of virus, but second attacks, which are uncommon, may be due to infection by a different strain.

Immune serum. After infection, antibodies present for many years:

1. Neutralize virus when mixed in vitro.

2. Intraspinal injection into monkeys before or shortly after inoculation with virus usually protects, but has no effect if any symptoms have appeared.

Morbid Anatomy

Changes in nervous system are widespread, a poliomyelo-encephalitis, always more extensive than clinical symptoms suggest: thus, in fatal cases with paralysis of limbs, lesions are present in bulb and often in cerebral hemispheres.

Large motor cells of anterior horn and of grey matter of brainstem specially attacked: sometimes large pyramidal cells of cerebral motor cortex. White matter not attacked.

Lumbar and cervical swellings of the cord most affected.

Spinal cord. In anterior horn, ganglion cells show degeneration and necrosis; foci of lymphocytes and polynuclear leucocytes, phagocytosis active. Slight changes in posterior horns. *Blood vessels*: hyperaemia, perivascular 'cuffing' with lympho-cytes; haemorrhages, thrombosis and rupture. *Glial tissues*: foci of cells, reaction secondary to changes in nerve cells. *Meninges*: congested.

Brainstem. Similar but slighter changes.

Extensive initial paralysis is due to nerve cells temporarily paralysed but recoverable; lesser permanent paralysis is due to nerve cells destroyed.

Cerebrospinal Fluid

Early stage: Clear; *pressure raised*; *cells increased*, 40–2000/mm^3, polynuclear leucocytes usually predominate; globulin raised. *Later*: Cells mainly lympho-cytes; globulin very high. *Throughout*: Glucose and chlorides normal; fine coagulum on standing. Normal in 3 weeks. Virus absent.

In a small proportion of definite cases CSF has been reported normal.

Blood

Polymorphonuclear leucocytosis: about 25 000/mm^3 in febrile stage.

Clinical Grades of Severity

Severity of manifestations depends on degree of infection. Three clinical grades recognized:

1. *Subclinical infections*. No clinical manifestations but characteristic changes in CSF. Only recognizable in extensive epidemics. (Abortive attack.)

2. *Non-paralytic infections*. Clinical manifestations as in *pre-paralytic stage*, but lesions do not produce paralysis. *Note*: Changes in CNS are similar to those in paralytic forms but of lesser degree: it is incorrect to regard this grade as an 'abortive' attack.

3. *Paralytic infections*

Symptoms

Incubation period. Four to twelve, and up to 35, days.

Pre-paralytic stage. Short febrile illness of a few days' duration. *Note*: So long as fever is present extension of paralysis is possible. At onset indefinite, suggesting influenza. Gradual development of symptoms due to involvement of nervous system, but often recognized only after appearance of paralysis or during epidemics. Headache, irritability, vomiting, drowsiness (rarely coma). *Hyperaesthesia of affected muscles*. Extreme tenderness on being touched: may be absent. Stiffness of neck and back often early and important sign: no head retraction; stiffness tested by directing subject to touch knees with lips. Kernig sign positive. Jerky involuntary movements. Reflexes flaccid.

May be interval of remission and apyrexia before stage of paralysis; or progress may be continuous.

Stage of paralysis. Sudden onset. Characteristics: (1) Degree of paralysis increases to maximum usually in first 3 days and all subsequent change is improvement; (2) Paralysis is flaccid; (3) Distribution often asymmetrical, e.g. one leg and opposite arm. The commonest frequency of affected parts in order is: legs, arms, back, thorax, diaphragm.

Cutaneous sensation: Normal.

Reflexes: Absent in affected limbs.

Sphincters: Unaffected, apart from occasional, early, and transient urinary retention.

Pain: Unusual; may be severe. General hyperaesthesia ceases at onset of paralysis.

By end of 3 weeks, extent of the paralysis usually much diminished: reflexes may be returning.

Stage of recovery. Recovery of movement may continue for 3 months.

Spinal form

Distribution of lesions: Most common is one leg: next one leg and one arm. In lower extremity, extensors of hip, knee and dorsiflexors of ankle are most affected: and in upper extremity, muscles of the shoulder. Abdominal muscles not uncommonly in young children. Marked paralysis of trunk muscles rare, but may be sufficient to produce scoliosis during subsequent growth.

Course and permanent results. All permanent paralysis is flaccid. During stage of recovery and as child grows, permanent results become obvious: (1) *Small size* and shortening of affected limb (bones do not grow if many attached muscles are paralysed); (2) *Deformities*, especially talipes, flexed knee, occasionally scoliosis, lordosis, mainly from action of unopposed muscles; (3) Muscles wasted; (4) Vasomotor changes. Skin usually cold.

Brainstem form. Medulla specially affected, but also pons and midbrain. Preparalytic stage usually brief. Bulbar, facial, ocular and other palsies. Extensive lesions of lower cranial nerves rapidly fatal. In surviving lesions of upper cranial nerves may be residual facial and ocular paralysis.

Clinical types. Spinal and brainstem forms are accepted as true poliomyelitis. Numerous other types described are now believed to have other aetiology, e.g. polioencephalitis, cerebral, cerebellar, meningitic, neuritic and ascending forms.

Prognosis

Acute stage. Deaths result from respiratory paralysis, either directly or secondarily from branchopneumonia; hence rare when these muscles are unaffected, and usually within first few days. Mortality varies in epidemics: may be over 10%, increases with age. Absolutely complete recovery is rare, usually one or two muscles being permanently affected. A large epidemic (Baltimore) gave: Complete recovery 50%; almost complete 29%; marked paralysis 18%; deaths 3%.

Recovery of power

1. Severity of 'preparalytic' stage is no guide to amount of permanent paralysis.
2. Complete recovery is rare.
3. Usually maximum paralysis in first few days.
4. Recovery of muscular power may continue up to 6 months. Further improvement is due to training of muscles.
5. Any return of reflex, superficial or deep, in early stages suggests recovery in muscles concerned.
6. If faradic response is present within 3 weeks, muscles will recover.
7. If reaction of degeneration present in muscles, *prognosis serious*. The sequel may be: (*a*) Gradually complete loss of galvanic response, denoting permanent paralysis; (*b*) Slow return towards normal response, showing possibility of improvement.

Diagnosis

Difficulties occur mainly in: (1) Preparalytic stage—stiffness of neck and back, and the CSF are helpful features; (2) Infants, especially with hyperaesthesia; (3) Abnormal types.

In Acute Stage, diagnosis from:

1. *Conditions with pain in limbs* simulating paralysis, e.g. *scurvy* (a painful swelling) *rickets* (other signs present), *rheumatic fever* (never under 2 years), syphilitic epiphysitis, osteomyelitis, dengue.
2. *Meningitis and encephalitis*. By: (*a*) CSF; (*b*) No early flaccid paralysis.
3. *Guillain–Barré syndrome*. By: (*a*) Sensory changes, (*b*) Sphincter disturbances. Protein elevated in CSF, cells absent.
4. *Multiple peripheral neuritis*. May be difficult. Onset gradual: distribution symmetrical: some sensory changes.

In Stage of Residual Paralysis. In central palsies, reflexes are spastic and reaction of degeneration absent: wasting and lack of growth may be present.

Laboratory

Throat washings, faecal samples should be collected early: may be kept at 0–4 °C for a short period; may be mixed with 50% glycerol in physiological saline and frozen for longer storage.

Paired serum samples may be taken 10 days apart and tested for complement-fixing antibodies.

Prophylaxis

Use of vaccines. Vaccine (Salk) containing the three strains of virus inactivated by formalin may be administered in three i.m. injections each of 1 ml. First two are separated by interval of 1 month, and the third is given 6 months later. Duration of acquired immunity is uncertain, and it is wise to give booster injection at time of outbreak of poliomyelitis to which the subject may be exposed. This vaccine probably stimulates antibodies preventing viraemia, but does not prevent virus replication in the intestine. The antibody response to Types I and III was not uniformly good and in the 1960s paralytic cases were ocurring among persons who had received 2 or 3 doses of this vaccine. Newer vaccines of this type produce higher rates of seroconversion to all 3 types.

Orally administered vaccine (Sabin) extensively used. It is a live attenuated virus vaccine which multiplies in the pharynx and ileal mucosa, stimulating local immunity. Transmission of the vaccine strains occurs. Rarely causes poliomyelitis in unvaccinated contacts. Vaccinate whole family or individual members of vaccination status uncertain.

This vaccine, preferably stabilized by the addition of magnesium chloride, is fed in a sugar lump. Three doses are given: 6–8 weeks between first two and 6 months between second and third. Oral vaccine has been extensively used in N. America and Europe since the mid-1960s and has proved very effective. Vaccine-associated cases of poliomyelitis have occurred, very rare. Failure of vaccination in the tropics may relate to failure of 'cold chain'; vaccine must be stored under refrigeration.

General measures

1. Notify all cases of major illness, i.e. paralytic and suspected non-paralytic polio.

2. Barrier nursing measures as for a faecal transmitted disease.

3. Children with family exposure kept at home for 2 weeks.

4. Adult contacts may move about freely but observe rigorous standards of personal hygiene and avoid handling foodstuffs outside the family.

5. During an epidemic avoid injections and elective surgery, and insist on thorough rest for all cases of febrile illness. Vaccinate with oral vaccine.

Treatment

Acute stage. Complete rest is essential, and no electrical or other active treatment is to be attempted at this stage. No drug is known to act upon the virus. Treatment as for any acute fever. Retention of urine may occur. Special measures in use are:

Affected limbs: wrap in cotton-wool. For pain: immobilization, aspirin. Warmth can be applied to affected areas and analgesics given to relieve muscle spasm. Barbiturates are contra-indicated.

Paralysis of respiratory muscles. In severe cases of spinal poliomyelitis the patient must be nursed in a cabinet respirator of the Drinker or Both type providing intermittent negative-pressure ventilation. With improvement a cuirass type of respirator may be used. Later still a rocking bed which tilts patient regularly, causing movements of diaphragm by movement of abdominal viscera, may be sufficient to assist respiration.

In cases of bulbar paralysis maintenance of clear airway is essential, and while postural drainage and suction of secretions from pharynx may be enough, often tracheostomy required. Cuffed endotracheal tube is now used and positive-pressure respirator supplying oxygen or oxygen and air required for intermittent positive-pressure ventilation. Antibiotic cover, adequate nutrition, and care over fluid and electrolyte balance make these methods of treatment the work of highly specialized teams.

Paralysed muscles. Essential principle: Paralysed muscles must be kept in position of relaxation and never be allowed to be stretched, actively or passively. Limbs kept at rest and in position for 3 weeks by pillows, sandbags and celluloid splints. Stretching may result from: (1) Gravity, e.g. drop-foot when lying in bed; (2) Overaction of unopposed muscles; (3) Limb placed in wrong position. This principle is of greatest importance. Subsequent treatment is: (1) Massage, light effleurage; (2) *Passive movements*, patient also to attempt movements daily; (3) *Electricity*, galvanic current.

Surgical treatment. Often necessary later, especially tenotomies, and transplantation of tendons.

Encephalitis Lethargica (*Epidemic Encephalitis*)

Acute disease of nervous system believed to have occurred in epidemic form in Austria in 1916, in France and Great Britain in 1917, and in USA in 1918.

Thought to be a virus infection but this is not proved. Believed to be followed in some patients (possibly 25%) by evidence of damage to extrapyramidal system forming syndrome known as 'post-encephalitic Parkinsonism'.

Chapter 10   *RABIES* (*Hydrophobia; Lyssa; La Rage*)

Acute, fatal, specific disease of nervous system due to neurotropic virus communicated to man through saliva of an infected animal either by bites, or licks of abraded skin. Corneal transplantation from donor dying of an obscure neurological disease, in fact rabies, has also transmitted rabies.

Distribution
Widespread. Common in Russia and France. Not uncommon in USA. Rare in Germany. Eradicated from Great Britain as a result of quarantine of dogs. Australia free. *Note*: In 1969 reported that since 1946 eight fatal cases were confirmed in UK, infection in each having been acquired abroad.
Animals. All mammals susceptible to inoculation, also birds. Dogs, wolves and jackals most frequent naturally: cats, cattle, horses rarely. Foxes spreading rabies across Europe. Propagation almost entirely by dogs; also by wolves, jackals, camels, and rarely horses and cattle; in Trinidad and S. America by bats (*see* p. 32).

Morbid Anatomy
Confined locally at bite site for 4 h. Enters skeletal muscle cells where initial virus replication takes place. Enters nervous system via muscle spindles and eventually reaches CNS. Travels at 3 mm/h along nerves. Nervous system only affected but secondary effects on respiratory and cardiovascular systems.
Macroscopic. Congestion and minute haemorrhages may be present.
Histology. Pathological changes are few compared with severity of clinical disease. Several lesions occur:
1. *'Negri bodies'*, 1903. Bodies present within nerve cells, especially large cells of *cornu ammonis* (hippocampus major): shape and size variable, 1–25 μm. With Romanowski stains, are eosinophilic. With Giemsa, structure visible; within bodies are small granules.
Nature of Bodies. Similar to inclusion bodies in other viruses.
Method of Examination (William and Lowden). Make smear from brain tissue, fix and stain with Giemsa.
Value in Diagnosis. Are diagnostic.
2. *Babes's 'rabic tubercles'.* Collections of round cells around the large cells of motor area in cord bulb; chromatolysis and degeneration of the motor cells follow. Are not specific of rabies.

3. *Van Gehuchten and Nélis*, 1900. In the peripheral ganglia of the central and sympathetic nervous systems, proliferation of endothelial cells occurs, destroying the nerve cells; final appearance not unlike sarcoma. *Method of examination*: Remove plexiform ganglion of the vagus nerve; stain paraffin sections with haemalum and eosin. Animal must be allowed to die of disease. *Value in diagnosis*: *Absence* of these changes *negative rabies*: presence not quite conclusive, occurring rarely in old animals, but sufficient if symptoms suggestive.

The Virus

An RNA-containing virus in the rhabdoviridae, 180×75 nm. Rapidly destroyed by sunlight, ultraviolet light, formalin, alcohol and quaternary ammonium compounds. Killed by $100\,°C$ for 3 min. If freeze-dried, and stored at $4\,°C$ retains activity for several years. Is neurotropic. Present in all nerve tissues, and in saliva, reaching latter through autonomic nerves. Spreads from site of inoculation entirely by nerves and nerve tracts. Absent from blood and solid organs.

Strains of virus. Naturally occurring, called Street virus, is uniform in pathogenicity with long and variable incubation periods.

After several passages in the rabbit pathogenicity increases and the incubation period is reduced to 6 days. These properties become constant and this is called 'fixed' virus. The process of animal passage to produce fixed virus may be done in other animals, e.g. dogs, monkeys, guinea-pigs, cats. Fixed virus has low pathogenicity for man.

Flury strain isolated in 1939 from a girl who died from rabies is one mostly used for preparing attenuated living virus vaccine.

Symptoms

Incubation and frequency of disease vary with:

Age: Shorter in children.

Site of infection: In order: (1) Face and head most severe, from richness of nerves and lacerated character of wounds; (2) Hands; (3) Other sites. Clothes protect considerably.

Severity of wounds: Punctures and extensive lacerations most serious.

Animal: In order: (1) Wolf—40% bitten by wolves develop symptoms; (2) Cat; (3) Dog.

Frequency of disease after bites from rabid dogs: 16%, if untreated.

Incubation period. Most often 40–50 days. Earliest 12 days. Rare after 3 months. Up to 2 years. No symptoms. Wounds heal naturally. Three subsequent stages are distinguished; often ill-defined, and develop rapidly.

Premonitory stage. Site of bite often becomes irritable, with pains in its neighbourhood. Depression, desire for solitude, intolerance of loud sounds and similar stimuli, with periods of irritability. Attacks of great *fear*. Insomnia. *Voice* becomes husky, and *difficulty in swallowing* commences. Temperature and pulse slightly raised. *Duration*, 1–2 days.

Stage of excitement. Extreme irritability. Expression of terror.

Spasms: Great severity and pain. Evoked by any stimulus. *Larynx and respiratory muscles* first affected. Laryngeal spasms especially caused by attempt to drink, by sight, or even mention, of *water*. Spasms evoked by fanning air across patient's face. Contractions of larynx may cause unusual noises. Often extreme dyspnoea. Later, spasms more general. *Saliva* abundant and viscid, cannot be swallowed and hangs from mouth. Between spasms, mentally clear. Maniacal attacks may occur.

Temperature, often up to 39·4°C (103°F) rarely normal. *Pulse*, rapid. *Duration*, 1½–3 days.

Stage of paralysis. Paralysis spreads and spasms cease. Paralysis may be of various types, resembling, e.g. Landry's ascending paralysis, myelitis, or hemiplegia. Unconsciousness, cardiac failure, death. *Duration*, a few hours.

Total duration. Usually 4–5 days.

Clinical types. (1) Furious rabies as above; (2) Paralytic or dumb rabies. Latter is very rare in man. Stage of paralysis alone present. May occur with extensive bites. Diagnosis only possible by inoculation in animals: no Negri bodies. Possibly due to toxins. Common experimentally in animals.

Diagnosis

Clinical. Usually simple in man, but history of bite concealed sometimes, or, with long incubation period, forgotten. Diagnosis from:

1. Tetanus: Trismus; spasms not completely relaxed, nor specially evoked by water.

2. Acute bulbar paralysis

3. Lyssophobia, pseudorabies: In persons bitten by animals. Incubation period usually short. No temperature. Hysterical manifestations. Long duration.

Pathological. (1) Detection of rabies antigen by direct immunofluorescence in brain, skin or corneal impression smears; (2) Inoculation of some saliva or, after post-mortem, of brain or cord into mice or rabbit brain. (3) Rabies Fluorescent Antibody test allows detection of virus in brains of white mice in 24 h, or in HeLa cell cultures in 3 h.

Examination of animal. Dogs or cats should not be killed, but chained, supplied with food and water, and watched. If the animal is alive in 10 days the disease is not rabies. If it dies, perform autopsy and examine brain, preferably using direct immunofluorescence.

Prognosis

Invariably fatal if symptoms develop. Rabies in cases bitten by rabid dogs, 16% (without inoculation). Efficient, immediate first aid measures reduce chances of infection.

Prophylaxis

Muzzling of dogs and destruction of stray dogs, together with 6 months' quarantine of all entering dogs will prevent the introduction of rabies. Vaccination of all dogs using live attenuated virus vaccine confers immunity for 3 years or more.

Post-exposure Treatment

Wounds. Early and thorough treatment most important. Wash with soap and water and then with clean water to remove all soap prior to irrigation with either alcohol, iodine or 0·1% quaternary ammonium compounds such as Cetavlon. Necrotic tissue should be removed. Wounds should not be sutured immediately unless absolutely necessary. Tetanus prophylaxis should be commenced.

Indications for inoculation. (A) Dogs and cats (1) if healthy at time of contact and through 10-days' quarantine, no prophylaxis; (2) if healthy at time of contact but become rabid, give rabies immune globulin (RIG) and start vaccination; (3) if rabid at time of contact or state unknown and cannot be observed, give RIG and start vaccination. (B) Wild animal suspected of carrying rabies in that area give RIG and start vaccination.

Vaccines

1. Human diploid cell vaccine (HDCV). Now the vaccine of choice. Mild local reaction and no allergic neuroparalytic incidents. Dose 1·0 ml subcutaneous on days 0, 3, 7, 14, 28 and 90.

2. To allow the most economical use of HDCV in the tropics, antibody responses to 0·1 ml doses given intradermally being studied. Not yet in routine use. 0·1 ml i.d. at 8 different sites on day 0; 4 sites on day 7 gives good neutralizing titres even if rabies immunoglobulin used as well.

Rabies Immunoglobulin (RIG)

1. Horse RIG: 40 i.u./kg body weight. Half infiltrated into the wound and half given i.m. Test for allergy to horse serum first.

2. Human RIG: 20 i.u./kg body weight given locally and i.m. as above.

Symptomatic of Clinical Cases. Palliative only. Avoid all stimuli. Opium and chloroform to ease spasms. Rectal injections.

Rabies in Dogs

Two types:

Furious type ('Street rabies'). Stages practically correspond to human type. Early change in disposition, alternate excitement and desire for solitude, with increasing excitement. Voice alters, bark ending in *high plaintive note*: very suggestive. *Progress*: difficulty in swallowing food, not specially marked in regard to water. *Furious stage*: dog attacks everything, usually *runs straight*, may travel great distance. Paralysis and death follow. *Duration*: 4–5 days.

Paralytic or dumb rabies. Rarer. Early changes in disposition as above. No fury. Paralysis commences in jaw muscles, lower jaw falls; hence unable to bite, and less dangerous. Paralysis extends. Death in 2–3 days. Not uncommon in rabbits killed with 'virus fixé': also occurs in dogs in Turkey.

Paralytic Rabies transmitted by Bats

Distribution. Widely in S. America. Also formerly in Trinidad. Twenty-five of 36 species of bats in USA have been found infected. Bats appear to be true carriers, remaining healthy though infected. Possibly they cause the appearance of rabies in areas previously considered free.

Mode of transmission. By 'vampire bats' (*Desmodus rotundus*). Bat bites cattle usually and laps (not sucks) blood. Bite painless, often unobserved. Man is rarely bitten. Transmission via respiratory tract has occurred in persons going into caves with large bat population.

Incubation period. Fairly constant, 3–4 weeks.

Symptoms. Always paralytic type. Acute onset with pyrexia and malaise. Numbness and paresis of legs, commencing unilaterally. Ascending paralysis follows in a few days, fatal when respiratory muscles reached. Hydrophobic symptoms absent. *Duration*: 4–8 days.

Chapter 11   **ARBOVIRUS DISEASES**

A large group of viruses, all RNA viruses, some showing neurotropism, is transmitted by arthropod vectors. These are often termed arboviruses. They have been classified (Casals, 1957) into certain immunologically related groups:

Group A

Viscerotropic: Semliki forest virus. O'nyong-nyong virus.

Neurotropic: Western equine encephalitis. Eastern equine encephalitis. Venezuelan equine encephalitis.

Group B

Viscerotropic: Yellow fever. Dengue. West Nile virus. Russian spring/summer complex including Omsk haemorrhagic fever. Kyasanur forest disease.

Neurotropic: St Louis encephalitis. Japanese encephalitis. Murray valley fever. Russian spring/summer complex.

Group C. A group of about 70 viruses obtained from mosquitoes which possibly infect man though clinical features are not known.

Ungrouped

Viscerotropic: Sandfly fever. Colorado tick fever. Rift valley fever.

General Characteristics

1. There is no complete cross-immunization between the different viruses.
2. Viraemia occurs at some stage in the case of the arthropod-borne virus diseases.
3. Immunity of high degree and long duration characteristically follows infections. Second attacks very rare.
4. Virus infections in general do not respond to chemotherapy.

The more important of these are considered at greater length.

Group A: Viscerotropic

Semliki forest virus. Like some others has been isolated from mosquitoes; in this case in Uganda. No clinical illness in humans caused by it has been recognized, but neutralizing antibody against the virus has been found in the blood of a number of apparently healthy people in parts of Uganda.

O'nyong-nyong virus. An outbreak of a disease, characterized by joint pains (the name O'nyong-nyong is an Acholi word meaning looseness of the joints), morbilliform rash, and lymphadenopathy, especially affecting the posterior cervical glands, occurred in 1959 beginning in north-western Uganda and spreading across the country to the south-east, extending into Kenya. It is estimated that about 750 000 people were affected.

> *Clinical features*. Sudden onset often with rigor, sometimes with epistaxis, followed by symmetrically distributed mild to severe pains involving most often knees, elbows, wrists, fingers and ankles, and usually severe enough to prevent the person standing up.
>
> Morbilliform rash usually appears about the fourth day, and is most on neck and face, then down trunk. The palms but not soles are occasionally affected. The rash is itchy, and pruritus may be present where there is no rash. The rash lasts 4–7 days and then fades without desquamation.
>
> Lymphadenopathy is very striking and affects posterior cervical glands, but sometimes axillary and inguinal glands also. The glands are rubbery and discrete.
>
> Recovery is complete.

> *Transmission*. A virus has been isolated and has been identified in anopheline mosquitoes *A. gambiae* and *A. funestus*.
> *Treatment*: Symptomatic.

Chikungunya virus. Infection characterized either by a dengue-like illness, or by a haemorrhagic fever (the name, an African one, implies 'doubled-up' and indicates patient's posture).

Outbreaks recognized in Tanganyika (1952–3), Thailand (1958), Calcutta (1963).

Transmission of virus possibly among forest monkeys in Africa by *A. africanus, C. fatigans* and *Mansonia* mosquitoes. Patient-to-patient transmission by *Aëdes aegypti*. In Thailand the virus isolated from *A. aegypti, C. fatigans* and other mosquitoes.

> *Clinical*. (1) In Africa a dengue-like illness (*see* p. 45). Note, however, absence of orbital pain. (2) In East a haemorrhagic fever, chiefly in children, like dengue haemorrhagic fever (*see* p. 46).
> *Diagnosis*. Specific diagnosis only by virus isolated in tissue cultures and by inoculation into newborn mice.
>
> Serological diagnosis is obscured by cross-rections with Semliki forest virus and O'nyong-nyong.
> *Treatment*. Must be symptomatic.
> *Prevention*. As yet only by measures to eradicate the main vector (*A. aegypti*), and use of mosquito nets and insect repellents.

Neurotropic
Western equine encephalitis. Disease of horses and mules occurring in the summer in western USA. Epidemics in humans have occurred.

> *Clinical features*. Incubation period 4–21 days. Onset of headache, drowsiness, fever, followed by more definite signs of encephalitis: disturbances of speech, ataxia, nystagmus. There may be slight leucocytosis, and the CSF shows pleocytosis of 10–400 cells/mm^3, predominantly poly-morphs at first, later mononuclear cells. There is usually a slight increase in protein content.
>
> Most patients make a complete recovery. Post-mortem examination of those who die shows a diffuse encephalitis with perivascular lymphocytic infiltration.
> *Transmission*. Virus will cause disease in a large range of experimental animals. *Culex* mosquitoes, particularly *Culex tarsalis*, have been shown to harbour the virus in nature. A reservoir host of infection is not known, but fowls are suspected. It is thought possible that some other arthropod vector—mite or tick—may transmit the infection among fowls.

Eastern equine encephalitis. Disease occurring during the summer in the eastern and some southern states of America, and affecting horses. Outbreaks in horses may be associated in time with human cases, and mortality among these patients has been very high.

Clinical features. Usually there is an initial phase of illness with nausea, vomiting, headache and fever of 24–36 hours' duration followed by a period of improvement. The second phase is associated with high temperature, gastrointestinal disorder, and symptoms and signs of severe meningo-encephalitis. Most of those affected have been children, and patients who recovered from the acute illness have, in many cases, suffered from severe sequelae. However, neutralizing antibody against the virus has been found in the blood of people who have not suffered from the clinical manifestations of the infection, so that subclinical infections must occur.

Transmission. Virus seems to be more pathogenic than that of Western equine encephalitis, and the two viruses are serologically distinct. During an outbreak in Massachusetts in 1938 the infection was found in pheasants and a pigeon in the area, and pheasants have been found infected elsewhere. Virus has been found in species of *Aëdes* mosquitoes, and also in mites and lice which may infest fowls.

Venezuelan equine encephalitis is a virus infection distinct from the Western and Eastern types of equine encephalitis. It is especially a disease of horses and mules, but infections in humans have occurred in Colombia and Venezuela, Ecuador, Trinidad and Panama.

Clinical features. In laboratory workers who became infected the disease is mild and influenza-like: headache, fever, gastrointestinal upset, muscle pains and tremor sometimes with diplopia occured. It seems possible that man may aquire the infection by droplet transmission.

Transmission in nature is uncertain, though mosquitoes of the *Mansonia* group have been suspected in the outbreaks among animals.

Group B: Viscerotropic

Yellow fever (*see* p. 40).

Dengue (*see* p. 45).

West Nile virus was isolated from an African woman with a mild febrile illness by intracerebral inoculation of blood serum into mice. Neutralizing antibody against this virus has been found in the sera of people in various parts of Africa. *Culex* mosquitoes are believed to be involved in transmission, and birds may be the normal hosts of the virus. Serological surveys show evidence of a widespread infection: S. Africa, to Egypt, Israel, and S. India.

Russian spring/summer complex is a group of clinical conditions found in the Far Eastern parts of the Soviet Union, but sometimes also in northern Europe, due to virus infection transmitted by ticks. The disease appears most often in May and June.

Clinical features. Incubation period of 10–14 days, and sudden onset of headache, nausea and vomiting, photophobia and fever. Signs of meningoencephalitis will appear, particular neurological signs depending upon which part of brain or spinal cord is most affected. Flaccid paralysis of shoulder-girdle muscles is distinctive feature. Complement-fixing and neutralizing antibodies appear in the blood, usually 2–3 weeks after onset of illness. This infection results in antibodies which may show cross-reaction with the virus of louping ill, a disease of sheep but one in which humans are sometimes affected.

Transmission is believed to be by the bite of a wood tick of the group *Ixodes*, and Russian workers believe small mammals and birds may be natural reservoirs of infection.

Kyasanur forest disease. In 1956 a disease broke out in the south-western part of India in Kyasanur forest. A few months earlier numbers of dead monkeys were found in the forest, from the nose and anus of which blood was found to be oozing. On the bodies of live monkeys in the forest, many ixodid ticks were found.

Clinical features. Onset of the disease in man was sudden with fever lasting 5–12 days, headache and great prostration. There was usually stiffness of the neck and back, and about the third day of illness bleeding occurred from the gums or from the bowel. Among early cases mortality rate was approximately 28%. At post-mortem examination focal areas of necrosis in the liver were found. There was no encephalitis.

Transmission. Virus isolated from larvae and nymphs of *Haemaphysalis* species of ticks, and found to be closely related to the viruses of Russian spring/summer complex.

Neurotropic
Ilheus virus infection
1947 Virus isolated from forest mosquitoes in Brazil.
1962 Clinical infections described from Trinidad.
This infection has been demonstrated in Brazil, Trinidad, Colombia, Central America. Probably a short fever and antibodies develop. Possible that encephalitis may occur.

St Louis encephalitis. Virus infection causing encephalitis in epidemics in the summer, in central and western USA. Large outbreak occurred in St Louis and Kansas City, Missouri, in 1933.

Clinical features. Three clinical groups were described in the 1933 outbreak:
1. *Acute encephalitic.* Sudden onset with fever, signs of meningeal irritation, and then evidence of bulbar involvement with ataxia, tremor and difficulty with speech.
2. *Influenza-like onset.* Here there were prodromata like influenza for a few days before the more typical signs and symptoms of meningoencephalitis appeared.
3. *Mild and abortive cases.* These would normally not have been diagnosed, except during an epidemic, when CSF was examined.

Infants are more severely affected than older patients, and the mortality and the severe neurological sequelae are more in them.

Diagnosis is usually of some form of encephalitis, but only detailed studies to isolate the virus, or the demonstration of antibodies in the blood, can confirm the nature of the illness.

Transmission. Culex mosquitoes, especially *C. tarsalis* and *C. pipiens*, are believed to be vectors. Chickens and other birds are readily infected, and while their health does not appear affected they develop viraemia. Mites which feed on the birds have been found infected with the virus.

Treatment. Symptomatic.

Japanese encephalitis is a summer encephalitis caused by a virus, found in the Far East and especially in Japan. In 1924 an epidemic in Japan caused 60% mortality among 6000 patients, and since that time outbreaks have occurred each summer. True mortality rate much lower. Many more inapparent than apparent cases.

Clinical features. Incubation period probably 1–2 weeks.

Prodromata: for 1–4 days anorexia, nausea, gut symptoms, respiratory symptoms, headache and fever. A range of severity of clinical illness follows: mild with headache and fever to severe aseptic meningitis or meningo-encephalitis. Signs of meningeal irritation may be present with tremors, difficulties with speech, and sometimes convulsions. Spastic or flaccid paralysis may occur. This acute phase may last 2 weeks, and if recovery occurs it is usually complete.

Abortive type: All the signs and symptoms are transient, and in some people the only evidence of infection is the development of antibody in the serum.

Diagnosis. Blood may show polymorphonuclear leucocytosis, and CSF will show increased pressure with rise in protein content, and increase in number of cells most of which are lymphocytes.

Clinical diagnosis is of encephalitis, but special tests are necessary to define the cause. Virus can be isolated from CSF, and rising titre of antibody in serum may be demonstrable. Haemagglutination-inhibiting and neuralizing antibodies appear in first week and complement-fixing antibodies in second week. Paired serum samples obtained 10 days apart show rising titre, CSF virus-specific IgM detected by enzyme-linked immunosorbent assay are useful diagnostically.

Pathological changes. Meninges: congestion, perivascular cuffing and infiltration with lymphocytes and some polymorphs.

Nervous tissue: neuronal degeneration in basal ganglia, cerebral and cerebellar cortex, and horns of spinal cord. Typically destruction of Purkinje cells in cerebellum.

Transmission. Virus is a small one of the order of 15–22 nm. *Culex* mosquitoes have been shown to be capable of transmitting, and one species found naturally infected during an epidemic in Japan. Natural reservoir of infection may be chickens, or some common animals: horses, cattle, pigs, sheep, or dogs which may be found infected. It is of interest that before epidemics of the disease in Japan intense transmission has been demonstrated in nestlings in colonies of herons in that country.

Treatment. While there is no specific treatment for established cases prevention may be obtained by vaccination with a killed vaccine prepared from suckling mouse brain or tissue culture. In epidemics vector control by application of organophosphate insecticides.

Australian X disease. Also known as Murray valley fever, is probably due to same virus as causes Japanese encephalitis.

Ungrouped Arthropod-borne Viruses
Sandfly fever (*see* p. 52)
Colorado tick fever. Tick-borne virus disease found in some western states of America, particularly in Colorado.

Clinical features. Sudden onset of feelings of coldness with generalized aching of the body. Temperature rises rapidly and is sustained at about 38·9–40 °C (102–104 °F) for about 48 h. During this time there is headache, pains in eyes and backache. In addition there may be anorexia, vomiting, photophobia and hypersensitivity of skin. Pulse rate is increased with temperature. Remission then occurs for 2–3 days when patient feels well except for weakness. There is then a relapse with symptoms like those of the initial phase but which may last a little longer. Convalescence is slow. In children encephalitis can occur, usually mild, rarely severe and fatal. Main pathological finding is a leucopenia of 2000–3000 leucocytes/mm^3.

Diagnosis. Patient is usually an adult man who has been into wooded areas, and who has found a tick or ticks attached to his body some days before the illness begins.

The pattern of fever with its saddle-back form associated with leucopenia is suggestive. A complement-fixation test is possible.

Transmission. The wood tick, *Dermacentor andersoni*, has been found infected in nature, and transovarian transmission of the infection from the female tick has been demonstrated. The natural reservoir of infection, other than ticks, is the golden-mantled ground squirrel. A prolonged viraemia occurs also in chipmunks and porcupines.

Treatment. Symptomatic only. Second attacks do not occur.

Rift Valley Fever

Epidemic disease of sheep and cattle in many parts of Africa, from Egypt to S. Africa. Man is highly susceptible both to direct transmission and laboratory infections. Transmitted by mosquito; mainly *Culex theileri* and some *Aëdes*, having been found infected in nature.

Virus
60–75 nm in diameter. Survives at low temperatures but is killed by heating to 56 °C for 40 min. Can be cultured on a range of cell lines and in infant and adult hamsters, mice and rats inoculated intracerebrally or intraperitoneally. Virus may be isolated by injecting blood from a patient taken within the first 3 days of illness into the peritoneal cavity of a mouse. Typical lesions (focal midzone necrosis with haemorrhages) are found in the liver.

Incubation Period
Four to six days.

Symptoms
'Three-day fever'. Headache, nausea, rigors, muscular pains, profuse sweats. Liver may be tender. *Blood*: Initial leucocytosis; later leucopenia. Complete recovery is the rule, though fatalities occur in patients with haemorrhagic or encephalitic features. One attack protects. Neutralizing antibodies can be demonstrated by a mouse protection test.

Treatment
Symptomatic. Prevention by administration of vaccine to animals. A formalin-inactivated vaccine gave protection in man and further vaccine development is proceeding.

Bwamba Viruses

Bwamba virus isolated 1937 in Uganda, probably associated with a short febrile illness in man.

Pongola virus has been isolated from *Aëdes* mosquitoes in S. Africa, and *Mansonia* mosquitoes in Uganda. Antibodies have been identified in the blood of wild monkeys.

Bunyamwera Viruses

This group of viruses named and isolated as listed, have been shown by experimental infection in man to produce encephalitis which was not fatal. Vectors are not yet known and probably natural infections form part of the clinical picture of 'short fevers' in the tropics.

Bunyamwera virus reported from Uganda, S. Africa and Nigeria.
Ilesha virus isolated in W. Nigeria.
Germiston virus isolated in S. Africa.
Guaroa virus isolated from man in Colombia.

Argentinian Haemorrhagic Fever (AHF); (Junin Fever; O'Higgins Fever; Mal de los Rastrojos)

Virus disease occuring in epidemic form in Argentina and possibly Bolivia, with fever, leucopenia and haematuria.

Virus
Virus first isolated from patients 1958. Called Junin virus. Reservoir in a range of wild rodents esp. *Calomys spp.* which develop persistent inapparent infection.

Obtained from blood of patient between 6th and 10th day of illness and maintained in HeLa cell culture.

Injection by any route into 1–4 day-old white mice causes death of the animals in 15 days.

Junin virus is antigenically related to Tacaribe virus which was isolated from bats and mosquitoes in Trinidad.

Epidemiology
Epidemics in Argentina in May during maize harvesting. Sex ratio of patients, male : female 4 : 1. Man infected by direct contact with rodents or rodent contamination of food during maize harvesting in the fields.

Clinical Features
Incubation period: 8–12 days. Onset with chills, headache, vomiting, fever. Painless enanthem of pharynx characteristic. Exanthem. Conjunctival suffusion and injection; swelling of face, neck and upper chest. Progressive oliguria, dark urine with much protein, rising blood urea. May be tremors, delirium or stupor. There is marked hypotension (fluid leaking out of vascular compartment), and haemorrhages from mucosae, including haematuria. Death may occur with severe circulatory collapse. Polyuria heralds improvement.

Diagnosis
Easy during epidemics. Enanthem of pharynx is typical.
Blood shows marked leucopenia, with thrombocytopenia.
Urine contains protein, granular casts and characteristic cells with cytoplasmic inclusion bodies.

Virus Isolation
In newborn mice.

Serology
Antibodies detected relatively early using indirect fluorescent techniques.

Treatment
Replacement of fluid lost into the interstitial compartment. Immune plasma given in first 8 days of illness. Vaccine development is progressing.

Prognosis
Mortality in epidemics probably 3–4% but reported up to 30% in some outbreaks. Prolonged convalescence in those who recover.

Chapter 12   ## YELLOW FEVER
(International Nomenclature: *Amaryl*)

Infectious disease due to a flavivirus, transmitted by *Aëdes* mosquitoes, and characterized by jaundice, albuminuria, haemorrhages, especially from stomach ('black vomit') and slow pulse with rising temperature.

Virus

Yellow fever virus is small, 38 nm in diameter. Killed by mild disinfectants, ether and sodium deoxycholate. In frozen, dried state in vacuo survives 10 years or more.

Vectors

Jungle yellow fever. S. America: a cycle of infection between mammals, especially monkeys and probably opossums, and forest mosquitoes of the genus *Haemagogus*. These feed at midday on resting monkeys. Men clearing the forest by tree-felling bring down forest canopy mosquitoes which bite man and may cause sporadic cases. In shady coffee plantations *Haemagogus* species may occur and spread the infection indiscriminately to men, women and children (Rural Yellow Fever). *Sabethes* drought-resistant mosquitoes may maintain transmission in dry seasons.

Africa: Infection among monkeys and bush-babies (*Galagos*) is spread by *Aëdes africanus*. It lives at 50–60 feet above ground in the forest canopy. Infected monkeys raid plantations near the forest and may be bitten by *Aëdes simpsoni*, a day-time biter which may convey infection to humans. Virus isolated from *Amblyomma* ticks; significance of this uncertain as yet.

Urban yellow fever. Aëdes aegypti, a house-haunting mosquito, is the important vector. *A. aegypti* breeds in small collections of water around houses. Once infected it remains so for life (2–4 months). There is no transovarian transmission of infection in the mosquito.

Geographical Distribution

Endemic and epidemic in W. Africa, W. Indies, and S. America, including Brazil, Bolivia, Peru, Ecuador, Venezuela and Colombia. Occasionally imported into Europe, but no epidemics. Ships were specially liable to epidemics (from conveyance of mosquitoes and length of incubation). *A. aegypti* usually keeps to low altitudes with warmth and moisture, i.e. near sea coast and big rivers, and thus determines general distribution. Modern animal 'protection tests' reveal wide belt in Africa from W. Coast to S. Sudan; also 'jungle yellow fever' in S. America and in Africa. *A. aegypti* is prevalent in Egypt and India, but there is no source of infection. Freedom of India and Far East with susceptible population and suitable mosquitoes is remarkable.

Mode of Transmission

Principal factors:

1. *A. aegypti* conveys infection by bite after feeding on blood of infected persons.

2. An infected mosquito cannot convey infection until an interval usually of about 10 days (at high temperatures may be 4 days); virus possibly passes through some developmental stage.

3. Blood of infected persons becomes infective in incubation period and ceases after first 3 days of illness—due to development of antibody. Infection conveyed by subcutaneous inoculation of 1 ml or less of blood.

4. The fomites and clothes of infected persons never contain virus.

5. Immunity after attack persists throughout life; due to antibodies in blood. Relative immunity of those born and living in endemic areas is due to some degree of cross-protection from previous infection with related flaviviruses.

6. Epidemics. Commence about 2 weeks after primary cases, i.e. 12 days for development in mosquito, and 2 days in man. Epidemics require mean temperature over 24 °C (75 °F); cease in cold weather.

7. Virus. Present in blood, liver and other organs. Virus can possess two qualities, 'viscerotropic' and 'neurotropic': alterable by passage through animals; when both present, known as 'pantropic virus'.

Freshly isolated virus is pantropic. In susceptible animals causes severe infection and necrosis of liver. If passaged intracerebrally in monkeys or mice the neurotropic quality only remains. If given by subcutaneous inoculation it causes an antibody response but is not likely to cause severe disease.

Pantropic virus grows on chick embryo and slowly loses much of its viscerotropism but retains its neurotropism.

17D Strain: In 1928 Mahaffy isolated from an African named Asibi a pantropic strain which underwent chance mutation to give the 17D strain. This has lost its viscerotropism and most of its neurotropism. It is now used for vaccination since it stimulates antibody formation.

Morbid Anatomy
Cutaneous and visceral haemorrhages; stomach contains black blood; blood in vessels clotted.
Liver. Size about normal. Friable, red or yellow in colour and greasy in consistency, with loss of the normal lobular pattern. Microscopic changes (Councilman lesions) usually sufficient for diagnosis: (1) Lobules show mild infiltrate with mononuclear cells. (2) In mid-zonal region of lobules (less at periphery) cell changes are: (*a*) cloudy swelling and necrosis of hepatocytes; (*b*) eosinophilic degeneration of liver cells produces Councilman bodies and intranuclear, eosinophilic Torres bodies; (*c*) preservation of reticulin framework.
Kidneys. Haemorrhagic foci; fatty degeneration, cloudy swelling, and marked changes of acute tubular necrosis.
Spleen. Slightly enlarged. May show superficial haemorrhages.

Clinical Types
Mild. Previously recognized only in epidemics, but now by serum tests. Symptoms as in onset only: few days' pyrexia: jaundice may be absent; mistaken for malaria, etc. Probably constitute majority of cases.
Severe. As described below.
Malignant. Death in rapid toxaemia: symptoms slight.

Duration of Infectivity
Not exceeding 5 days from onset of symptoms.

Isolation
From bite of mosquitoes by mosquito net or screening on doors and windows for at least 5 days after onset of symptoms.

Symptoms
Incubation period. Three to six days.
Onset. Sudden, with rigor, often in early morning. Usual early symptoms: *severe headache*, often frontal, marked *prostration*, pains in back, rapid pyrexia, skin dry. Three stages are often distinctly marked.

Stage 1. Initial Fever. Duration 1–3 days. Temperature high from onset 37·8–41 °C (100–106 °F), remains steady or rises. Four important features are:

1. *Facies*: face flushed, eyes red and injected, may be icteroid tinge.
2. *Pulse rate* at first rapid; commences to fall with steady or with rising temperature; may continue to do so in following stages (Faget's sign).
3. *Albuminuria* early and increasing, with diminution in urine volume.
4. *Jaundice* shows in sclerae about third day. In severe cases ecchymosis may appear.

Other symptoms: *Vomiting*: first of food, then of acid and blood towards end of period. *Constipation*. Headache. Epigastric pains. *Pains* in body and limbs of varying severity; may be intense. *Tongue* remains clean at edges, but white fur forms on dorsum. Jaundice of skin usually commences at end of stage.

Stage 2. Stage of Calm or Remission. Duration 1–3 days. Change from previous stage rapid. Temperature falls nearly to normal, pulse slows further, and symptoms diminish. In mild cases convalescence may now set in. Rarely, anuria and black vomit occur: death then almost invariable.

Serious cases more frequently pass into next stage.

Stage 3. Stage of Reaction of Secondary Fever. Onset about fifth day. Duration a week or more. This is the critical period. (1) Temperature rises gradually to 40 °C (104 °F); (2) Pulse rate continues to fall, 40–60; (3) Jaundice becomes more pronounced; (4) Vomiting recurs with 'coffee-grounds' ('black vomit'). Tarry stools. Petechiae; (5) Urine diminishes, albuminuria increases. Abdominal pains. Prostration and weakness extreme.

In favourable cases symptoms commence to subside gradually about 8 days from onset.

In unfavourable cases: (*a*) Vomiting and jaundice increase; or (*b*) Suppression of urine occurs, with delirium, uraemic convulsions, coma, and death. Groups (*c*) and (*d*) often occur together.

Summary of Symptoms

Jaundice. Appears mildly about third day. May become profound in third stage. Liver not enlarged.

Temperature. (1) In first stage high from onset, usually 39·4–40·5 °C (103–205 °F); steady or rises. (2) In second stage falls to 36·7–37·8 °C (98–100 °F); (3) In third stage rises to 38·3–39·4 °C (101–103 °F); in favourable cases after about 3 days commences to fall by lysis, but in unfavourable cases usually rises continuously until death.

Pulse rate. On first day 100–110, then falls to about 75 at end of first stage. Subsequently falls lower, to about 50. *The falling pulse rate with steady or rising temperature is characteristic* (Faget's sign).

Urine. Onset of albuminuria usually early, even in mild cases. In second stage may be absent. In third stage as in severe acute nephritis; anuria frequent. Haemoglobinuria rarely.

Vomiting. In first stage, nausea and vomiting of food, acid, and blood. In third stage, 'black vomit', black fluid containing blood pigment. Amount very large.

Spleen. Not enlarged except with malaria.

Constipation. Stools not clay-coloured until late. May be 'tarry' from blood.

Mental condition. May remain clear. Delirium in severe cases.

Haemorrhages. Skin, mucous membranes, venepuncture sites.

Blood. Usually leucopenia without lymphocytosis. Clotting time greatly prolonged. May be hypoglycaemia and, in later stages, high blood urea. Bile present.
Transaminases elevated. Hypoglycaemia with severe hepatic damage.

Progress

Relapses are uncommon. *Convalescence* usually surprisingly rapid, and strength
returns quickly.
Mortality. Under good conditions should not be more than 15%. High mortality
among alcoholics and debilitated subjects.
Malignant form. All severe symptoms developed by third day. Delirium, extreme
toxaemia, rapid death.

Diagnosis

In early stages. Easy in epidemics. Leucopenia usual about third to fifth day. With
certainty only by animal inoculation: blood taken during first 3 days of fever,
intracerebral inoculation of susceptible mice with 0·03 ml.
In convalescence (or subsequently). By mouse protection test. If antibodies
absent in blood taken early in illness but develop later, the disease is yellow fever.
In fatal cases. By liver changes. If autopsy refused, small portion removed by
'viscerotome' through puncture wound.

Differential Diagnosis

Mild cases resemble infective hepatitis, malaria, or simple pyrexias. In epidemics
simple.
Blackwater fever. No headache, no falling pulse, haemoglobinuria constant,
haematemesis very rare.
Malaria. Protozoa in blood; enlarged spleen.
Dengue. Difficulty occasionally caused by coexistence.
Relapsing fever. Borrelia present in blood; enlarged spleen.
Leptospirosis. By laboratory tests. Leucocytosis. Jaundice often later in
appearing—about fifth day.

Control of Yellow Fever

   1. Immunization of all persons proceeding to or on entry to endemic areas.
   2. Quarantine of all non-immunized persons leaving endemic area: period 6
days, for India 9 days.
   3. Prevention of export of mosquitoes in sea, land, or air transport.
Aerodromes rendered 'anti-amaryl' (very difficult). Interior of ships and aircraft
sprayed with aerosol pyrethrins and DDT.
   4. Local elimination of *Aëdes* mosquito. *Aëdes* is highly domestic, living in
houses and depositing eggs in small collections of stagnant water: may be present
on ships and dhows. Mosquito surveys important. Larval control measures most
important. Adult mosquitoes destroyed by sprays.
   5. Provision of mosquito nets.
   6. Recognition and screening of cases of the disease. Early isolation urgent:
virus present in first 3 days of fever.

Active Immunization by Vaccine

Live vaccine used: consists of attenuated virus grown in chicken embryo, and
dried in vacuo: kept in sealed ampoules at 0°C (very sensitive to heat);

reconstituted with cold sterile distilled water immediately before use. One injection subcutaneously. Immunity probably complete by tenth day: India requires fifteenth day. International certificate valid from 4 days after primary inoculation and immediately after reinoculation for 10 years. Although live vaccine used, mosquitoes do not become infective after biting immune person.

Usually no reaction to vaccine: occasionally slight malaise about fifth day. Encephalitis reported in a few cases in infants under 1 year given the vaccine. Hence vaccination is best delayed until after this period. Pregnancy is a contraindication to vaccination. Yellow fever vaccination and oral polio vaccination should either be done at the same time or separated by 3 weeks. French workers have used neurotropic mouse-brain virus in association with vaccinia given by scarification. Some cases of encephalitis have deterred others from its use.

Treatment.
Intensive supportive treatment.

Chapter 13   **DENGUE** *(Break-bone; Dandy or Seven-day Fever)*

Specific infectious fever, lasting 6 or 7 days, due to a virus conveyed by mosquitoes, and characterized by severe pains, an initial fever, a remission, and a terminal fever and eruption, or by a haemorrhagic fever.

Geographical Distribution
In tropics and subtropics only. Largely related to the distribution of main vector, *Aëdes aegypti*. Mainly a coast disease, following trade routes, but epidemics reach considerable altitudes.

Virus
Virus is 50 nm in diameter. 4 types (1–4) showing antigenic overlap with viruses causing yellow fever, Japanese encephalitis, and West Nile fever.

Transmission
Aëdes mosquitoes, mostly *A. aegypti*, transmit. Man's blood infective for 18 h before and 3 days after onset of illness. Mosquito will become infective 11–14 days after the blood meal, and remains so for the rest of its life. Disease tends to occur in epidemics. Acquired immunity is type specific and life long. Subsequent attacks caused by infection with other serotypes.

Classic Dengue

Symptoms
Incubation period. Variable: probably 5–9 days.
Initial fever. Sudden onset: chill, severe headache and aching of eyeballs, *intense pains in joints and muscles. Temperature* 39·4–41 °C (103–106 °F), often maximum on first day. *Pulse* rapid: usual febrile symptoms. *Face* suffused, often

swollen; mucous membranes congested, causing sore mouth and conjunctivitis; skin erythematous; this general condition forming so-called *initial eruption*. Nausea and vomiting not uncommon (may be severe).

Period of remission. Between second and fifth day (often third) temperature falls, with sweating, cessation of pains in joints, and of headache, epistaxis often occurring: congestion disappears. May occur by crisis or less rapidly. Duration 2–3 days.

Terminal fever and eruption. Fever and pains recur, usually milder than initial stage; duration 25–36 h. *Eruption*: may be absent; earliest on palms and back of hands: later on trunk, thighs and legs. Commences as reddish, erythematous areas, fading on pressure, finally may coalesce; but varies in different epidemics, resembling measles or scarlet fever, and is not characteristic in type. Often persists several days. *Miliary desquamation* follows. *Bradycardia. Leucopenia. Total duration*. Usually 7–8 days.

Character of pains. Great severity. *Knees most constant site, also back*, but none immune. Localization of pain very difficult and cause uncertain: joint is not swollen, and can be palpated or moved passively without discomfort, but intense pain follows movement by patient: nor are muscles tender, though probably are cause of pain.

Convalescence. Protracted, from mental and physical weakness. Pains in one or more joints often occur intermittently for long periods.

Complications
Rare. Cervical glands may be enlarged. Rarely haemorrhages, orchitis, boils.

Varieties
Temperature typically shows 'saddle-back' curve. Inoculation experiments prove temperature may be continuous for 5–7 days, explaining certain 'five-day' and 'seven-day' fevers of tropics.

Mortality
Direct mortality nil. Debility resulting may predispose mental depression.

Diagnosis
In epidemics simple. Main symptoms are intensity of pains, period of remission, and terminal eruption. Diagnosis from:
Influenza. Occurs in cold seasons.
Malaria. Protozoa in blood.
Yellow fever. Jaundice, haemorrhages.
Rheumatic fever. Not epidemic; effects of salicylates.

Treatment
Symptomatic. Adequate time for convalescence is needed.

Prophylaxis
Anti-mosquito precautions.

Haemorrhagic Fever Caused by Dengue Viruses

Aetiology
Appears to occur in some individuals when experiencing a second infection with a

different serotype. Some cross-reacting but non-neutralizing antibodies seem to promote the growth of virus and may do this in the host to produce a high viral load. Haemoconcentration related to increased capillary permeability is a cardinal feature. Immune complexes and complement activation may contribute to this.

Epidemiology
Similar to that of dengue. Cases latterly reported from Philippines, Thailand, Singapore, Malaysia, S. Vietnam and Bengal. Usually only affects children.

Pathology
Thrombocytopenia and haemoconcentration (haematocrit by 20%). Hypotension. Low output state with cold, clammy periphery. Evidence of disseminated intravascular coagulation.

Clinical Features
Onset abrupt with nausea, fever, and on or about fourth day circulatory collapse and shock occur and last up to 24 h during which temperature becomes normal. Petechiae develop on second to fourth day, especially on face, extremities, and trunk. Slight melaena and/or haematemesis may occur.

Only rarely have haematuria, marked albuminuria, or oliguria occurred.

Diagnosis
On clinical features with confirmation by isolation of virus in sample of typical cases at regional virus laboratory. Blood inoculated intracerebrally into suckling mice or cultured; often difficult, isolation of Chikungunya virus easier.

Treatment
Symptomatic. Replacement of fluid depletion intravenously. Normal saline, Ringer's lactate, plasma or plasma expanders. Haematocrit or central venous pressure monitoring guide in fluid administration. Fresh blood or fresh, frozen plasma given to try to counter haemorrhagic manifestations.

Prognosis
Mortality rate 5–50%.

Chapter 14	VIRAL HEPATITIS

Condition produced by viral infection with one or at least 5 and probably more separate agents: (1) hepatitis A virus (HAV); (2) hepatitis B virus (HBV); (3) delta agent (δ), and (4) at least 2 separate organisms causing non-A and non-B hepatitis (NANB). These organisms are entirely separate from Epstein–Barr virus (EBV), cytomegalovirus (CMV), toxoplasmosis and yellow fever, all of which may damage the liver.

Hepatitis A Virus Infection

Aetiology
HAV is a 27 nm RNA-containing virus. Now grown in cell culture.

Epidemiology
Faecal-oral transmission. Less commonly via urine. Occurs world-wide. Specially common where personal and public hygiene inadequate. Common in tropics and subtropics. High proportion of cases subclinical, occurring in children. Cases in homes for the mentally retarded. Europe and N. America cases more common in teenagers and adults. Sporadic and epidemic cases. Relatively common cause of hepatitis among homosexuals. Pregnant women with hepatitis have a high mortality.

Incubation Period
3–6 weeks.

Duration of Infectivity
Latter half of incubation period and first 3–7 days after jaundice appears.

Pathology
Liver cell necrosis in a predominantly centrilobular distribution, multifocal throughout liver. Swollen, ballooned cells. Others shrunken. Variation in nuclear size. No fatty change. Reticulin undamaged except in fulminant cases which show collapse of reticulin. Variation in severity of hepatocyte damage; mild in subclinical cases. Cellular infiltrate of lymphocytes in portal tracts and proliferation of Küpffer cells. Bile thrombi obstruct bile canaliculi in cholestatic cases. Regeneration of cells from remaining hepatocytes. Does not progress to cirrhosis.

Biochemical changes in blood reflect liver cell damage. Alanine and aspartate transaminases rise during the prodromal phase. Enzymes released by damaged hepatocytes. Peak levels occur usually by the end of the first week of the icteric phase. Total and conjugated bilirubin levels rise in icteric cases. Moderate elevation of alkaline phosphatase. Prothrombin time prolonged. All changes revert to normal with resolution. Cholestatic cases show marked elevation of total and conjugated bilirubin and alkaline phosphatase. Bile readily detected in urine. Leucopenia seen in blood count. Atypical mononuclear cells may be found.

Symptoms
Prodromal features. Fever (up to 104 °F). Headaches. Shiveriness. Rarely macular or papular rash. Anorexia. Spleen enlarged in less than 20%. Symptoms persist for 5–6 days. Then nausea and vomiting at time of appearance of jaundice. Lethargy. Fever settles at this time except in fulminant cases.
Jaundice. Eyes yellow. Skin yellow. Urine dark. Stools pale. May be softer than normal. Pruritus in cholestatic phase.
Liver. Enlarged. Smooth. Tender.
Fulminant cases. Progress rapidly to hepatic coma. Liver small in cases with massive hepatic necrosis.
Anicteric cases. Elevation of transaminases after febrile prodrome. Serology for HAV gives diagnosis.

Course

Anicteric and most icteric cases settle rapidly within 2–4 weeks of the prodrome. A small number of patients have prolonged cholestasis which regresses spontaneously. High mortality in fulminant cases. Persistent hepatitis (PH) with elevated transaminases and normal bilirubin in a few cases. Settles spontaneously without sequelae. No chronic carrier state.

Diagnosis

Differentiate from other viral hepatitides, drug-induced jaundice (chlorpromazine, methyl dopa, isoniazid). Also paracetamol overdose in patients with impaired consciousness and liver function. Also infections: EBV; CMV; toxoplasmosis; malaria; leptospirosis; very rarely, yellow fever. Fever persists in those infections causing jaundice and deranged liver function. Defervescence occurs at the time of appearance of jaundice in viral hepatitides presently being discussed.

Confirmation

HAV infection confirmed by finding specific anti-HAV IgM in patient's serum.

Treatment

No specific treatment. Adequate rest to combat the debilitation. Normal diet but fat avoidance if the patient wishes it. No indication for steroids. Avoidance of alcohol for 3–6 months after hepatitis traditionally recommended. Management of fulminant cases requires maintenance of fluid and electrolyte balance; low protein diet; oral neomycin or lactulose administration; correction of clotting defects.

Prevention

1. Hand washing and adequate disposal of faecal wastes.
2. Prophylactic anti-hepatitis immunoglobulin (AHG) (0·02 ml/kg body weight) in short-term travellers (3 months or less) to tropics and subtropics.
3. Prophylactic AHG (0·02 ml/kg body weight) given i.m. as soon as possible to household contacts. May not prevent infection.
4. Active vaccination not available yet.

Hepatitis B Virus Infection

Aetiology

HBV is a 42 nm DNA-containing virus. Small spherical and tubular structures found in serum from infected patients represent excessive production of the HBV surface antigen (HBs) by infected hepatocytes. HBV distributed widely through body fluids: blood, saliva, semen, tears, colostrum, breast milk, serous fluids. HBV genome may be incorporated into host-genome.

Epidemiology

Predominantly spread by blood and blood products. Plasma infusions, transfusions. Needle stick accidents and minor cuts from used scalpel blades among medical, nursing and laboratory staff. Shared syringes in drug addicts. Numerous injections from same syringe and needle in tropics and subtropics. Instruments and needles used in ritual and medicinal scarification. Acupuncture. Tattooing.

Common among homosexual men. Transmission common in other situations where parenteral route seems less likely, e.g. homes for mentally retarded, suggests that HBV transmission via oral route occurs. HBV infection may result in a carrier state that can be lifelong. Marked geographical variations in carrier state: 0·1% of population in N. Europe, USA to 20% in Asia. Intrauterine or perinatal transmission occurs and may be a factor in encouraging chronic HBV carriage.

Incubation Period
45–160 days.

Duration of Infectivity
Blood infective for weeks prior to symptoms. Infectivity declines in most persons with resolution of illness.

Pathology
HBV-infected hepatocytes large with ground glass appearance of cytoplasm. Necrosis of hepatocytes is focal. Scattered through centrilobular zones. Severe cases may show a line of cell necrosis from portal tracts to centrilobular veins, (bridging necrosis). Lymphocytic infiltrate of portal tracts. HBV carriers may show chronic inflammation of portal tracts. HBV infection can progress to chronic active hepatitis (CAH); portal and periportal inflammation with piecemeal necrosis and loss of limiting plate hepatocytes. This may progess to cirrhosis and eventually to primary hepatocellular carcinoma (PHC). PHC is commonest cancer in males in many tropical countries with HBV as underlying cause. Cell-mediated immune responses may terminate HBV infection by destroying cells with virus markers on their surfaces and an aberration of this response may lead to continuing hepatocyte damage in CAH.

Symptoms
Prodromal features. 1–3 weeks before jaundice. Similar to HAV but less marked and more gradual in onset. Urticarial skin rash and arthritis occur occasionally. Prodromal illness more like HAV infection does occur.
Jaundice. Gradual onset. Biochemical features similar to those for HAV.
Liver. Enlarged, smooth, tender.
Fulminant cases. Uncommon. Progress to hepatic coma.
Anicteric cases. Probably common. Only detected by serology.

Course
Many more anicteric cases than icteric. Majority resolved with eradication of infection. HBV carrier state may last several months. Chronic persistent hepatitis; elevated transaminases, normal protein—no lasting sequelae. CAH elevated transaminases; raised globulin; piecemeal necrosis on liver biopsy (these features must be present more than 6 months after acute HBV infection); can lead to cirrhosis and PHC.

HBV Serological Markers
Hepatitis B Surface Antigen (HBs). Produced by infected hepatocytes. A marker of the presence of virus. Detected in acute or chronic hepatitis or the carrier state. Cleared in 2–3 months in uncomplicated cases.

Antibody to HBs (Anti-HBs). Appears with clearance of HBs. Associated with lasting immunity to reinfection with HBV only. HBs/anti-HBs complexes occur and cause vasculitis occasionally.

Hepatitis B 'e' Antigen (HBe). Presence highly correlated with infectivity.

Antibody to HBe (Anti-HBe). Presence indicates minimal risk of infectivity in patient who is HBs positive.

Hepatitis B Core Antigen (HBc). Antigen present early in the course of infection.

Antibody to HBc (Anti-HBc). Anti-HBc IgM indicates recent HBV infection. Found 2–4 weeks after HBs. Anti-HBc IgG indicates past infection with HBV (more than a few months before).

HBV Carrier State. Factors which predispose to this are infection at an early age; male sex; immunosuppression.

Perinatal Transmission. Occurs particularly where mother has had HBV infection in 2nd or 3rd trimester or within a few months of delivery. Intrauterine infection does occur but is rare. HBe antigen positivity correlates with risk of infection of infant. Anti-HBe positive mothers have a much lower infectivity. HBV infection rates may be as high as 70% among infants of HBe positive mothers. Prevention discussed below.

Diagnosis
Acute hepatitis, as for HAV. CAH: diagnosis lies between cryptogenic and drug induced (oxyphenisatin, isoniazid, α-methyldopa and nitrofurantoin), HBV markers usually indicate the association. Cryptogenic occurs most often in young females (LE cells present; antinuclear factor +, smooth muscle antibody +).

Confirmation
Detection of HBs and anti-HBc IgM in serum in acute hepatitis. HBs in CAH and carrier state.

Treatment
No specific treatment. Steroids contraindicated.
Acute hepatitis, as for HAV.
Fulminant hepatitis, as for HAV.
CAH: steroids of no benefit, cf. cryptogenic CAH where they are valuable.
HBV carrier: a variety of antiviral drugs and interferon currently under trial. No conclusive recommendations.

Prevention
1. Volunteer blood donors.
2. Screening of blood and blood products for HBV.
3. Single use of disposable syringes and needles.
4. Adequate sterilization of non-disposables.
5. Avoid accidental injury with blood-contaminated sharps among medical personnel.
6. Administer anti-HB immunoglobulin (anti-HBIg) to those who have had needle sticks etc. (0·04–0·07 ml/kg i.m.).
7. Avoid direct contact with body fluids from HBV-infected persons.
8. Vaccination: a vaccine derived from pooled, inactivated high titre HBs containing serum given in 3-dose vaccination schedule highly effective in evoking anti-HBs protective responses. Should be offered to groups at risk: patients

requiring multiple infusion (e.g. haemophiliacs); patients with immunodeficiency; patients and staff of haemodialysis, transplantation and oncology units; staff and residents of homes for the mentally handicapped. Other groups at risk of infection are workers in health-related jobs; male homosexuals; drug addicts; prostitutes. In those areas of the world where HBV carriage is common and PHC is common, vaccination would prevent this risk in susceptibles.

Note:
HB vaccine alone reduced perinatal transmission considerably (70% to 20%) to the offspring of Chinese HBe+ mothers. HB vaccine with a single injection of anti-HBIg reduced transmission further to 6% and HB vaccination plus monthly anti-HBIg for 7 months reduced it to 3%.

Delta-agent Infection (δ)

This is an agent capable of causing hepatitis only in the presence of HBV which has essential helper function for δ. δ can cause hepatitis in (1) a person with acute HBV infection; (2) a HBV carrier; and (3) in patients with HBV CAH. δ is associated with parenteral transmission. It probably has a wide geographical distribution, perhaps occurring with and paralleling the prevalence of HBV infection.

Non-A Non-B Hepatitis

Due to 3 agents at least.
(1) Parenterally transmitted: 2 agents; (i) Causes hepatitis after whole blood transfusion. Donors may have no history of parenteral exposure so parenteral is not sole route of infection. Causes anicteric and icteric disease of varying severity; can be fulminant. May progress to PH or CAH. (ii) Causes hepatitis in recipients of factors VIII or IX. Milder disease than (i). Range of severity of attacks. Can cause chronic hepatitis.

Evidence for transmissible agents: (i) parenteral transmission to chimpanzees; (ii) Prevention of transmission by treatments known to kill viruses; (iii) Absence of cross-immunity in chimpanzees.

(2) Enteral: Single agent so far. Convalescent faecal concentrates caused hepatitis in volunteer without evidence of HAV, HBV, EBV, CMV, etc. Epidemics in Asia. Waterborne transmission, possibly person to person as well. Range of severity. Higher mortality than HAV, HBV, EBV, CMV. Particularly severe in pregnant women, fulminant hepatitis and fetal loss.

Virus Identification
Not yet achieved for NANB.

Chapter 15   **PHLEBOTOMUS FEVER** (*Sandfly Fever; Papatasi Fever; Three-day Fever*)

Acute specific fever of short duration caused by viruses conveyed by bite of sandfly (*Phlebotomus papatasi*). Twenty-three viruses make up the phlebotomus fever serogroup.

Distribution
E. Mediterranean, India, Brazil, N. Argentina.

Mode of Infection
Infection conveyed by bites of sandflies. Sandfly infectious 6 days after biting infected man and remains so for life. Females bite at sunset and dawn in summer and early autumn and transovarian transmission of infection can occur in the fly. Males do not suck blood. Patient's blood infectious for 24 h preceding the onset of fever.

Symptoms
Bites cause papules with intense itching. *Incubation*: 4–6 days. *Invasion*: Rigor, severe headache, face swollen, conjunctivitis, photophobia, orbital pain and general pains. Bradycardia. Temperature 39·4–40 °C (103–104 °F), rising in 24–36 h for 3 days. *Crisis* on fourth or fifth day; may be accompanied by sweating, vomiting, or diarrhoea. *Blood*: early leucopenia; later polynucleosis. No eruption. No recrudescence. No complications. No sequelae, except some weakness. Never fatal. Severe cases may suggest benign lymphocytic meningitis.

Diagnosis
Clinically difficult, especially from dengue, also malaria and influenza.

Prophylaxis
Outdoor and indoor spraying with DDT. Small size of fly enables it to pass through mosquito netting: spray net with DDT. Repellent, dimethylphthalate to exposed parts.
  Since sandfly cannot fly above 3 m from ground an upper-storey bedroom protects.

Chapter 16   **HAEMORRHAGIC FEVERS**

Epidemic Haemorrhagic Fever (*Songo Fever;* *Nephropathia Epidemica; Korean Haemorrhagic Fever*)

Definition
Acute fever occurring in epidemics and characterized by prostration, proteinuria, renal failure and haemorrhagic manifestations.

Epidemiology
First received close attention by western observers during Korean war in 1951 but described by Japanese in Manchuria in 1930s. Particularly common in late spring and autumn among persons camping in fields, especially those near forests. Thought to be transmitted to man in virus-contaminated rodent excreta, but causative agent not isolated. Seems probable that Asian and European forms of haemorrhagic fever are similar infections.

Aetiology
Russian workers have reproduced disease in human volunteers by parenteral injection of serum and urine obtained from patients prior to fifth day of illness. Infective agent passes through grade N Berkefeld filters. Attempts to isolate the agent in culture so far unsuccessful.

Pathology
Internal organs congested and haemorrhagic. Kidneys swollen and haemorrhage limited to medulla. Skin, heart, brain, adrenals and serous surfaces most affected.

Clinical Features
Febrile period lasts 3–8 days and limbs ache and loin pain common. As fever defervesces, haemorrhages and proteinuria develop and clinical condition deteriorates. Hypotension and shock-like condition supervene. Haematocrit increases as fluid enters tissues; nausea, backache and abdominal pain become severe as result of local oedema. Proteinuria increases.

Stage of oliguria and renal failure follows and as fluid returns from tisues to plasma haematocrit decreases, lasts 3–5 days and death not uncommon at this time.

If patient recovers, diuresis occurs. Potassium deficiency and hypernatraemia may develop. Patients often very dehydrated.

Secondary infections, especially of lung bases, not uncommon.

Diagnosis
On clinical features. Serological (IF) test using lung of infected Apodemus as antigen.

Prognosis
In different outbreaks fatality rate varies from 2 to 5%.

Treatment
Symptomatic. Careful regulation of fluid and electrolyte balance. Nutritional support. Circulatory support as needed.

Omsk Haemorrhagic Fever and Kyasanur Forest Disease

Epidemiology
These diseases are conveyed to man by ticks from wild vertebrate hosts. Vectors of Omsk haemorrhagic fever are *Dermacentor pictus* and *D. marginatus*, but vertebrate hosts not identified. Kyasanur forest disease thought to be conveyed by *Haemaphysalis spinigera* and the reservoirs include monkeys in the region, especially langurs and bonnet monkeys, various birds and rodents. Latter thought to be those most important for transmission to man.

Aetiology
Both diseases caused by arboviruses of group B. They are closely related to Russian spring-summer encephalitis which is also a tick-borne group B arbovirus infection.

Pathology, Clinical Features and Treatment
Similar to epidemic haemorrhagic fever but alimentary tract more markedly
involved. Haemorrhagic manifestations often develop during a second febrile
period which follows an afebrile interval.

Lassa Fever

Definition
An acute and sometimes very severe infection with Lassa virus which is an
arenavirus.

Aetiology
The virus is of the RNA type, of diameter 110 nm and contains a number of
granules from which the group takes its name (arenosus, Latin, sandy). The first
described member of the group is the virus of lymphocytic choriomeningitis which
has been known for many years and is of widespread distribution. Lassa virus is
limited to West Africa; all other members of the areno group have only been
found in the Americas.

Epidemiology
The only animal known to be a reservoir of infection in nature is the
multimammate rat *Mastomys natalensis*. This rat is widely distributed in tropical
Africa. Initial infections of Lassa fever in man result from *Mastomys* entering
dwellings and contaminating food. From the index case the virus is transmitted in
body secretions, particularly vomit, urine and faeces. Droplet spread appears to
be relatively uncommon. Subclinical and mild cases can occur and exceed
numbers of severe cases.

Pathology
Virtually all tissues of body contain small foci of necrosis surrounding which there
is little or no inflammatory change. Inclusion bodies not uncommon in damaged
cells.
Shock. Increased capillary permeability is associated with shock, hypotension,
oliguria and peripheral vasoconstriction. Renal changes minimal.
Haemorrhagic changes. Usually slight.

Clinical Features
Onset. Incubation period 5–17 days. Insidious over 2 or 3 days with increasing
malaise and often a sore throat. Aching of limbs usually severe.
Established disease. Marked by prostration usually more severe than the degree
of fever would suggest though temperature often rises to 40 °C. Erosions usually
present on pharynx and sometimes a gelatinous adherent membrane. Nausea,
diarrhoea and vomiting common. Localized haemorrhages occur in skin of those
more severely affected. Pulse at first slow but later tachycardia supervenes and
results from myocardial damage. Oliguria may occur. In those who recover some
degree of nerve deafness and dizziness from labyrinthine damage may occur.

Diagnosis
Suspect Lassa fever in patients with pyrexia for which malaria has been excluded

as a cause and who are in or who have been in West Africa within the preceding three weeks. Particularly suspect in those severely ill.

Immunological diagnosis. Antibodies, detectable by complement-fixing and fluorescent techniques appear at the end of the second week of illness or in the case of the fluorescent antibody test even earlier than this.

Virus isolation. In Vero cell cultures after 72 h.

The highest degree of laboratory security is necessary before work can be done with Lassa virus and currently only the laboratory at the CDC Atlanta, Georgia, USA and the Microbiological Research Establishment, Porton, England are working with this virus. Specimens of blood, urine, faeces for diagnosis should be collected and transmitted to one of these centres with maximal security.

Management

Patients to be isolated with maximal security and attendants to wear fully protective clothing, masks and gloves. Plasma from a patient who has recovered from the disease may aid recovery. Criteria for use not well defined, serum glutamic oxaloacetic transaminase 3 times normal is one indication. Treatment with interferon may be tried.

Full supportive measures for shocked and dehydrated patients necessary.

Virus may continue to be secreted in urine and faeces for up to five or six weeks following clinical recovery.

Haemorrhagic Fevers of South America

Aetiology and Epidemiology

This group is caused by related viruses now designated arenaviruses of which the first described was from the Argentine and named Junin virus. In Bolivia, Machupo virus is causative factor. Both related to Tacaribe virus isolated from bats in Trinidad and to other members of the areno group recently identified in S. and Central America, i.e. Ampari, Pichinde, Panama, Tamiami and Latino.

Pathology

Bolivian haemorrhagic fever (BHF): widespread reticulo-endothelial cell proliferation. Eosinophilic inclusion bodies in Küpffer cells and free in sinusoids. Haemorrhages in gut wall and CNS. Argentinian haemorrhagic fever (AHF): focal liver necrosis. Küpffer cell hyperplasia. Renal tubular necrosis.

Clinical Features

Petechial haemorrhages appear on or about fourth day of initial fever. Hypotensive phase commences on sixth to eighth day, at which time temperature becomes normal.

Neurological complications not uncommon and include tremor, delirium and convulsions.

Diagnosis

BHF: virus isolation difficult, serological diagnosis in 20% of proven cases. AHF: virus isolation in newborn white mice, and in a range of cell lines. Serological testing with indirect immunofluorescent test.

Prognosis
Serious. Up to 20% mortality.

Treatment
As for epidemic haemorrhagic fever.
(*See also* Haemorrhagic Fever caused by Dengue Viruses, p. 46.)

Chapter 17   **MARBURG AND EBOLA VIRUS INFECTIONS**
                   (*Vervet Monkey Disease; Green Monkey Disease*)

Definition
Disease caused by specific virus or group of viruses of RNA type and of pleomorphic shape. Virus has not yet been fully classified.

Aetiology
Virus is of unusual morphology being of variable length up to 665 nm, often tortuous in shape and ends are often in shape of a hook or horseshoe. Marburg and Ebola viruses, though they produce similar clinical disease and are morphologically identical, are immunologically distinct.

Epidemiology
Reservoir in nature is not known although rodents are suspected. First human cases were described in 1967 in laboratory workers in Marburg. Infection was transmitted to man from vervet monkeys which had recently been imported from Africa. Vervet monkeys are not now thought to be reservoir of infection but are likely to be infected from the suspected rodent reservoir. Once the disease has occurred in man, human transmission is in much the same way as Lassa fever, i.e. in various secretions and particularly when patients with pyrexia of unknown origin are admitted to hospital and not suspected of having an infectious disease. In latter part of 1976 there were over five hundred cases of Ebola virus infection in southern Sudan and Zaire and much transmission occurred in this way. Mortality in this outbreak was in excess of 50%. Venereal transmission has occurred.

Pathology
Widespread necrotic changes occur in all organs and in these, as in the skin, haemorrhagic manifestations may develop. In infected cells intracytoplasmic inclusions resembling Negri bodies may be found. The central nervous system is commonly involved.

Clinical Features
Onset. Incubation period is 3–10 days following which onset is sudden with nausea, headache and aching eyes. Fever rapidly develops and is associated with bradycardia.
Established disease. Bradycardia may be replaced by tachycardia as myocardial damage develops. Vomiting and diarrhoea are common and a rash develops between the fifth and seventh days. Rash is most marked on buttocks, trunk and outer aspects of arms. Fever commonly subsides about seventh day but may recur

from twelfth to the fourteenth day. Tonsillar inflammation and meningeal irritation may occur. Bleeding occurs from gums and from needle punctures and there may be haematemesis and/or melaena; the rash itself, however, is not usually haemorrhagic. Marked thrombocytopenia develops and transaminase levels are increased.

Diagnosis
Suspect in persons who are resident in or who have been in tropical Africa, particularly central and eastern tropical Africa, within the preceding 14 days and for whom malaria has been excluded as a cause of the fever. Antibodies detectable by complement-fixing or fluorescent techniques appear during the second or third week of the illness. Tissue culture and/or animal inoculation enable the virus to be isolated from body secretions and blood but maximal security in collecting and transporting specimens and in working on them is necessary—*see* Lassa fever.

Management
Isolation and handling of specimens as for Lassa fever. Supportive treatment important. Plasma from a patient who has recovered from the disease may be of benefit and can be given in amounts of 250–500 ml. Treatment with interferon has been employed and may be of some value.

Chapter 18	**ACQUIRED IMMUNODEFICIENCY SYNDROME (AIDS)**

Disease characterized by impaired cell-mediated immunity (CMI) with consequent susceptibility to opportunistic infections that require CMI for their control. This definition excludes those patients immunosuppressed by chemotherapy or radiotherapy and those who have any known disease associated with impaired CMI.

Aetiology
Caused by infection with the human immunodeficiency virus (HIV), previously called human T-cell lymphotropic virus III (HTLV-III). Virus invades T-helper cells and can destroy them. In a proportion of those infected with HIV this results in impaired CMI and these patients have a high risk of developing life-threatening opportunistic infections with one or more pathogens. Also a considerably increased risk of developing a highly aggressive form of Kaposi's sarcoma.

Epidemiology
AIDS was first recognized among male homosexuals in the USA but the disease has a worldwide distribution. Passive anal intercourse with numerous sexual partners was a major risk factor. Later studies showed other high-risk groups: haemophiliacs, intravenous drug abusers, Haitian males, prostitutes and infants born of HIV-positive mothers. Haitian males may have been infected by sexual contact with visiting infecting males. Transmission of the disease among heterosexuals of both sexes occurs in Africa with peak prevalence among sexually active age groups. Infection uncommon below 20 years and over 60 years.

Major routes of infection appear to be: (*a*) semen introduced into rectum, and (*b*) blood and blood products, particularly factor VIII concentrates. Also evidence of transmission from males to females. HIV positivity in both sexes from the Congo basin area of Africa and occurrence of AIDS in African women who have not been transfused or received blood products. Overall infection rate in Africa 6%.

It should be emphasized that while 80% of patients with AIDS have antibodies to HIV not all those infected with HIV virus develop AIDS. Many remain asymptomatic while others have self-limiting illness. Studies in the next decade needed to show how many of these will develop AIDS.

Incubation Period
6–36 months (from transfusion related cases). May be longer.

Period of Communicability
May be lifelong once infected.

Immunopathology
Usual features are lymphopenia, hyperglobulinaemia, and large numbers of B-cells which secrete immunoglobulin without stimulation in vitro. Lymphopenia is result of reduction in T-helper cell population.

Clinical Features
1. AIDS prodrome (AIDS-related complex) lasting from 4 weeks to a year, comprising fever, night sweats, weight loss, anorexia and intermittent diarrhoea. Oral candida may be present. Generalized lymphadenopathy may also be present.
2. AIDS is characterized by development of opportunistic infections and Kaposi's sarcoma. Considerable range of pathogens involved—viral, bacterial, fungal and protozoal. Often infection with more than one pathogen. Viral pathogens include *herpes simplex*; *cytomegalovirus* affecting CNS, lungs or gut; *papovavirus* causing progressive multifocal leucoencephalopathy; HIV itself neurotropic causing dementia. Atypical mycobacteria, non-typhoid salmonellae and *Listeria mono-cytogenes* (causing meningitis) are possible bacterial pathogens. Fungi include candida causing oral, pharyngeal, oesophageal or disseminated infections; *cryptococcosis* causing CNS or disseminated infections; aspergillus causing CNS or disseminated infections. Pneumocystis pneumonia; toxoplasmosis (CNS); *Isospora* and cryptosporidium (gut); leishmaniasis are protozoal pathogens. *Giardia lamblia* should also be considered as cause of diarrhoea. Disseminated strongyloidiasis may occur.

Lungs most common site of infection and infection with more than one pathogen is common. Pneumonia common cause of death in AIDS. Pneumocystis causes 50% of all pulmonary infections in AIDS.

Kaposi's sarcoma usually begins with a flat, red macule which persists and becomes raised. Finally it develops a purplish colour. Gut is commonly involved. Kaposi's sarcoma much more aggressive in AIDS (cf. slowly progressive form seen in Africa). It has been suggested that this tumour is due to infection with another virus.

Diagnosis
DiGeorge and Wiskott–Aldrich syndromes rare causes of impaired cell-mediated

immune responses. Treatment for malignancies of various sorts with chemotherapy or radiation is readily recognizable. History of homosexuality, intravenous drug abuse, haemophilia or transfusion together with pulmonary, CNS, disseminated infection or chronic gut infections suggests AIDS. Presence of oesophageal candida also suggests this condition. In Africans none of the above risk factors may be present.

Management
Vigorous treatment of infections is necessary and presence of several pathogens should be anticipated. Intensive care with respiratory support may be needed. Pneumocystis pneumonia is treated with co-trimoxazole or pentamidine; antifungal drugs are used for superficial and deep mycoses; acyclovir can be used topically, orally or parenterally in herpes simplex infections and spiramycin reported to be effective in chronic diarrhoea due to cryptosporidium. Azidothymidine shown to be of value against HIV in early clinical trials. Further studies awaited.

Isolation
Patient should be isolated in hospital only with regard to the immediate infective episode, plus standard precautions as for HBV for specimen handling.

Prognosis
Overall mortality is 42% in AIDS. Those who have Kaposi's sarcoma have mortality of 22%, rising to 47% in those with pneumocystis pneumonia and 59% in those with both conditions. Long-term outlook of asymptomatic HIV carriers uncertain at present but it seems likely that they may remain well. Natural history of HIV infection associated with lymphadenopathy is not clear but there is evidence that progression to AIDS is not an invariable sequela.

Prevention
Anyone who is a known carrier or who might recently have been infected should not donate blood. All blood donated should be screened for presence of anti-HIV antibodies (anti-HIV). Effective screening and confirmatory tests for anti-HIV available. Blood products made from pooled sera made safe by heat inactivation and alcohol treatment. Public education about the virus, its transmission and the disease caused is needed. Awareness of these factors may help to reduce transmission. General public needs to know that HIV carriers and AIDS cases are not infectious to others in family, workplace, school or social contact. Additional advice on the use of condoms during anal or vaginal intercourse by infected persons and advice on avoidance of intercourse with prostitutes is also needed. Drug abusers in Europe and North America are a possible source of infection for heterosexuals. Addicts should not share syringes. Research on vaccine development proceeding, but HIV is a poor immunogen.

Chapter 19   **KURU**

Definition
A 'slow virus' infection. A remorselessly progressive and invariably fatal

degeneration of the CNS affecting people of the Fore tribe in New Guinea and marked by ataxia and incoordination.

Epidemiology
Only affects members of Fore tribe and those who have had very close contact with this tribe. Young children not affected; sexes equally affected in youth but among older patients predominates in women. Thought to be transmitted by ritualistic cannibalism in which portions of brain of dead relatives are eaten. No new cases since cannibalistic practices stopped.

Aetiology
Formerly thought to be genetic, but recent evidence implicates a slowly developing virus infection. Incubation period up to 20 years. Intracerebral inoculation of chimpanzees with brain tissue from kuru patients has been followed in 3–4 years by development of the diseases in the animals.

Kuru and Jakob–Creutzfeldt disease are the only known slow virus infections in man though scrapie in sheep is now known to be a slow virus infection. Motor neurone disease in man and some other demyelinizing diseases are suspected of being slow virus infections.

Pathology
Widespread neuronal degeneration especially of cerebellum and extrapyramidal tracts. Less marked degeneration of anterior horn cells, inferior olives, thalamus, and pontine nuclei.

Clinical Features
Initial locomotor ataxia and in 1–2 months tremor of extremities, head and trunk develops and is aggravated by fatigue. Wild athetoid movements later, and later still patient becomes bedridden. After 3–6 months mental faculties become impaired and there is strabismus and incontinence. Emotional lability a feature.

No nystagmus, no changes in blood, cerebrospinal fluid, or urine.

Treatment
Unavailing, symptomatic only.

Chapter 20   # SMALLPOX

Highly infectious disease causing an exanthematous eruption due to variola virus, a DNA-containing virus in orthopox group. Disease eradicated by speedy case finding and containing outbreaks locally by vaccination.

Transmission
This was by droplet infection.

Clinical Features
Incubation period of about 11 days (range 7–17 days). Then fever, headache,

backache and malaise were usual prodromal features, 2–4 days. Rash appeared on face and arms with all lesions of roughly the same age and evolving through stages macule, papule, vesicle, pustule and scab. Pustules were umbilicated. Scabs separated by 3 weeks. Fevers settled after the prodrome, recurring at the pustular stage.

Mild forms in persons who had been vaccinated. Severe forms of infection characterized by extensive coalescing lesions (40% mortality) and haemorrhagic form (almost uniformly fatal).

Vaccination and Control

Vaccine was highly immunogenic and evoked very effective protective immunity. Early efforts at attempted mass vaccination of populations not effective but efforts to find cases and vaccinate local populations was highly effective. Last natural case of smallpox occurred in Somalia in 1977.

2

Diseases Due to Rickettsia and Chlamydia

Chapter 21　　**TYPHUS FEVER**

The typhus group of diseases is caused by various strains of *Rickettsiae*. The group varies in clinical severity and in epidemiological and serological factors.

Rickettsiae

Very small bacteria. Pleomorphism common, may be diplococcal or long forms. Obligate, intracellular parasites; grow better in cells not undergoing rapid multiplication. Hence the more serious nature of typhus diseases in the aged, debilitated, or starved. Radiation damage to cells may similarly predispose. The rickettsiae have been grown in chick embryo tissue and a variety of cell lines.

Provisional Classification of Typhus Fevers

No systematic classification at present possible. Same vector may transmit different strains of *Rickettsiae*. Specific rickettsial serology, now available, will distinguish between species. Weil–Felix reactions no longer used in many laboratories.

1. *Epidemic typhus* ('True or Exanthematic Typhus'). *Insect vector*: louse (*Pediculus humanus*). Conveyed man to man. No animal reservoir. Classic type. Distribution universal. *Causal organism*: *R. prowazeki*. Weil–Felix reaction: positive to OX 19, negative to OXK, positive to OX 2.

2. *Endemic typhus*. Primarily diseases of lower animals, especially rodents, conveyed from them to man by bites of: (2.1) ticks, (2.2) mites, and (2.3) fleas: never from man to man. Endemic and sporadic, but never epidemic.

> 2.1. *Tick-borne*: Types: (*a*) Rocky Mountain spotted fever. *Reservoir*: rodents, especially ground-squirrels. *Insect vector*: *Dermacentor andersoni* (wood-tick) and others. *Causal organism*: *R. rickettsii*. (*b*) Fièvre boutonneuse. *Reservoir*: dogs. *Causal organism*: *R. conori*. (*c*) Tick typhus of S. and E. Africa. *Vectors*: various cattle ticks. *Causal organism*: *R. conori*. In these diseases the Weil–Felix test positive to OX 19 in lower titres than in louse-borne typhus, and to OX 2.
>
> 2.2. *Mite-borne*: Tropical 'scrub' typhus, Japanese river fever. *Insect vector*: larvae of *Trombicula akamushi* and *Trombicula deliensis*. *Reservoir*: rats and mice. *Causal organism*: *R. tsutsugamushi*. Weil–Felix reaction: negative OX 19 and OX 2, positive OXK.

2.3. *Flea-borne* (*Murine*): Tropical 'urban' typhus. *Reservoir*: rats. *Insect vector*: *Xenopsylla astia* and *cheopis* (rat-fleas). *Causal organism*: *R. mooseri*. Weil–Felix reaction: positive OX 19 and OX 2 negative OXK.

Other rickettsial diseases. The following gives no Weil–Felix reactions:

Rickettsialpox, caused by *R. akari*, transmitted by a mite, normally an ectoparasite of mice.

Methods of Diagnosis

1. *Weil–Felix reaction*. Serological test. Certain bacilli of proteus group, known as *Proteus OX* strains, are agglutinated in high titre by serum of typhus patients: but are not cause of typhus. Agglutinins appear about fifth day, titre then rises to maximum from eighth to twenty-eighth day. Convenient test in many ways but does not distinguish typhus and spotted fever infections. False positive reactions in proteus infections and relapsing fever, leptospirosis, vibrio infections. Two strains principally used: (*a*) *Proteus OX 19*: positive for epidemic (louse-borne) and flea-borne types; (*b*) *Proteus OXK*: positive for mite-borne types; reactions of tick-borne types vary and usually lower titre. *Proteus OX 2* also in use. Titre above 1–100 positive: *rising titre* especially important. 'O' antigens now in common use: reactions recorded as OX 19, etc.

2. *Agglutination*. Agglutinins to *Rickettsia* develop in serum during typhus, both epidemic and endemic: can be thus diagnosed and type differentiated. Rickettsial suspensions obtained from infected egg yolk sac or mouse lung.

3. *Complement-fixation test* is now possible in several rickettsial infections, in which a pure culture of the organisms is used to make an antigen.

4. *Indirect fluorescent antibody test (IFAT)* Widely used. Applicable with all rickettsial infections. IgM and IgG titres can be determined. Species- or group-specific tests available.

5. *Isolation and culture of rickettsia*. Hazardous to laboratory personnel so not a routine procedure. Pure strains obtained by intraperitoneal injection of blood of patient into guinea-pig: killed during pyrexia; organism in brain and spleen. Cultured on egg yolk sac.

Active Immunization

Numerous vaccines under trial: results uncertain. Unsettled if endemic strains immunize against epidemic and vice versa. Vaccines may be: (*a*) Live: some deaths have resulted and method dangerous. (*b*) Killed: *Rickettsia* grown in yolk sac of fertile egg (Cox) and in mouse-lung preparations (Durand and Giraud).

Epidemic Typhus Fever (*Exanthematic, Louse-borne, or True Typhus*)

Conveyed by lice, characterized by sudden onset, marked nervous symptoms and toxaemia, rash and pyrexia, terminating by crisis about fourteenth day. Typhus and typhoid fever only distinguished in the nineteenth century.

Aetiology

Epidemics of enormous extent occur. Endemic in Russia and the Balkan States.

Ireland has suffered heavily. Also in Mexico and Eastern States of America. Principally in temperate regions. War, famine, poverty and dirt favour outbreaks. Spreads more rapidly than any of the other great epidemic diseases; mortality among attendants is high.

Morbid Anatomy
Vasculitis affecting small vessels in skin, brain, lungs, liver, kidneys, etc., due to replication of organism in endothelium leads to occlusion of small vessels. Rash is visible after death.

Mode of Infection
From man to man by body or head lice: crushed on the skin in scratching: never water-borne. Conclusive evidence of animal reservoir other than man (*see* Brill's Disease, p. 67) not yet obtained.

Blood infective in febrile stages, also shortly before and after.

Organism. Rickettsia prowazeki: occur as minute intracellular bodies in stomachs of typhus-fed lice and in blood of typhus patients.

Lice most infective 5–7 days after feeding, and hence probably some development occurs. Transmitted from excreta of gut scratched into skin, but not by bite. Louse dies in 10 days. Louse faeces remain infective for 60 days.

Monkeys and guinea-pigs can be infected.

Epidemics can be controlled by measures directed against lice.

Serum from convalescent patients is protective for a short time, but has no curative power.

Weil–Felix reaction. Strongly positive to *Proteus OX 19*, negative to *OXK*.

Duration of Infectivity
Four weeks from onset.

Quarantine Period
Fifteen days.

Symptoms
Incubation period. Usually about 12 days, but very variable. Limits 5–14 days: possibly 3 weeks. Occasionally slight malaise for a day or two.

Clinical stages. (1) Early. (2) Late.

1. Early
Onset. Abrupt.

Rigors. Common. Chills may recur in 24 h.

Pains. In back and legs, especially thighs.

Headache and nausea. Vomiting not uncommon.

Mental symptoms. Onset early, commence with sleeplessness. *Early prostration.*

Expression. Dull, becoming vacant. Face flushed, with earthy hue (*facies typhosa*).

Temperature. High at onset, rises steadily to maximum on fifth day. Pulse rapid; tongue furred; constipation; bronchial catarrh.

2. Late
Fifth to tenth day. Characterized by restlessness, rash and delirium.

Rash. Onset: Usually fourth to fifth day. Commences in axillae and then abdomen: spreads to chest and extremities. *Rare on face and neck*. Absent in 5–10% of cases.

    Character: two elements.

        2.1. Subcuticular mottling, diffuse, irregular and dusky.

        2.2. Papular spots. Very irregular size and shape, and indefinite outline. Slightly elevated. Pink or dusky colour. In early stages, disappear on pressure; later, some spots become petechial, *resembling flea-bites*. Usually very numerous. Continue to appear for 2 or 3 days. (In children, close resemblance to measles, owing to coalescence of spots into blotches.) Rash has so-called 'mulberry' appearance.

Delirium. Replaces headache towards end of first week; most marked at night. Often restless, alert and very violent: in other cases comatose.

    Prostration increases, tongue dry, sordes. Temperature high, 40·5 °C (105 °F). Pulse rapid.

    Tenth to fourteenth day. *Extreme nervous prostration*, incoherence, stupor, passing to unconsciousness and coma; muscular tremors, *subsultus tendinum*, and coma vigil common (adynamic typhus). The earlier the onset of this typhoid state the worse the prognosis. Cranial nerve lesions.

Rash. Darkens, and spots become petechial in centre, like remains of flea-bites. Duration of rash usually 7–10 days.

    Cardiac weakness frequent. Pulse rapid and soft. Tongue dry and shrivelled. Sordes. Deafness.

    In severe cases pin-hole pupils and 'ferret' eyes. Incontinence. Hiccup serious.

    In unfavourable cases: (1) Coma vigil: vacant gaze, open eyes, dilated pupils, complete unconsciousness; almost always fatal. (2) Hypostatic congestion of lungs. (3) General exhaustion and cardiac failure.

    Most often on fourteenth day, patient falls asleep, and wakes extremely weak, but conscious; temperature drops in a few hours; symptoms clear; convalescence rapid. Abatement may occur by lysis.

Complications

Pneumonitis; otitis media; parotitis; thrombosis of large arteries causing, e.g. hemiplegia; cutaneous gangrene.

Variations in Type

Mild cases occur, with convalescence on tenth day, especially in children: blood infective. Malignant forms, *typhus siderans*, fatal in 2 or 3 days.

Prognosis

General mortality 12–20%, but varies greatly with treatment, age, and in different epidemics and surroundings. Varies directly with age. In children 2–4%; after 40 years over 50%. Death most frequently in second week from toxaemia; in third week from pulmonary causes.

Diagnosis

In epidemics is simple. Difficulties usually in first few days before eruption. (*See* Methods of Diagnosis, p. 64.)

1. Typhoid. In typhus: sudden onset, rigor, early prostration and mental symptoms, with absence of diarrhoea, abdominal tenderness and enlarged spleen; aspect dull; character of rash distinctive, but not invariably. Cultures and Widal negative. Diagnosis often very difficult.

2. Measles. Catarrhal symptoms. Koplik spots. Rash brighter, edges more defined, marked on face.

3. Cerebrospinal fever. CSF distinctive.

4. Purpura. Common mistake in sporadic cases.

5. Flea-bites. May resemble petechiae in later stages of rash.

6. Severe smallpox. Difficulty from initial scarlatinal rash. True rash affects face early.

7. Relapsing fever. Examination of the blood.

Control and Prevention
Measures against lice can control epidemics, viz. spraying of houses and clothes with DDT. Decontamination of clothes, blankets best by heat (kills lice and rickettsia). After decontamination and delousing isolation not necessary. Insecticide resistance patterns guide choice of effective agent.

Vaccine
No longer available.

Chemoprophylaxis
Not routinely recommended.

Treatment
Single dose doxycycline, 200 mg, best. Defervescence within 48–72 h. Occasional mild, self-limited recrudescences. Severe recrudescence needs more antibiotic. Tetracycline 25–50 mg/kg/day in divided doses for 2–3 days. Chloramphenicol may also be used.

Brill's Disease
Symptoms mild. Previous history of epidemic typhus usual. Is now regarded as recrudescence of infection latent for many years.

Rocky Mountain Spotted Fever

Acute infective, endemic fever of the typhus group, conveyed by bites of a tick, resembling epidemic typhus in fever, constitutional disturbances and petechial eruption.

Distribution
Montana and Idaho. Also fairly common in some of the eastern states of America. Commonest in spring months.

Epidemiology
Reservoir: rodents, especially ground squirrels and woodchucks. *Vector*: *Dermacentor andersoni* (wood-tick); *D. variabilis*. Organism develops in all tissues. Bite conveys infection. Eggs infected. *Organism*: *R. rickettsii*. Domestic animals, bears, etc. are hosts of ticks, but are not infected. One attack protects.

Symptoms
Resembles epidemic typhus.
Incubation period. 3–12 days.
Onset. Sudden: rigor, general pains, myalgia. Temperature high by second day.
Eruption. On third to fifth day. Commences at wrists: extends to trunk and limbs: face mainly escapes. At onset: pink macules disappearing on pressure: becomes petechial: may be discrete or confluent.
In second week. Temperature high. Pulse rapid. Spleen may be palpable and tender. Typhoidal state in severe cases. Myocardial involvement common. Acute tubular necrosis after prolonged hypotension.
At beginning of third week. Temperature begins to fall and rash to fade. Normal temperature and convalescence in fourth week. Constipation usual. May be vomiting in second week. Slight leucocytosis.

Complications
Gangrene may follow.

Prognosis
Main determinant in fatal cases is delay in starting correct antibiotic. Increasing age also adverse prognostic feature. Death rates 10–60%.

Diagnosis
From measles and meningococcal disease.

Treatment
As for epidemic typhus but daily dosing for 6 days. Supportive care in severe cases.

Fièvre Boutonneuse (*Tick-bite Fever; Marseilles Fever*)

Distribution
Shores of Mediterranean. African coasts.

Epidemiology
Reservoir: dog. *Vector*: *Rhipicephalus sanguineus* (dog-tick). *Organism*: *R. conorii*. *Weil–Felix reaction*: usually negative to all strains of *Proteus OX*, but may be positive to OX 19. Guinea-pigs inoculated with patient's serum become immune to epidemic typhus.

Symptoms
Primary sore forms at site of bite with local lymphangitis. May be no other symptoms. Fully developed forms resemble Rocky Mountain fever but milder: fever 8–10 days, headache, rash on fifth day is a papular type spreading from extremities in towards trunk. Low mortality.

Other Tick-bite Fevers
Many types including:
Indian tick fever. Described by Megaw in 1917. Transmitted by *Haemaphysalis leachi* var. *indica*, *ixodes*, *ricinus*, and *R. sanguineus*. Agglutinins to proteus OX

19 or OX 2 appear after tenth febrile day, maximum 2–4 weeks after defervescence. Responds therapeutically to broad-spectrum antibiotics.

North Asian tick-borne rickettsiosis. Transmitted by various *Ixodid* ticks. Caused by *R. siberica*—closely related to *R. conorii* from which it is distinguished by cross-immunity tests.

Kenya tick-typhus. Transmitted by *H. leachi* and *R. simus* vectors, the former found on dogs. Serological evidence of infection found in rodents and *R. conori* have been isolated from eight rodent species.

South American tick-bite fever. Reservoir: rats and rodents. Resembles *fièvre boutonneuse.*

South African tick-bite fever. Reservoir: probably dog. *Vector*: various larval ticks. Resembles *fièvre boutonneuse*.

Scrub Typhus (Tsutsugamushi Fever; Japanese River Fever)

An acute infective, endemic fever of the typhus group, conveyed by the bite of a mite. Characterized by a local eschar, followed by inflammation of lymph glands, fever and a typhus-like eruption. Considerable range of clinical severity, mild to severe and even fatal.

Distribution
Originally recognized on river banks in Japan and later in Malaya. Now known to have wide distribution, but areas often sharply circumscribed.

Epidemiology
Reservoir: rats and mice. *Vector*: a mite, larva of *Trombicula akamushi. Organism*: *Rickettsia tsutsugamushi* (*R. orientalis*), *Weil–Felix reaction*: negative to OX 19, positive to OXK. One attack does not protect.

Symptoms
At the site of bite, black eschar with red areola forms: separates about fourth week, leaving ulcer. Site of bite may be inapparent.

Incubation period. Five days to 2–3 weeks. Then lymph glands draining area of eschar become enlarged and tender, temperature rises rapidly, with rigors and general malaise.

Eruption on fourth to seventh day: red macules fading on pressure later becoming petechial: commences on trunk and extends to limbs: face may be affected. Lasts 4–7 days.

With eruption, general symptoms increase. Conjunctivitis. Pneumonitis common. Abdominal discomfort and constipation. Spleen may be palpable. Leucopenia distinct.

Temperature falls after 2–3 weeks and convalescence commences.

Prognosis
Varies greatly. Mortality in Japan 20–50%.

Diagnosis
From plague.

Prophylaxis

Repellent for mites: DBP (dibutylphthalate) rub into clothing every 2 weeks. DDT no effect. Cotton-rat vaccine: no evidence of protection.

Treatment

As for epidemic form. Doxycycline should be repeated after 5 days, to prevent relapse.

Murine Typhus *(Flea Typhus; Urban Typhus)*

Now regarded as the primitive endemic form of the epidemic type. Protective cross-immunity with louse typhus.

Distribution

World-wide.

Epidemiology

Reservoir: rats (also squirrels, shrews). *Vector*: rat fleas, *Xenopsylla astia* and *cheopis*. *Weil–Felix reaction*: positive to OX 19, negative to OXK. Never conveyed from man to man, and never becomes epidemic, although mode of infection resembles plague: ascribed to fact that rats do not die of the disease, and infection is transient and hence fleas do not migrate.

Symptoms

As in epidemic typhus, but milder.

Treatment

As for epidemic type.

Chapter 22   TRENCH FEVER

Disease transmitted by the excreta of lice, and characterized by an initial febrile period, tendency to relapses and periodic pyrexia, and frequently by hyperaesthesia of the shins. Never fatal.

History

Occurred during the 1914–18 war to an enormous extent among troops on active service. Few cases among civilians, and disease disappeared. Seen again in 1942 on Polish-Russian frontier.

Mode of Transmission

Organism: Rickettsia-like organism: *Rochalimaea quintana*.

1. Organism is present in blood of patients: can be transmitted by inoculation of blood. Not present in faeces.

2. Transmission by lice fed on trench-fever patients: (*a*) Bites do not convey infection; (*b*) Excreta of lice inoculated by scarification convey the infection.

3. Lice after feeding are not infectious for 5 days, i.e. a cycle occurs in body.

4. Lice are infective for at least 23 days.
5. Rickettsiae are present in excreta of lice fed on patients.
6. Rickettsiae never found in material obtained from man.
7. Organism has been transmitted from a patient a year after attack.

General Course
(1) Initial fever, lasting 3–20 days; (2) Recurrent pyrexia, lasting 1–2 days—may continue for many months. Initial sustained pyrexia not always present in experimental infections.

Symptoms of Primary Fever
Incubation period. About 2–3 weeks under ordinary conditions. By scarification: about 8 days. By simple transference of lice to healthy persons: 14–38 days.
Onset. Sudden. Often previous malaise is present for 2–3 days.
General symptoms: (1) *Headache* severe: frontal and at back of eyes; (2) *Giddiness*; (3) *Pains in back and legs*; (4) *Sweats*, often profuse; (5) *Face* flushed; (6) *Conjunctivitis* common; (7) General febrile symptoms: anorexia, constipation, shivering, but no definite rigors; vomiting occasionally; (8) Herpes labialis occurs occasionally; (9) *Spleen*: enlarged in about one-third of the cases. Usually tender; (10) *Tenderness and pain in shins*: *most characteristic* symptom; often very acute. Usually not present in first few days. Especially lower half of shins. Pain, also severe, may occur in thighs and knees; sometimes in calves, but this often entirely absent; (11) *Rash*: pale pink irregular erythematous or roseolar spots, do not project, disappear readily on pressure. Do not occur in more than one-third of the cases, and usually not until relapses or the periodic rises. Formerly mistaken for enteric spots; (12) *Blood*: may be moderate leucocytosis.

Pyrexia
1. *Initial fever* Duration usually 3–6 days, occasionally up to 20 days; often fluctuates; then falls to normal. *Relapses* very frequent. *Temperature* may be irregular, subsequently, sometimes for long periods, even in absence of definite relapses.
2. *Relapsing pyrexia*. *Periodic rises* occur, usually at 5-day intervals: feels well in intervals. *Febrile period* 1–2 days: temperature 38·9–40 °C (102–104 °F); pulse rapid. Symptoms as in initial fever.
   Occurs in small proportion of cases. May follow directly on initial fever or after interval of weeks. Initial fever may be overlooked.
   Attacks tend to diminish: duration of pyrexia may be very short, a few hours only, may be unnoticed (or possibly absent), while malaise, increased pulse, and other symptoms occur.
   Identical febrile attacks may occur many months after infection.

Sequelae
(1) Slight febrile attacks; (2) Myalgia; (3) Tachycardia; (4) Debility may result from the constant shin pains and pyrexia. Endocarditis never results.

Progress
Never fatal. Shin pains often persist after other symptoms have subsided. Complete recovery finally.

Treatment
Antibiotics probably specific as in typhus.

Chapter 23   Q FEVER

An infection acquired by the respiratory route in dusts or aerosols from infected animals. May cause acute or chronic infection in man.

History
First recognized in 1935 among meat-workers in Brisbane. Was discovered to be cause of epidemic of 'primary atypical penumonia' in Italy. Distribution now known to be widespread.

Epidemiology
Causal organism: *Coxiella burneti*: grows on yolk sac and in guinea-pigs and mice. *Insect vector*: certain ticks. *Vertebrate reservoir* (in Australia); bandicoot and many other hosts. Cattle, sheep and goats and probably other mammals are susceptible. *C. burneti* is highly infectious. Man-to-man infection has been reported but is rare. Spread by fomites important. Organism endures for months on clothing and implements.

Laboratory Tests
Complement-fixation test: highly specific.

Symptoms
Subject to considerable variation. Inapparent to prolonged febrile illness.
Incubation period. Usually 16–18 days: limits 13–32 days.
Onset. Sudden. Temperature rises to 40 °C (104 °F) in few days.
  Headache: very severe. Sweats. Prostration. Resembles mild typhus. *No rash.*
Pulmonary involvement. Little sputum. May be chest pain. Crackles in chest. X-rays show lower zone involvement usually.
Hepatitis. Q fever causes granulomatous hepatitis. Persisting fever, liver may be enlarged and tender. Liver biopsy not always abnormal.
Acute epididymo-orchitis. May occur in acute Q fever.
Endocarditis. Occurs usually on abnormal valves, though some patients not known to have abnormal valves before. Fever, anaemia, finger clubbing, splenomegaly, embolic phenomena.

Diagnosis
Q fever enters differential diagnosis of atypical pneumonia (mycoplasma, psittacosis), granulomatous hepatitis (sarcoid, TB, lymphoma), causes of prolonged febrile illnesses, e.g. brucella. Causes of blood culture negative endocarditis.

Laboratory Confirmation
A rising Coxiella phase II antigen (CFT) complement-fixation test found in acute infections. High levels of phase I CFT suggest endocarditis.

Treatment
Tetracycline in standard doses is effective in acute Q fever. Fever settles promptly, co-trimoxazole has also been effective. Prolonged antibiotic therapy with tetracycline for months in endocarditis. Combination therapy of doxycycline with trimethoprim or rifampicin has been used.

Prognosis
Excellent in acute cases but mortality in Q fever endocarditis remains high.

Chapter 24   **LYMPHOGRANULOMA VENEREUM**
**(Tropical or Climatic Bubo; Lympho-
granuloma or Lymphopathia Inguinale;
Poradenitis)**

Venereal disease characterized by inflammatory enlargement of lymph glands draining genitalia, resulting in males in inguinal bubo and haemorrhagic proctocolitis (anogenital syndrome) in females and homosexual males. Caused by *Chlamydia trachomatis* (immunotypes LGV 1, 2 and 3). Chlamydiae are in a separate order from viruses and bacteria.

Aetiology
Distribution. Originally recognized on coasts in the tropics. Cases have occurred lately in many countries, including Great Britain.
Organism. Organism estimated by filtration to be 125–175 nm in size. Elementary bodies found in human infections are 200–400 nm in size. Communicable to guinea-pigs by subcutaneous and to monkeys by subdural inoculation with sterile pus.

Morbid Anatomy
Necrotic, granulomatous lesions. Late fibrosis.

Incubation Period
A few days to 3 weeks after coitus, and a further 2 weeks to glandular enlargement.

Primary Lesion
Papule or herpetiform lesions on penis, labia or posterior vaginal wall. May be urethral discharge or cervicitis.

Glandular Enlargement
Glands affected are those draining genitalia, and differ in males and females.
Males. Inguinal glands involved: draining anogenital region. Enlarge insidiously: commences 2–3 weeks after primary lesion. Pain variable. Periadenitis follows; glands fuse to skin, which becomes reddish-violet. *Multiple* areas of softening appear, suppurate, and produce multiple sinuses. Groove where inguinal

ligament crosses involved inguinal glands. May heal in few months or longer. *Iliac glands* may enlarge, but never suppurate. Stricture of rectum occurs rarely. Urethral stricture may follow urethritis.

Females. Deeper pelvic glands and those around lower part of rectum are affected. Haemorrhagic proctocolitis. *Sequelae*: Stricture of rectum in lowest few inches; with or without elephantiasis and ulceration of external genitalia. Fistulae, especially rectovaginal.

General Symptoms
Fever of several weeks, lassitude, malaise. Occasional erythema nodosum, erythema multiforme, general glandular enlargement, arthritis.

Diagnosis
From gonorrhoea, syphilis, chancroid, actinomycosis, from other causes of stricture and from other tropical buboes.

Serology
High or rising complement-fixation test titre. Indirect immunofluorescent antibody tests. IgM antibody indicating recent infection.
Frei test. Delayed hypersensivity skin test. Rarely used.

Treatment
Tetracycline 2 g daily in divided doses for 2–4 weeks is effective and will improve rectal stricture in its earlier stages. Sulfisoxazole 1 g q.d.s. × 3 weeks. Aspirate fluctuant buboes to prevent discharge. Surgical repair of late lesions, strictures, fistulae, etc. after a prolonged course of antibiotic.

Non-LGV Chlamydiae

Common cause of urethritis (non-specific urethritis, NSU) and female genital tract infections.

Aetiology
Chlamydia trachomatis (immunotypes D–K).

Epidemiology
Common in sexually active young adults. Commonest cause of urethral discharge in Europe and N. America.

Symptoms
Scant chronic urethral and less commonly vaginal discharge. Dysuria, fever, lower abdominal pain, pelvic peritonitis in females. Adhesions may follow. May cause salpingitis. Perihepatitis (Fitz-Hugh–Curtis syndrome).

Diagnosis
From other causes of urethritis, etc., i.e. gonococcal and ureaplasma infections. Pus cells in discharge, non-gonococci on gram stain, culture for chlamydia available.

Treatment
Tetracycline 250 mg q.d.s. for 2–3 weeks. Erythromycin also effective.

Trachoma and Inclusion Conjunctivitis

Follicular conjunctivitis due to infection with *Chlamydia trachomatis*. Recurrent acute infections over many years caused entropion with consequent abrasion of cornea causing ulceration, scarring and eventual blindness. Trachoma common in tropics and subtropics, 700 000 000 infected and 20 000 000 blinded by it.

Aetiology
Chlamydia trachomatis, immunotypes A, B, Ba or C. Repeated acute infections.

Epidemiology
Overcrowding, lack of sufficient water for washing eye secretions from face, shared applicators for eye make-up.

Symptoms
Trachoma itself causes very little. Minor eye discharge. More marked symptoms of conjunctival irritation, inflammation and discharge related to secondary bacterial infection. Signs in trachoma relate to development of pannus, acutely inflamed conjunctival follicles. Follicles are lymphoid aggregates. Heal with scarring causing Herbert's pits. Eventually scarring causing inversion of eyelids and traumatic keratitis with appropriate signs and symptoms follows. Blindness when cornea trauma has progressed to fibrous scarring.

Confirmation
Clinical. Any two of tarsal follicles, tarsal scarring, pannus, Herbert's pits.
Laboratory. Giemsa stain of conjunctival scraping shows characteristic blue-stained intracytoplasmic inclusions in epithelial cells. Culture in embryonated hens' eggs.

Diagnosis
Viral infection. Toxic, follicular conjunctivitis with molluscum contagiosum, prolonged use of topical drugs, allergy to eye cosmetics. Scarring of eyelids—trauma, severe bacterial conjunctivitis.

Treatment
Medical. (1) Topical: 1·0% tetracycline eye drops or ointment 2–4 times daily for 2–3 weeks. (2) Systemic: non-pregnant adults and children over 8 years—tetracycline 250 mg q.d.s. for adults and a reduced dose for children for 3 weeks; Sulphonamides or co-trimoxazole for 3 weeks.
Surgical. Operations to counter entropion. Not entirely successful but worthwhile as trauma to cornea reduced.

Control
Measures to improve housing, water supplies, personal cleanliness and hygiene.

Chapter 25   # PSITTACOSIS

Acute infective disease due to *Chlamydia psittaci*. Characterized by fever, constitutional disturbances and pulmonary complications. Primarily a disease of birds.

Bird Infections
Parrots and budgerigars most susceptible, especially from S. America. Also canaries, gulls, pigeons and some other birds. Affected birds exhibit general malaise, sneezing, and signs of a 'cold', and often intractable diarrhoea and vomiting.

Organism
Relatively large (220–235 nm). Elementary bodies present in specific lesions and tissue cultures. Maintains virulence for considerable periods. Infection occurs from bird to bird, from bird to man, and from man to man. Chlamydiae present in blood up to twelfth day. Bird after recovery from illness may remain carrier for many months (at least 8). Laboratory infections occur readily. One attack protects: recovered parrot resistant to re-infection.

Morbid Anatomy
Areas, scattered or confluent, of haemorrhagic pneumonia. General septicaemia.

Symptomatology in Human Beings
Incubation period. Usually 7–14 days.
Onset. Usually rapid. Temperature high from onset. Resembles atypical enteric: malaise, headache, anorexia, nausea, apathy. Also vomiting, sweating, shivering, photophobia.
Pulmonary symptoms. Cough from the onset, or later in the first week: often spasmodic. Respiration not increased in frequency. In second week, consolidation of lungs: physical signs very variable. No pleural effusion.
Intestinal symptoms. Abdominal distension may be marked. Constipation obstinate. Spleen not palpable. May be slight diarrhoea, but rarely prominent.
   Eruptions occasionally present: no constant character: may suggest enteric. *Leucocytosis* is absent. *Diphtheroid stomatitis* develops from mouth-to-mouth feeding of sick parrots.

Progress and Prognosis
In favourable cases, fever lasts 15–20 days: lungs clear gradually. Long convalescence. Mild forms also occur, especially in children and young adults. In fatal cases lungs show thrombosis and haemorrhagic pneumonia. Mortality about 20%, due to pulmonary complications.

Diagnosis
Usually by record of association with sick parrots. Especially from influenza and enteric. Serological diagnosis with complement-fixation test.

Treatment
Tetracycline effective, 500 mg q.d.s. × 14 days. Chloramphenicol also effective.

Chapter 26

RELAPSING FEVERS

A. Louse-borne

Acute infectious disease caused by spirochaete conveyed by lice, and characterized by alternate periods of fever and apyrexia of 5–10 days' duration.

Distribution
Occurs in all continents, with slight differences in spirochaetes, mode of transmission and symptoms. Widespread in Egypt and India. Occurred in N. and E. Africa (particularly Ethiopia) in recent years and S. America.

Spirochaete
Spirochaeta (Borrelia) recurrentis discovered in blood by Obermeier in 1873; invariably present during febrile periods, but not in intervals. Length 15–40 µm: numerous spirals: actively motile, by lashing movements and action of spirals. Visible with dark-ground or phase contrast microscopy. Cultured on Noguchi's medium.

Epidemiology
Transmitted from man to man, conveyed by lice (*Pediculus corporis* and *capitis*). Spirochaetes undergo developmental cycle in louse and become present in all body fluids after 5–16 days. Infection by crushing infected lice over a bite or skin abrasion and not by bites. Louse infective for 28 days: no transovarian transmission. Human blood also directly infective. Laboratory infections common. Prevalent in winter months. Epidemic, especially in times of famine and civil unrest.

Morbid Anatomy
No special changes except enlargement of spleen and liver.

Symptoms
Incubation. From 2 to 15, usually 5–7 days.
Invasion. Sudden onset: rigors, headache, sweats, intense pains in long bones, giddiness, and often vomiting. *Temperature* 39·4–40 °C (103–104 °F) on first day. Pulse 110–180. *Spleen* enlarges, also liver. Slight jaundice; constipation or diarrhoea. Occasionally herpes. *Eruption* (not constant): erythema or rose-

coloured spots, commencing on neck and spreading downwards. *Blood*: spirochaetes present, polynuclear leucocytosis.

Crisis. Usually fifth to seventh day of fever. Sweating: rapid apyrexia. Death at crisis may occur in weakly persons.

Apyrexial period. Duration about the same as fever. Spirochaetes absent or scanty (congregate in liver and spleen). Rapid improvement, followed by:

Recurrence. About fourteenth day. Similar to initial attack, but usually milder. Rarely more than one recurrence in European type: occasionally three or four. Absence of recurrence rare.

Convalescence. Slow, owing to exhaustion.

Complications
Not common. Delirium during fever. During convalescence: rarely iritis, meningitis, paralyses, convulsions.

Prognosis
In good conditions, mortality under 2%, especially with modern treatment. With overcrowding and bad hygiene, rises to 20 or 30%. One attack does not protect.

Diagnosis
From malaria, Weil's disease, typhus, yellow fever: in temperate zones from influenza, undulant fever. During febrile period, spirochaetes in blood. Wassermann reaction transient positive. A specific antiserum can agglutinate spirochaetes (rarely used).

Treatment
Tetracycline and erythromycin are effective. Tetracycline 500 mg as a single dose is the treatment of choice except in children under 7 years and pregnant women. Erythromycin can be used as an alternative, especially in the latter 2 groups of patients, in a single oral dose of 500 mg.

Most patients experience a Jarisch–Herxheimer reaction 2–3 hours after treatment, with coldness, severe headache and myalgia. The temperature rises abruptly, the pulse rises and blood pressure falls. Intravenous infusion to maintain blood pressure may be needed.

Delousing and insect repellants, together with bathing and washing of clothes, are effective in control.

General treatment of fevers, cold sponging, etc. At crisis, stimulants necessary, especially in old or weakly persons.

Prophylaxis. Factors promoting spread are similar to typhus: overcrowding and lice. Sterilization of clothes, cleanliness of dwellings, protection from lice.

B. Tick-borne
Closely allied, but conveyed by a tick.

Distribution
In endemic foci in N., Central and S. America, Southern Spain and Portugal, Africa, Middle and Far East.

Various species which cannot be reliably distinguished in the laboratory. *Borrelia duttonii* (Africa), *B. hispanica* (Spain), *B. persica* (Iran) and *B. hermsii* and *B. turicatae* (N. America).

Epidemiology
Transmitted by tick bites. *Borrelia duttonii* affects man who is also the reservoir and the vector is *Ornithodorus moubata*. Wild rodents are the reservoir of the other species of borrelia and man is infected when he is bitten by an infected tick. Transovarian transmission occurs in the tick.

Clinical Course
Resembles louse-borne relapsing fever. Differences: (1) Pyrexial periods short, 2–3 days; (2) Spirochaetes scanty (use thick film); (3) Relapses more numerous; (4) Tends to be more severe; nervous system may be affected—signs of meningitis, optic atrophy (may develop after attack), aphasia, and cranial nerve palsies; (5) No seasonal prevalence. Fulminating, meningitic, and in babies algid forms occasionally.

Prognosis
Mortality lower than in louse type. Infants and children tend to suffer more severe attacks than do adults.

Treatment
As for louse-borne disease.

Prophylaxis
Application of tick repellants to the skin. Mosquito net. Night-light deters ticks. Impregnation of soil floor or mud-plaster walls of infected huts with benzene hexachloride (Gammexane) 15 mg active base per square foot applied as a watery suspension gradually will eradicate ticks.

Chapter 27   # LEPTOSPIROSIS

Infection of man and many animals by organisms of the genus *Leptospira* is widespread throughout the world and these can be characterized serologically into a large number of serovarieties (serovars). The 170 serovars of the interrogans complex presently recognized are divided into 18 serogroups. There is only one species in the genus presently recognizable, i.e. *Leptospira interrogans*, and the species is divided into 2 complexes, interrogans and biflexa. The former contains all the pathogenic strains. Leptospires are parasites of animals, especially of rodents, and form colonies in the renal tubules of the host, so that it is by the urine of the animals that infection is spread. Leptospires may enter new hosts through the mucous membranes, including the conjunctiva, or through cuts or abrasions on the skin.

Leptospiral infections cause disease of varying severity from severe illness with hepatorenal involvement to self-limiting febrile illnesses.

Weil's Disease

Acute infection due to *L. interrogans* of several serovars including ictero-haemorrhagica and characterized by fever, jaundice, enlargement of liver, haemorrhages and frequently a secondary fever. Severity of disease may relate to infecting dose of organisms.

Distribution
Worldwide. In association with rats and wet environments.

The Spirochaete
Leptospira interrogans. Length 5–25 μm. In stained preparations, 4–5 waves (Fontana's silver method); with dark-ground illumination, numerous fine spirals; by special methods, characteristic flagellum with terminal hook resembling a question mark, hence 'interrogans'.
Cultivation. Grows in Fletcher's or Castaneda's medium.
Distribution in human body. In peripheral blood up to fifth, and rarely ninth, day of disease. Later, excreted in urine. Occurs in liver, adrenals and, later, kidneys, but scanty in all human organs. Absent in life from duodenal contents.

Mode of Transmission
Reservoir: Rats (may be apparently healthy). Transmission from urine of infected rats and human beings. Cattle shed the organisms. Infection through wet or abraded skin: farm workers and abattoir workers most often infected in temperate parts of the world. In the tropics, a wider range of the population is exposed to infection. Not from man to man.

Morbid Anatomy
Liver. Enlarged; proliferation of hepatocytes; mild focal necrosis: Küpffer cell hyperplasia: centrilobular biliary stasis. Poor correlation between the severity of changes and severity of disease in fatal cases.
Kidneys. Usually enlarged. Small haemorrhages throughout. Degenerative changes of variable degree affect epithelium of convoluted tubules and loops of Henle. Glomeruli little affected. Leptospires demonstrable in tubules by special staining techniques.
Voluntary muscle. Especially in gastrocnemius a typical non-inflammatory degeneration of small groups of voluntary muscle fibres occurs with loss of striations and hyaline change.
Lymph nodes. May enlarge.
Haemorrhages. Into organs: lungs, kidneys, stomach.
Spleen. Enlarged.
Blood. Some anaemia develops. Sedimentation rate increased. Neutrophil leucocytosis common by end of first week (90% of 20 000–30 000).

Incubation Period
Average 10 days, extremes 2–26 days.

Onset
Sudden. Chills, headache, fever (39–40 °C), marked prostration, conjunctival suffusion. Severe muscle pains and muscle tenderness. Anorexia, constipation, vomiting. Rarely diarrhoea.

Hepatorenal Disturbances
Evident between third and sixth days. Hepatic tenderness and enlargement.

Jaundice. Conjugated hyperbilirubinaemia with modest elevation of transaminases, rarely greater than 230 i.u./L. Renal disease evidenced by proteinuria, pyuria, haematuria and elevated blood urea. Renal tubular necrosis may cause renal failure. Haemorrhagic manifestations more likely in patients with renal dysfunction.

Atypical Clinical Forms

Not uncommon; diagnosis difficult because leptospirosis not usually suspected. May suggest influenza, tonsillitis, rheumatic fever, pneumonia. Haemoptysis. Jaundice often absent, also in mild forms.

Course

Defervescence after 4–9 days, with relapse of fever in second week. Resolution of the disease over 3–5 weeks.

Diagnosis

Clinical. The protean clinical manifestations lead to diagnosis often being unsuspected. In enteric, jaundice rare, especially before second week. From acute infective hepatitis, by late onset of jaundice, but often clinically impossible. In yellow fever there is usually leucopenia, bradycardia, and the early appearance of jaundice. A remission of symptoms is common about the third day. Black vomit is rare in leptospirosis. In falciparum malaria (bilious remittent fever) and blackwater fever and in relapsing fever the blood must be thoroughly searched for the causal organisms.

Pathological

1. *Blood.* Spirochaetes present until fifth day and rarely to ninth, and thus often present only in pre-icteric stage. (Culture using Fletcher's or Castaneda's medium).

2. *Animal inoculation: guinea-pig.* Intraperitoneal injection of 3–5 ml of patient's blood (or urine in later stages). Peritoneal fluid withdrawn by a capillary pipette in 3 or 4 days may show leptospires. Incubation period 6–13 days, then jaundice, collapse, and death in 24 h, may be petechial haemorrhages: spirochaetes present in blood and solid organs, especially liver, also kidneys and adrenals. Haemorrhages in lungs and intestinal walls: spleen enlarged: acute parenchymatous nephritis.

3. *Muscle biopsy* of gastrocnemius may show characteristic histological change.

4. *Agglutination reaction.* On a culture of spirochaetes. Positive about sixth day: increasing titre for 2–3 weeks: persists many years. Demonstration of a rising titre is of great value.

5. *Urine.* Spirochaetes present, not before tenth day, almost invariably present by twentieth day: rare after fortieth day. Centrifuge urine and examine deposit by dark-ground microscopy. They survive best when the urine is neutral or slightly alkaline.

The icteric patients seem to be those at risk of dying but the mortality rate in proved cases is under 10%. Mortality increases with increasing age. Liver failure or renal failure are the common causes of death.

Treatment
Sucessful antibiotic treatment seems to depend most on early treatment with large doses of the therapeutic agent, within 4, and preferably 2, days of the onset of disease. Penicillin G 600000 u intramuscularly 4-hourly for 7 days is effective, Jarisch–Herxheimer reaction may follow 6 hours after first injection. Streptomycin, tetracyclines, chloramphenicol and erythromycin are effective. General treatment of jaundice. Renal failure with anuria is recoverable so that urgent measures to avoid severe electrolyte disturbance may save life. Care regarding fluid and electrolyte balance and peritoneal dialysis or haemodialysis may be needed to counter renal failure.

Prophylaxis
Measures against rats.

Other Forms of Leptospirosis

1. Anicteric febrile illness without localizing signs.
2. Aseptic meningitis, with severe headache, photophobia and neck stiffness. Before the fifth day of the illness CSF may be normal, then cell count increased, polymorphs predominate, but by 12th day lymphocytes predominate. CSF protein raised, CSF sugar almost always normal.

Chapter 28   **TREPONEMATOSES**

Infections by treponemata have been found in all parts of the world. The most widespread and serious both in morbidity and mortality is syphilis, caused by *Treponema pallidum*. Other treponemal infections are: Yaws (*T. pertenue*); Pinta (*T. carateum*); Bejel or non-venereal syphilis (a trepenoma intermediate between *T. pallidum* and *T. pertenue*).

Syphilis
Specific infection by *Treponema pallidum*, acquired by sexual contact, or transplacentally by the fetus of an infected mother. Essential lesion is an infective granuloma.

Introduction into Old World from America in 1493 is generally accepted.

Name 'syphilis' appears first in 1530, in a poem by Girolamo Fracastoro. 'Syphilus' was the name of the infected hero.

Schaudinn, 1905, discovered the *Spirochaeta pallida*.

Wassermann, 1908, described the original serum test based on Bordet-Gengou reaction.

Ehrlich, 1910, produced salvarsan as a cure.

Efficacy of penicillin (1943) in treatment shown.

The Parasite

Morphology. Very delicate organism: often somewhat curved: length 4–14 μm, breadth 0·25 μm: numerous fine, sharp, regular corkscrew spirals, commonly eight to twelve in number, of 1 μm width and 1 μm between their apices, persisting at rest and after staining. Flagella stained by special methods, one at each end. Motile but not very active, movements being: (1) Rotary about long axis; (2) Backward and forward movements; (3) Bending movements. Change in position slight. Does not pass a Berkefeld filter.

Occurrence in the body. Spirochaetes are extracellular.

Primary lesions: Presence most numerous in primary sore.

Secondary lesions: In cutaneous eruptions: scanty. More in mucous patches and condylomas.

Gummas: Scanty: rarely found.

Nervous system: In tabes and general paralysis: very scanty.

Congenital infections: Often extremely numerous in tissues, especially in liver.

Have been found in placenta, umbilical cord and, with difficulty, in blood of infected persons.

Cultivation. In vitro cultivation has not been achieved.

Transmission to animals. In higher apes: by scarification and inoculation: subcutaneous inoculation negative. Primary lesions after 30 days: resembles human lesion with induration of glands. Secondary lesions mild: occur in about 50%. No tertiary lesions. Wassermann reaction positive. In *lower monkeys and rabbits*: local sore and some secondary symptoms. In rabbit's eye, produces iritis and keratitis.

Methods of obtaining spirochaetes

Chancre. Wash with normal saline and scrape edge: if painful, swab with 4% eucaine: squeeze with *protected fingers* to obtain deep fluid: transfer fluid to slide with platinum loop.

Glands. Puncture groin glands with hypodermic needle.

Method of examination. (Oil-immersion lens for all methods.)

Dark-ground illumination. Special paraboloid condenser. Morphology and motility of spirochaete well exhibited.

Sections: Levaditi's silver deposition method. Tissue impregnated with silver nitrate: then reduction by pyrogallic acid deposits silver on the spirochaetes: sections cut by microtome.

Identification of T. pallidum. Mainly by:

1. Number (8–12) and regularity of spirals. Parasite very fine.

2. With Giemsa, stains faint pinkish violet. Other spirochaetes stain deeper blue.

T. refringens, present in ulcerated lesions: (*a*) Thicker and coarser; (*b*) Few, irregular, and flatter spirals; (*c*) Stains deeper and more blue; (*d*) Greater motility.

Morbid Anatomy

The histological basis of a syphilitic lesion is the same at any stage: a collection of epithelioid cells with some scanty giant cells, plasma cells and fibroblasts and lymphocytes forming a granuloma, together with obliterative endarteritis of blood vessels. The picture varies with the site of the lesion.

Primary chancre. Consists of: (1) Central area relatively acellular but rich in mucopolysaccharides; (2) Surrounding cellular infiltrate of polymorphs and lymphocytes. Central necrosis occurs later and macrophages and plasma cells enter the surrounding area.

Gumma. An 'infective granuloma'. Consists, in early stage, of cells as above. *Early*: vessels scanty. *Later*: new vessels numerous. Then obliterative endarteritis occurs, followed by caseation of tissue, necrosis and rupture in certain situations.

Distinction from tubercle difficult. Main points: (1) In gumma, new vessels prominent, in tubercle absent; (2) In gumma, epithelioid and giant cells scanty, and later less definite than in tubercle.

Modes of Infection
Conveyed by secretion from syphilitic lesions, especially chancre and early secondary lesions. But semen may contain spirochaetes in absence of lesion of external genitals.

Sexual contact. Common sites of chancre: *Male*, sides of fraenum, glans, sulcus, prepuce; less commonly, within meatus, shaft of penis, scrotum, etc. *Female*, labia minora, os uteri, clitoris, meatus; occasionally labia majora; vagina rare.

Transmission by connection is unusual more than 5 years from original infection: but there is no time limit to infection of fetus by mother.

Congenital infection. Intra-uterine infection of fetus through placenta. Mother often has no signs, but Wassermann reaction is positive.

Extragenital sexual contact may produce chancres in the mouth and on lips, on nipples and in the rectum (females and male homosexuals). Usually painful, cf. genital chancres painless.

In medical practice, e.g. on fingers of back of hands.

Syphilis may be *Congenital* or *Acquired*.

Immunity
Infected persons are not susceptible to reinoculation but become susceptible again after cure. Antibodies produced are not protective. Two laws of last generation state: (1) *Colles' Law*—a syphilitic infant does not infect its own mother; (2) *Profeta's Law*—a mother with syphilitic symptoms may suckle her own infant without infecting it. Explanation is that mother and child respectively are in fact already infected.

Acquired Syphilis

Incubation Period
Interval between infection and appearance of primary lesion (chancre) usually 3–4 weeks with a range of 10 days to 10 weeks. Period often impossible to determine.

Note: Infection with spirochaetes is generalized within few days of inoculation, certainly before appearance of chancre. After inoculation of a rabbit by scarification, spirochaetes are present in nearest lymph nodes in 30 min.

Stages of Syphilis
Symptoms are referred to three stages, *Primary*, *Secondary* and *Tertiary*. A period of latency may follow the secondary phase lasting many years. The division between stages is empirical and stages may merge into each other.

Recent nomenclature is to count primary and secondary stages together as *Early*, and the other stages as *Late*.

PRIMARY STAGE

The Chancre
Initial lesion of syphilis is the 'primary', 'hard', or 'Hunterian' *chancre*, a local manifestation which commences as a painless, small, red papule: enlarges to size of pea: ruptures, forming small ulcer.
Characteristics. Raised, edges indurated, may feel like nodule of cartilage, floor often greyish slough, secretion slight, suppuration uncommon. Freely movable. Painless in a genital site.
Progress. Granulation occurs, and ulcer heals with or without treatment.
Scar. May be slight or absent.
Usually single, occasionally two or, rarely, more.
Site. See Modes of Infection, *above*.

Varieties of Chancre
On glans induration often absent. A tight prepuce becomes oedematous, chancre palpable below. In females, often obscured by oedema: frequently unnoticed.
Sepsis. With infection by septic organisms or bacillus of soft sore, acute ulceration occurs: very painful; diagnosis obscured.
Extragenital chancres. Induration less marked: ulceration greater. May be painful, cf. genital chancre.
Phagedaena. Rare: rapid ulceration, penis may be destroyed.

Lymph Nodes
In area of chancre (e.g. groin) enlarged, may form large 'bubo': suppuration only with septic infection.

Serological Tests
Non-treponemal antigen tests positive by time of presentation with chancre.

Diagnosis
Especially from:.(1) Genital herpes; (2) Chancroid; (3) Trauma; (4) Circinate balanitis in Reiter's Syndrome; (5) Behçet's disease; (6) Scabies.

SECONDARY STAGE
Is a period of manifestations of general infection, a long-drawn fever with constitutional symptoms, as opposed to the localized lesion of the primary stage.

Onset
Usually 5–12 weeks after chancre.

Duration
About 2 years, but no definite limit.

Principal Manifestations

(1) Rash; (2) Sore throat; (3) Mucous patches; (4) Condylomas; (5) General enlargement of lymph nodes; (6) Loss of hair; (7) Anaemia; (8) Fever; (9) Headache and insomnia not uncommon.

Other manifestations. Periostitis. Eyes (especially iritis). Nephrotic syndrome. Nails. Mild hepatitis. Acute myelitis. Joints. Testes. Effect on pregnancy. Secondary lesions possess a general tendency to be symmetrical.

Rash

General characteristics

1. *Polymorphic*: Macules, papules, etc. present simultaneously, yet spots tend to be of similar size: roundish; except roseola, are infiltrated.

2. *Roughly symmetrical*: Abundant. On flexor rather than extensor surfaces. Occasionally a few spots only. e.g. on flexor surfaces of forearms.

3. *Colour*: A coppery or raw-ham tint is specially suggestive.

4. *Does not itch*.

5. Disappears without treatment.

May resemble any known rash, e.g. seborrhoea.

Main varieties

Macular syphilide, syphilitic roseola: Commonest type and earliest onset. *Appears* about 6 weeks after chancre. *Duration*, 3–6 weeks. Rose-coloured spots, size about 10 mm; when well developed, do not disappear on pressure, no infiltration. On trunk and flexors of arms; very rare on face. May leave peculiar brownish discoloured areas, especially on neck. Recrudescence not uncommon, sometimes in late stages.

Papular or lenticular syphilide: Onset tends to be later than previous type. Raised, often coppery, shiny scales at margins, infiltrated. Desquamates. Abundant distribution, includes face. *Duration*, 1–3 months or longer.

Numular syphilide: Coin-like lesions with well-defined edges, on face or perineum, especially in dark-skinned races.

Papulopustular syphilide

Squamous syphilide (syphilitic psoriasis): Resembles psoriasis, but less silvery and scaly, infiltrated, and mainly on flexors: development rapid, often coppery tint, fissures common.

Rupia (crusts form over ulcers). *Ecthyma* (ulceration of pustules). These are rare forms developing in neglected pustular eruptions.

Differential diagnosis

Pityriasis rosea: Diagnosis from macular syphilide. Itches: covered with fine scales: glands and mucous membranes unaffected. Scaly syphilides are infiltrated and less pink.

Lichen planus: Diagnosis from papular syphilide. *Lilac tint*, flat-topped, polygonal, shiny. Itches.

Psoriasis: Mainly on elbows and knees. Shiny and scaly. Chronic. Itches.

Drug rashes

Sore Throat

Tonsils swollen: *ulcers*, small, grey, clear-cut, shape, (*a*) kidney or (*b*) 'snail track', often symmetrical. Entire mucous membrane of mouth and tongue (glossitis) often inflamed: also *larynx* (hoarseness).

Mucous Patches
Flat grey areas. *Site*: moist regions, especially angles of mouth, and also within mouth, e.g. on tonsils.

Condylomas
Papules, from hypertrophy of papillae; moist, round. Very infective; always syphilitic. *Sites*: skin surfaces in apposition, i.e. external genitals, perineum, toes, under breasts. Specially in women.

Lymph Nodes
Generalized slight adenitis, especially *epitrochlear* and *cervical glands*. Never suppurate.

Alopecia
Hair loses gloss and falls out: often in patches. Grows again after treatment.

Anaemia
Very common.

Fever
Usually slight. Very rarely severe. Night sweats occur.

Serological Tests
Always positive.

Other Lesions
Less frequent or characteristic:
Bones. (1) Wandering ('osteocopic') pains common, mainly at night; (2) Symmetrical subacute periostitis of long bones frequent: may result in '*nodes*', e.g. on edges of tibiae.
Eyes. *Iritis* common, usually in second year: iris muddy, pupil small and reacts sluggishly. Rarely, choroiditis and retinitis.
Nails. 'Syphilitic onychia': ulceration around and destroying nail: nails brittle.

Occasional Lesions
Nephrotic Syndrome. Tends to be very severe. *See* Renal Syphilis, p. 94.
Hepatitis
Acute Myelitis
Joints. Very rarely affected in acquired syphilis. Subacute painless symmetrical arthritis, usually knees.
Testes. Rarely affected. Epididymitis or orchitis.

Pregnant Woman
Usually aborts.

Late Secondary Syphilis
Certain symptoms tend to occur late in the secondary stage, or there may be recurrences of former symptoms. Such manifestations emphasize the fact that the division into stages is not absolute; these symptoms may even occur years after infection.
Rashes. Any type of secondary rash may occur, especially roseola.

Usually less characteristic in late stages. Rupia occasionally.
Iritis. Essentially a late secondary manifestation.
Superficial Glossitis
Acute Myelitis
Orchitis. Painless and symmetrical.

Some of these are variously regarded as late secondary or as tertiary manifestations.

TERTIARY STAGE

Occurrence
30% of those untreated.

Onset
Usually from 2 to 10 years after infection. Occasionally after 6 months. No absolute upper limit.

Duration
Unlimited. Recurrences common.

Fever
Rare.

Lesions of Tertiary Syphilis
A classification follows, but the pathological basis is the same throughout, with the gumma as its predominant expression with its sequelae and changes in the blood vessels. Gummas very uncommon since advent of penicillin.
1. Gumma.
2. Cutaneous and mucous-membrane lesions.
3. Visceral lesions: (*a*) Nervous; (*b*) Circulatory: (i) Mesaortitis (aneurysm); (ii) Obliterative endarteritis, etc.; (*c*) Liver; (*d*) Testis; (*e*) Bones; (*f*) Alimentary system (rectum); Rare: (*g*) Respiratory system; (*h*) Kidneys.
4. Various lesions: Miscarriages; effect on pregnancy. Amyloid disease.
Gumma. No tissue or organ immune (except possibly prostate): especially in skin, mucous membrane, subcutaneous tissue and muscles.

Clinical appearance (e.g. in subcutaneous tissue): Firm, painless swelling develops rapidly, enlarges, softens, ruptures, discharges contents: ulcer results.

Ulcer: Circular; deep, wall steep and 'punched-out'; floor, yellow 'wash-leather slough'; base infiltrated; foul discharge common.

Termination: Varies with site and treatment. Responds rapidly to treatment except in brain.

1. Absorption: With treatment, if gumma is unruptured, this may be practically complete (e.g. in testis). May be absorbed after fluctuation.

2. Ulceration, healing and scar: *Thin 'tissue-paper' scar, usually pigmented.* Almost, but not quite, pathognomonic of syphilis.

On bones: Hardens, producing osteosclerosis.
Recurrences: Frequent.
Scarring: In certain sites may cause serious deformities, e.g. larynx, rectum and liver.
Diagnosis: (1) Origin without cause, grows rapidly, softens, ulcer distinctive;

(2) History and signs of previous syphilis; (3) Serological tests positive; (4) Yields to antisyphilitic treatment. Spirochaetes rarely found.

Cutaneous and Mucous-membrane Lesions

Nodular cutaneous syphilide (*tertiary or tubercular syphilide, syphilitic lupus*): Essentially, collection of small gummas. Commences as small brownish nodules, which enlarge; area increases by coalescence with fresh outlying nodules, producing serpiginous syphilide. *Margins* round or roughly crescentic; diameter 2 cm and upwards. At edges raised nodules. Periphery extends, while in centre healing and scarring occur in various degrees. Skin thickens. *Site* usually single, especially forehead, neck, back and scrotum, also palms and soles. Resembles *lupus vulgaris*: distinguished by: (1) rapid growth, (2) no apple-jelly nodules.

Multiple cutaneous gummas: Condition more severe than last; numerous gummatous ulcers.

Mucous membranes: Gummas common: ulceration very rapid; destroys all tissues, e.g. nasal cartilage; heals with much scarring and deformity, whence strictures. *Sites*: nose; palate (perforations); larynx (strictures); pharynx; tongue, often with leucoplakia (*see* Syphilis of the tongue, p. 92).

Rare cutaneous conditions: Leucoderma is sometimes syphilitic (or parasyphilitic). Keratoderma of the soles.

Bone Lesions

Long bones: Localized gummas. Pain severe, especially at night. Discharge through skin.

Bones affected: Clavicle (especially sternoclavicular joint), sternum, ribs, tibia, femur. Dactylitis rare. No bone immune.

Flat bones: Lesions may be extensive, causing great disfigurement. Now rare.

Bones affected: Skull: bones of nose and palate; frontal and parietal bones (may penetrate skull). Gumma of inner layer of skull may press in brain. Vertebrae rare: may cause retropharyngeal, lumbar, or iliac abscess; or pressure on cord.

Diffuse osteitis and periostitis not common.

Testis. Lesion may be:

1. *Diffuse interstitial*. Testis enlarged, smooth, painless. May shrink later.
2. *Nodular gummas*. May discharge through skin.

Note: Epididymis, prostate, ovaries rarely affected.

Visceral Lesions. *See* p. 91 and elsewhere.

Amyloid Disease. Common formerly in chronic syphilis.

Effect on Pregnancy. *See* Congenital Syphilis, *below*.

QUARTERNARY STAGE (PARENCHYMATOUS SYPHILIS)

Diseases occuring usually many years after infection: (1) Tabes dorsalis; (2) Dementia paralytica.

Congenital Syphilis

General Principles

Inheritance of syphilis and effects on pregnancy.

1. *Effects of syphilis on pregnancy*. May cause *repeated* miscarriages. The liability diminishes with the interval since infection, and with treatment. Typical results are: (*a*) *Repeated miscarriages*. (*b*) Waning effects in successive pregnancies (Kassowitz's law), e.g. sequence in 6 consecutive pregnancies: (i) early abortion;

(ii) miscarriage in later months; (iii) syphilitic infant, death in few days, (iv) healthy at birth, syphilis in few weeks (typical 'congenital syphilis'); (v) malnutrition only, possibly interstitial keratitis later; (vi) healthy life. May be a healthy child between syphilitics. This progressive sequence is doubtful.

2. *Congenital syphilis*. Always inherited from mother, in whom Wassermann reaction is positive even if no symptoms are present; this explains Colles' law (*see* p. 84). Mother may have ceased to be sexually contagious. Chances of transplacental infection decrease with increasing duration of untreated maternal infection.

3. *Effect of treating mother*. Adequate dosage of penicillin given to the mother at any stage of pregnancy will secure an uninfected child in the great majority of cases.

4. *Congenital syphilitic child* shows: (1) Wassermann reaction positive; (2) Immunity to acquired syphilis—this explains Profeta's law; (3) Response to treatment.

5. *Syphilitic father*. Has syphilitic child only if his lesion can infect the mother.

6. *Transmission to third generation* doubtful.

Symptoms

1. *Present at birth*, death occurring within a few days. Emaciated and feeble: bullous eruption on palms and soles, syphilitic pemphigus neonatorum; snuffles; epiphysitis and disease of skull bones; enlarged liver and spleen. Rarely, syphilis haemorrhagica neonatorum.

   Syphilitic foetus has large spleen and liver, teeming with spirochaetes, bone changes and various syphilitic lesions. The placenta shows cirrhosis and arterial changes. Hydramnios common.

2. *Appear a few weeks after birth* ('congenital syphilis'). Healthy at birth. Symptoms divisible into: (1) Early symptoms; (2) Late symptoms. Both groups suggest long-drawn secondary stage, lesions similarly tending to be symmetrical; (3) Tertiary and para-syphilitic lesions. Any symptom of acquired syphilis may occur.

Early Symptoms

Wasting without cause, muddy complexion.

'Snuffles'. Onset 3–8 weeks. A syphilitic rhinitis causing: (1) Contagious discharge, whence 'snuffling'; (2) Necrosis of nasal bones, whence later characteristic depressed bridge of nose.

Cutaneous lesions. Onset 3–12 weeks. Protean: may be erythema, macules, papules or vesicles. (1) Scaly macular eruption: commonest, yellow to coppery or raw-ham tint; scanty or profuse, especially on buttocks; may be eczematous in napkin area; (2) Pemphigus: rare, may be present at birth; bullae on palms and soles, may become generalized and fatal; (3) Mucous patches in mouth and fauces. Condylomas around anus; (4) Inflammation of larynx: hoarse cry; (5) Ulceration at angles of mouth ('rhagades'), whence later radiating scars; (6) Hair loses gloss and falls out, especially *eyebrows*.

Enlargement of liver and spleen. May be jaundice.

Bone affections. (1) *Syphilitic epiphysitis*: ends of long bones; often symmetrical or multiple. Occurs within first few months. Rapid loss of movement (syphilitic pseudoparalysis). Epiphyses may suppurate or separate. Diagnose from rickets by (*a*) early age, (*b*) localization of thickening; (2) Bossing of frontal prominences of skull; (3) Craniotabes (not confined to syphilis); (4) Syphilitic

dactylitis: phalanges, metacarpals, metatarsals. From second year onwards. Swelling may rupture. Diagnosis from tuberculosis difficult.
General glandular enlargement is uncommon.
Occasional symptoms. Iritis, onychia, various rashes, orchitis.

Progress
Improves under treatment. Development is slow: may be 'infantilism'.

DELAYED CONGENITAL SYPHILIS
Onset during second dentition or puberty.
*Eye. Interstitial keratitis** bilateral; may cause blindness; cornea steamy (ground glass); duration 1–2 years. Prognosis good: clears from periphery to centre, where opacities may remain. Commonest late symptom; may be sole syphilitic lesion.
Iritis, disseminated choroiditis: not uncommon, often with keratitis; prognosis worse, vision permanently affected. Rarely, optic atrophy.
Synovitis (Clutton's Joints). Painless, symmetrical, with effusion. Usually in *knees*. Synovitis of this type is always syphilitic.
Bones. Symmetrical periostitis, especially of *tibiae*. Result: inflammatory thickening, mainly in middle, whence '*sabre-shaped curvature*'. Syphilitic dactylitis.
Ear. Causeless, rapid, permanent, bilateral deafness:* probably labyrinthine. Age 11–20 years. Females predominate.
*Hutchinson's teeth.** Upper central *permanent* incisors stunted, peg-shaped, cutting edge smaller than base: edge deeply notched, exposing dentine. Rarely recognizable in adults owing to rapid erosion of cutting edge. Canines may be notched, and first molars domed (Moon's molar).

Tertiary Lesions
Gummas; not common, but may occur as in acquired syphilis and at any age or site (especially testes).

Parasyphilis
'*Juvenile general paralysis*'. Rare. Occurs at about 16 years.
    Tabes dorsalis is considerably rarer. *See* Syphilis of the Central Nervous System.

Residual Symptoms
(1) Pallor, malnutrition; (2) Depressed bridge of nose; (3) Radiating scars at angles of mouth; (4) Square or asymmetrical skull; (5) Liver and spleen may be palpable; (6) Wassermann reaction positive; (7) Thickening of tibiae; (8) Corneal opacities; (9) Hutchinson's teeth.

Visceral Syphilis

SYPHILIS OF THE LUNGS
Very rare. Most important is the fibrosis at the root of the lung, the frequency of which is not yet fully known.

A. Congenital Syphilis
White pneumonia of the foetus: large areas airless, grey and smooth (not granular,

---

*Hutchinson's triad.

as in 'grey hepatization'): alveolar walls thickened, filled with desquamated cells: numerous *T. pallida*. Pathological interest only: life not exceeding few hours.

B. Acquired Syphilis
1. *Interstitial pneumonia* (fibrosis) at *the root of the lung*; fibrosis spreads outwards along bronchi and vessels. May be associated with gummas and with bronchiectasis. Characters: (1) Symptoms in general resemble pulmonary tuberculosis, tubercle bacilli absent; (2) Changes mainly at root of lungs, noticeable in radiograph; (3) Improves with antisyphilitic treatment; (4) Syphilitic history and other lesions may be present; (5) Wassermann reaction positive. No spirochaetes in sputum.
2. *Gummas*. Very rare. Then several and encapsulated: may be caseous and bronchiectatic cavities.

SYPHILIS OF THE BRONCHI

Secondary
May be hyperaemia, causing cough ('syphilitic bronchitis').

Tertiary
Gummas in or near large bronchus: tend to fibrose, producing bronchial stenosis or bronchiectasis. Invasion of lung rare.

SYPHILIS OF THE TONGUE
Lesions frequent; some characteristic. Carcinoma may follow.

Primary: Chancre
Site: Usually near tip on dorsum. Indurated. Ulceration may be deep.
Diagnosis: (1) Epithelioma, at sides of tongue, painful. (2) Tuberculous ulcer, painful, pulmonary disease advanced.

Secondary
Shallow ulcers.

Tertiary
Leucoplakia: Mucous membrane thickened and white, especially in smokers. Proof of syphilis not invariable. Carcinoma may follow.
Syphilitic glossitis: Diffuse gummatous infiltration: results in *deep fissures*, large hard tongue, leucoplakia common. Very characteristic. Carcinoma may follow.
Localized gummas: Infrequent.

SYPHILIS OF THE PHARYNX
Lesions frequent.

Primary: Chancre
Uncommon. Usually tonsil. Induration slight.

Secondary
1. *Erythema*: Dusky red rash. Palate or tonsil. Diffuse or localized.

2. *Mucous patches*: On tonsils, pillars, or soft palate: produce 'snail-track' ulcers: often symmetrical. Often late secondary stage. Symptoms slight.

Tertiary
Gummatous ulceration, often rapid and extensive. Frequent sites: posterior pharyngeal wall; posterior wall of soft palate. Dysphagia usual. Perforation of soft palate common; also adhesions of soft palate to posterior wall.

SYPHILIS OF THE LIVER (Syphilitic Hepatitis)

A. Congenital Syphilis
1. *Diffuse hepatitis*. Occurs in infants born with disease, or developing signs within a few weeks. Present in most early fatal cases.
   Macroscopic: Liver large and tough, of yellow or flinty colour.
   Histology: Pericellular cirrhosis. Spirochaetes in enormous numbers. (In early stages in fetus, a diffuse, small round-cell infiltration.)
   Physical signs: Liver enlarged, below navel. Spleen also enlarged. Ascites rare. May be jaundice.
2. *Later congenital syphilis*. Liver changes similar to acquired forms. Jaundice not common.

B. Acquired Syphilis
Secondary
Tertiary. Lesions important, usually 10–20 years after infection. (1) Gummas; (2) Scarring of liver. May coexist.
   Gummas: *Size*: from a pea to a fist or larger. Often multiple. *Site*: any part, most commonly anterior surface, junction of right and left lobes. *Appearance*: firm, greyish, roughly spherical. Three zones present in early gummas, especially when large: (1) Caseous centre; (2) Surrounding fibrous-tissue zone; (3) Outer zone of small round-cell infiltration, where condition is advancing. *Progress*: caseation; then absorption partial or complete, resulting in *scarring*. Rarely softening or calcification. Local peritonitis may occur.
   Scarring of liver: Depressed scars on surface of live: fibrous-tissue strands run inwards; may be gummatous or caseating areas. Scarring of all degrees from small superficial linear scars up to extreme deformities (*hepar lobatum*).
   Amyloid disease: Now rare. Other organs also affected.
Symptoms. Three principal groups:
   1. *Tumour of the liver (gumma)*: Palpable mass: liver usually large and tender. Pain in right hypochondrium or epigastrium common. *Spleen* may be palpable. Often no other syphilitic signs. *Diagnosis* from neoplasm difficult. *Wassermann reaction* positive. Antisyphilitic treatment effective. Jaundice rare.
   2. *Resembles atrophic cirrhosis of liver (scarring)*: Fever and ascites: may be jaundice. Liver edge irregular, if palpable. Portal obstruction probably mechanical from gumma or scarring in the portal fissure. May be no syphilitic signs. Haematemesis unusual.
   3. *With enlargement of spleen*: May simulate splenic anaemia, and many conditions with splenomegaly.

SYPHILIS OF THE ALIMENTARY TRACT
Syphilitic lesions are very rare between pharynx and rectum.

Stomach. Syphilitic lesions very rare at autopsy. Occasionally diagnosed during life. Symptoms may resemble carcinoma: severe pain after food, vomiting, wasting and achlorhydria; haematemesis rare. Radiographs: diffuse involvement of walls with stiffening and diminished mobility; pylorus may be incompetent or obstructed. Wassermann reaction positive. Rapid improvement with antisyphilitic treatment; hydrochloric acid returns.

Intestines. Lesions very rare. Stenosis has resulted from gummas.

Syphilis of rectum. Early: syphilitic proctitis or anal chancre in homosexual men, occasionally in women. Late: slow gummatous growth immediately above internal sphincter; usually surrounds rectum. *Stricture of rectum* subsequently develops: may be extreme; distinguished from neoplasm by hard fibrous ring.

   Note: Many cases previously ascribed to syphilis were probably due to gonorrhoea or lymphogranuloma venereum.

Spleen. Enlargement not uncommon. Gummas and scarring not infrequent; liver usually involved also (*see above*).

SYPHILIS OF THE CIRCULATORY SYSTEM

The heart. The principal effects on the heart are due to syphilitic lesions of the coronary vessels, resulting in fibroid myocarditis, and to syphilitic lesions of the aorta, resulting in aortic valve disease, and aneurysm.

   Gummas are very rare, but some recorded cases are of special interest owing to their position in the bundle of His and functional tissues of auricle and ventricle, producing disturbances of cardiac rhythm and Stokes–Adams' syndrome.

RENAL SYPHILIS

A. Secondary Syphilis
Mild simple albuminuria. Not uncommon. Prognosis good. Formerly ascribed to mercury, erroneously.

Nephrotic syndrome
   Onset: commonest 2–4 months after chancre, viz. at time of rash.

B. Tertiary Syphilis
Little importance.
   1. Amyloid disease.
   2. Gummas of the kidneys: very rare. Undiagnosable in life.
   3. Interstitial nephritis. Only with arterial disease.

SYPHILIS OF THE NERVOUS SYSTEM
See textbook on diseases of the nervous system.

Diagnosis

General Diagnosis
Lesions often distinctive and simplified by multiplicity. History and signs of earlier disease often present, viz.:

Primary chancre. Scar may be present. Difficulties due to: absence of scar, urethral and extragenital chancres, masking by gonorrhoea or soft sore; in females, presence on os uteri.

Secondary lesions. Inquire and examine for these.

Tertiary lesions. Examine for results of gummas, e.g. 'pigmented tissue-paper' scars on legs, perforations of palate, etc.
In women. Repeated miscarriages.
Congenital syphilis. Residual phenomena (*see* p. 89), especially depressed nose, radiating scars from mouth, history of interstitial keratitis and blindness at puberty.

Specific Diagnosis
Treponema pallida. In chancres, condylomas, and mucous patches. For methods, *see under* 'Parasite', p. 83.
Serological tests
Cerebrospinal fluid

Serological Tests
1. Tests for reaginic or antilipoidal antibodies. The Wassermann Reaction (WR) was the first serological test available. The original workers used a saline extract of syphilitic tissues as antigen but later work showed that saline extracts of normal tissue worked just as well and alcoholic extracts of normal tissue were even better. Cardiolipin extracted with alcohol from ox heart together with lecithin and cholesterol forms an antigen that will have complement-fixing properties when mixed with syphilitic sera. The Venereal Disease Reference Laboratory (VDRL) and Rapid Plasma Reagin (RPR) tests demonstrate the presence of antibodies in syphilitic sera by producing flocculation. These tests may be titred out. Biological false positive reactions occur. These tests detect IgM and IgG and *not* IgE antibody.
2. Tests for antitreponemal antibody
>*2.1. Group Specific Tests*
>The Reiter's strain of *T. pallidum* which is avirulent and cultivable in vitro provides a source of antigen which can be used to detect antitreponemal antibodies in the Reiter Protein Complement Fixation Test (RPCFT). False positive reactions occur.
>*2.2 Specific Treponemal Tests*
>*Treponema pallidum* Immobilization Tests (TPI) use a virulent strain that is maintained in rabbits. The test demonstrates the presence of complement-fixing antibodies to the organism which immobilize >50% of the organisms in a positive test.
>
>   *Treponema pallidum* Haemagglutination Test (TPHA) detects antitreponemal antibody by haemagglutination of tanned red cells to which is fixed an antigen derived from ultrasonically disrupted *T. pallidum*.
>
>   Fluorescent Treponemal Antibody Absorption Test (FTA-Abs). This is an indirect fluorescent antibody technique in which Reiter protein antigen is first mixed with test serum and then this mixture is put on a slide to which *T. pallida* are fixed. Any syphilitic antibody bound to the Reiter protein will also bind to the antigen on the slide and its presence is shown by positive fluorescence when a fluorescein-labelled anti-human globulin is added to the slide. Total antibody and IgM antibody can be detected.

Interpretation of Results

Stage		WR	RPCFT	TPI	TPHA	FTA-Abs
PRIMARY	Early	Neg.	Neg.	Neg.	Neg.	+ (80%)
	Late	Pos.	Pos.	Pos.	Pos.	Pos.
SECONDARY		Strongly pos.	Strongly pos.	———— Strongly pos. ————		
LATENT		Pos. (Falling titre)	Pos.	Pos.	Pos.	Pos.
TERTIARY		Pos. (May be neg.)	Pos.	Pos.	Pos.	Pos.

Note: These tests do not differentiate between syphilis, yaws, endemic syphilis and pinta.

Biological False Positive WR: Occurs in acute infectious diseases, including malaria and infectious mononucleosis, as well as chronic diseases like leprosy and disseminated lupus erythematosus. Specific tests for treponemal antibody are negative.

Congenital syphilis: serological diagnosis is difficult as IgG antibody from the mother crosses the placenta in the 3rd trimester. IgM antibody does not cross the placenta and so antitreponomal IgM in an infant's blood indicates congenital infection.

Syphilis of nervous system. Positive in 80–90%.

Parasyphilis. Dementia paralytica: always positive (also CSF). *Tabes dorsalis*: positive in 70%

Cerebrospinal Fluid

In lesions of nervous system, examine CSF: (1) Cells; (2) Globulin; (3) Antibody reaction. In neurosyphilis:

Cells. Small lymphocytes present. Over 20 cells/mm^3 is pathological. This is diagnostic in chronic conditions, but also occurs in tuberculous meningitis, benign lymphocytic meningitis, and to some extent in acute poliomyelitis and encephalitis lethargica.

Globulin. Increased (Pandy's test). Albumin: globulin ratio altered.

Antibody reaction. Tertiary syphilis, may be positive or negative; *dementia paralytica*, always positive: *tabes dorsalis*, positive in 70–90%. Specific antitreponemal tests positive.

Treatment of Primary, Secondary and Early Latent Syphilis (<2 Years)

Treatment must be commenced immediately on diagnosis—e.g. by examination for spirochaetes in primary lesions—and must not await serological tests. Drug of choice is penicillin. Penicillin is highly effective, spirochaetes disappearing in 12–24 h. Chancre and mucous lesions of secondary stage rapidly resolve. Wassermann reaction usually negative in 3–4 months.

Penicillin

Dosage: Benzathine penicillin G 2·4 million units give i.m. once; or Aqueous procaine penicillin 6·0 million units once daily i.m. for 10 days.

Serological Reaction after Treatment
The WR becomes negative by 6–12 months post-therapy. Specific treponemal tests remain positive for life and so are not helpful in assessing response.

Test reaction at intervals of 3 months for a year, and then at intervals of 6 months. Cure may be assumed if negative at end of 2 years. Do CSF examination if still positive 18–24 months after treatment.

Complications following Penicillin Therapy
Jarisch–Herxheimer reaction. Patient should be warned of possibility in the 12 h following the first dose of penicillin there may be a rigor with pyrexia of up to 38·4 °C (101 °F) and exacerbation of the signs and symptoms. It can be serious in tertiary or late syphilis and may then necessitate steroids to cover the first few penicillin injections.
Penicillin hypersensitivity. When penicillin allergy is documented, tetracycline (500 mg q.d.s. × 15 days) or erythromycin (500 mg q.d.s. × 15 days) may be given orally. Tetracycline should not be given to children under 8 years and in pregnancy.

Treatment of (1) Late Latent and (2) Tertiary Syphilis
Procaine penicillin i.m. (1) 9 million u/day × 15, (2) 12 million u/day × 20 days.

Pregnancy
The pregnant woman should be given procaine penicillin 6 million u daily, for 10 days.

Treatment of Congenital Syphilis
Good results on same general lines as for adults. The infant dose is calculated as 50 000 u of procaine penicillin/kg body weight/day. The course of injections is 10 days.

In older children or adolescents the penicillin course is as for adults with acquired disease, but is adjusted for the weight of the patient.

Chapter 29   # YAWS (Framboesia)

Contagious inoculable disease characterized by raspberry-like granulomas, caused by *Treponema pertenue*.

Distribution
Widespread in tropics. Children most often.

Mode of Infection
Direct contact with sore of an infected person. Wound-feeding flies may act as mechanical carriers.

Relation to Syphilis
T. pertenue indistinguishable morphologically from *T. pallidum*. General clinical resemblance, especially in late stages. Wassermann and treponemal serology positive early and persistently in blood but never in CSF. But note: (1) Never

congenital; (2) Primary lesion extragenital, and infection not conveyed sexually; (3) Primary lesion is distinctive; (4) No visceral or central nervous system lesions; (5) Mucous membranes in general not affected; (6) Mothers are often inoculated from children. Identity of yaws and syphilis much discussed: yaws claimed to be primitive and tropical form of syphilis: syphilis being communicated by sexual connection and not by contact becoming more virulent and neurotrophic.

Incubation Period
Two to four weeks.

Symptoms
Often described as having primary, secondary and tertiary stages (but must not be correlated too closely with stages of syphilis).

Primary lesion. Papule forms: gradually enlarges, forming granuloma from which the surface epidermis becomes eroded producing the raspberry-like warty lesion, the surface of which is usually covered by yellow crust. This is 2–5 cm in diameter, constitutes 'mother yaw': nature often overlooked: usually heals in about 6 weeks. *Site*: lower extremities commonly: any site where skin is broken: genitals rare. Constitutional disturbances moderate: fever and joint pains.

Secondary eruption. Usually before primary yaw has completely healed secondary eruption appears. Commonest clinical manifestation. Skin loses gloss, patches of furfuraceous desquamation form. Multiple papules appear in these areas: any site, but most profuse in perspiring areas. Papules, often in clusters, enlarge and coalesce: skin desquamates, leaving reddish surface resembling raspberry, the 'yaws' papillomas which are teeming with spirochaetes. Grows for 2 weeks, then stationary several weeks, projecting up to 1 cm. Then shrinks: crust forms from secretion and forms scab. Finally drops off, leaving patch of paler skin.

Successive crops of papillomas appear, with fever and rheumatic pains.

Foot yaws: Papules on feet, often painful owing to thick epidermis: may ulcerate and form cracks slow to heal. (Crab Yaws.)

Other clinical manifestations:

Skin: May be circinate groups of small cone-shaped acuminate papillae on extensor surfaces. Tend to appear in cooler conditions of climate. Plantar and palmar hyperkeratosis.

Tendon sheaths: Ganglion may occur especially near wrist. Contains some granulation tissue.

Periosteum: Several proximal phalanges: multiple dactylitis—never suppurates.

Periostitis of long bones: may resolve or may leave irregularities due to new bone formation.

Such a change on the nasal bones leading to new bone deposition causes Goundou: facial deformity which led to the description by early explorers in Africa of seeing 'horned men'.

Tertiary stage. May follow in direct sequence from secondary stage, but may only appear after a latent period lasting months or years.

Skin and subcutaneous tissue:

Gummatous swelling common. Usually ulcerates to produce chronic granulomatous indolent ulcer. *Sites*: often leg, or dorsum of wrist and hand. Healing eventually with tissue-paper-like scars.

Hyperkeratosis of palms and soles, difficult to distinguish from that of secondary stage, but usually associated with more scarring and depigmentation. Note increased incidence of Dupuytren's contracture in yaws areas.

Depigmentation in irregular map-like areas may occur called a pinti-form lesion, since it resembles late pinta.

Bones: Destructive osteitis usually associated with sinus formation and small sequestra, and with some sclerosis of surrounding bone.

Common sites: 'Cold abscess' of brow with involvement of outer table of frontal lobe. Single suppurative dactylitis, closely resembling tuberculosis. Femora, with resulting thickening and irregularity. Nasal septum and bones of hard palate resulting in gangosa—destructive lesion causing gross deformity of face.

Joints: Bilateral painless hydrarthrosis of the knees: not common. Juxta-articular nodes are fibrous tissue nodules forming in the tendinous expansions over articular capsules.

Common sites: Knees, elbows, hips.

Diagnosis

In a known yaws area usually easy in primary and secondary stages by seeing the lesions. Tertiary lesions sometimes difficult to differentiate from leprosy, cutaneous leishmaniasis, espundia and other types of chronic ulcers or osteitis.

The isolated case of yaws may be most difficult to diagnose since almost every yaws lesion can be matched by some lesion occurring in syphilis. History is the main guide, and sometimes the age of the patient.

Serological tests for syphilis, including the Treponemal Immobilization Test, become strongly positive in late primary and early secondary stages of the disease. They continue less strongly positive during periods of latency.

Organisms morphologically identical with *T. pallidum* can be obtained from serous exudate in primary and secondary eruptions.

Mortality

A deforming disease but not a killing disease.

Treatment

Penicillin causes speedy regression of primary and secondary manifestations. More prolonged treatment is needed for late cases.

Mass treatment campaigns, supported by WHO have been based upon the following:

1. Every campaign must be associated with an effort at improving the whole health of the population, and building up treatment centres which can serve after the mass treatment campaign is finished.

2. A census of the population based upon visiting dwellings is made.

3. While it is being made all the people are examined to look for obvious lesions of infectious yaws.

4. Immediate treatment is given by the i.m. injection of 1·2 megaunits of procaine penicillin with aluminium monostearate (PAM) of known potency.

5. All household contacts of the patient with infectious yaws are given 0·6 megaunits of PAM at once.

6. The population is re-surveyed and treatments on the same plan are given again in an interval of 6–12 months.

Pinta

An infection due to *Treponema carateum* resulting in alterations in the pigmentation of the skin.

Geographical Distribution
The headwaters of the Amazon, S. America.

Transmission
Probably by direct contact.

Clinical Manifestations
Commonest: tertiary stage skin lesions: map-like areas of loss of pigment; may be anywhere on the body but common sites are hands, feet and genitalia.

Less common: secondary stage or pintids. Widely spread, small, sometimes confluent, maculopapules, the early ones reddish in colour, the later ones purplish-brown. Tend to be on exposed skin areas.

The primary lesion, a single pintid, has only been seen after experimental inoculation.

Pathology
Chronic inflammation of the dermis with round-cell infiltration, and progressive destruction of the melanin-carrying cells.

Diagnosis
By recognizing the skin lesions.

T. carateum, morphologically identical with *T. pallidum*, may be obtained in the tissue juice obtained by squeezing an affected area of skin in the secondary stage, using the blades of a haemostat forceps.

Eosinophilia is found in the early stages of the disease.

Serological tests for syphilis are positive.

Treatment
In early cases, and in mass treatment campaigns, penicillin, as in yaws. No treatment will restore lost pigment to the depigmented areas of the late stage.

Intermediate Treponematoses

The following is a list of intermediate treponemal diseases:

Sibbens or Button scurvy (Pollock, 1953) was known in Scotland in the seventeenth century.

Radesyge was known in Scandinavia.

Bejel, occurring among Bedouin Arabs, is probably the best known of these diseases (Hudson, 1928).

Njovera (Willcox, 1951) is found among the Karanga people of Rhodesia.

Dichuchwa (Merriweather, 1953) occurs in Botswana, and seems to be identical with njovera.

Endemic syphilis of Bosnia (Grin, 1953) has been the subject of considerable investigation.

Siti (McFadzean and McCourt, 1954) is the local name in the Gambia of a condition resembling yaws, but believed to differ in several respects from it.

Irkintja has been described among Australian aborigines.

Clinical Features

These diseases are all associated with the presence of a treponeme identical with *T. pallidum*, and the serological tests for syphilis are positive in those suffering from them.

A primary lesion is almost never seen.

Secondary lesions resemble framboesiform papillomas but tend to be confined to the perspiring areas. Commonly papules are seen at the angles of the mouth (split papules), and condylomatous lesions in other areas such as armpits, and perineum.

Tertiary lesions resemble those of yaws. It is unsettled whether in some of these diseases, e.g. endemic syphilis, changes in the CSF may occur.

Transmission

Direct contact may be involved, and in some, sexual contact may be the means of transmission. In endemic syphilis and bejel it is believed that the common use of utensils in a household spreads infection.

Treatment

With penicillin, as in yaws.

Chapter 30   *RAT-BITE FEVER*

Relapsing febrile disease, transmitted to man by bites of infected rats, rarely cats and ferrets, and characterized by fever, lymphangitis, eruption and tendency to relapses.

Bacteriology

Two different infecting organisms: (1) *Spirillum minus*: first described in Japan. (2) *Streptobacillus moniliformis*: more recently described, probably commoner: caused 'Haverhill fever', a milk-borne epidemic: difficult to culture, use Loeffler's medium.

Symptoms

No essential distinction between the two infections. *Bite heals normally*.

Incubation Period

S. minus longer than 10 days; *S. moniliformis* less than 10 days.

Onset

Pain returns at site of bite, scar breaks down; becomes an ulcer with surrounding inflammation and vesicles: lymph nodes draining area enlarge. This onset may not occur.

Course

After further interval, patient suddenly becomes acutely ill.

Temperature rises to 39·4 °C (103 °F): rigors, vomiting, general pains.
Rash: S. minus macular, red brown, spreads from initial lesion. *S. moniliformis* petechial rash, morbilliform.
Arthritis: S. moniliformis common. *S. minus* rare.
Temperature falls in 3 or 4 days: often crisis with sweating: symptoms improve.

Relapse
Interval, 3–6 days (variable). Temperature rises again, with return of lymphangitis, glandular enlargement, and rash. Relapses last 1 or 2 days. Relapses may occur for weeks or months in absence of treatment.

Blood
Polymorphonuclear leucocytosis or leucopenia.
  Suppuration does not occur. Spleen rarely palpable.

Mortality
Low. No fatal cases in Great Britain.

Diagnosis
From relapsing fevers. Wassermann reaction positive in at least 50% of cases *S. minus*; positive in less than 25% of cases *S. moniliformis*. Spirilla difficult to find in peripheral blood: inoculate white rats or mice.

Treatment
Penicillin: Specific for both organisms. Procaine penicillin 1 megaunit daily is given for 5–7 days. Endocarditis can occur in *S. moniliformis* infection and treatment requires 10–15 million units of penicillin/day for 4 weeks.

Section 4 Bacterial Diseases

Chapter 31   *TYPHOID FEVER*

Acute disease due to infection by specific organism, *Salmonella typhi*, characterized clinically in typical instances by: (1) Fever; (2) Rose-coloured eruption; (3) Enlarged spleen; (4) Abdominal tenderness; (5) Diarrhoea or constipation; and (6) Toxaemia.

Enteric group of fevers. Includes typhoid and paratyphoid fevers caused by infection with organisms of the group *Salmonella*. This group includes numerous strains of *S. typhi* and *S. paratyphi*.

Clinical description. Typhoid is here described as it occurs in uninoculated persons.

Epidemiology

General prevalence. Typhoid fever exists throughout the world. Prevalence has fallen but continues to be significant in most developing countries. *Death rate* in England and Wales per 100 000 persons in 1910, 4·6, in 1931, 0·6 in 1949, 0·2, and by 1963, 0·0. In most developing countries mortality persists at a significant (2–3%) level. Increased mortality followed emergence of chloramphenicol-resistant strains of *S. typhi* in 1970s in Mexico and Far East. In Mexico mortality rates around 13% occurred. Fortunately few isolates in these regions are now chloramphenicol resistant.

Season. Most prevalent in autumn: probably due to effect of temperature on existence of organisms outside the body.

Sex. Males and females equally liable.

Age. Most frequent in youth and early adult life. At extremes of life, course tends to be atypical. Infants rarely attacked. Very rare over 50 years of age.

Immunity. One attack usually protects.

Bacteriology

Morphology. Short, thick, actively motile bacillus with rounded ends. Length 2–4 μm, thickness 0·5 μm. No spores. Flagella, 8 to 12 in number: need special stains. Stains with all ordinary stains, but is *Gram-negative*. These charactistics are common to the coli-typhoid group.

Growth optimum 37 °C. Killed at 60 °C in 15 min, rapidly at 100 °C; can survive in ice, sterile water and drying.

S. typhi fulfils Koch's postulates: (1) Constantly present in the disease; (2) Can be isolated and cultivated outside the body in successive generations; (3) The isolated organism reproduces the disease.

Cultural characters. Grows readily on all usual media. No gas produced in any carbohydrate media. Special characters: (1) Lactose, saccharose: no change. (2) Dextrose, mannitol, maltose: acid. (3) Litmus milk: acid, but no clot (after 10 days often returns to alkaline). (4) No indole formation. (5) Gelatin: no liquefaction. (6) Neutral-red broth: no change, or slightly yellow. (7) Special media: (*a*) MacConkey—neutral-red bile-salt peptone lactose agar—yellow colonies, (*b*) Fluid enrichment media, e.g. tetrathionate or selenite broth; ox bile. (*c*) Solid selective media, e.g. brilliant green, desoxycholate citrate agar, bismuth sulphite. (8) Certain strains grown on plates give colonies smooth (S) and rough (R), and such differ in agglutination properties.

> *'Non-lactose fermenters'*. The pathogenic bacilli, typhoid, paratyphoid, dysentery, do not ferment lactose. *E. coli* and most of the non-pathogenic bacilli ferment lactose, but some only slowly ('late lactose-fermenters').
>
> *Vi-phage typing*. Bacteriophages act on Vi antigens, a phage being specific for a given antigen. Hence phage typing can be used, by special techniques, to differentiate strains of *S. typhi* which cannot be distinguished by any serological method. At present 72 strains of typhoid bacilli so identified. By such typing, connection may be traced between cases during investigations in epidemics. Phages are viruses which destroy bacilli.

Differentiation of coli group. E. coli communis: (1) Produces red colonies on MacConkey's medium; (2) Produces acid and gas in lactose and most carbohydrates; (3) Acidifies and clots milks. Also other differences. *B. proteus* produces yellow colonies on MacConkey's, but liquefies gelatin.

> *Identification by agglutination*. Final identification depends on agglutination by specific sera.

Bacteriological examination. For identification, bacillus must be isolated and cultural characters ascertained. Final identification depends on agglutinations.

> *1. From the blood*. Blood cultures are positive in first week in 90–95%; in second week incidence falls rapidly; in fourth week rarely positive and in relapses only occasionally. Earliest absolute proof of infection. Antibiotics may sterilize blood in 2 h but occasionally cultures positive at end of full course. *Method*: A few ml blood taken into broth or desoxycholate medium. Incubate 12 h or longer. Subculture on selective media and identify growth.
>
> *Clot culture* in which portion of blood clot is mashed in broth, often positive when blood culture negative. Reason for this is that serum in typhoid is bactericidal.
>
> *2. From faeces*. Bacilli not present in first few days, but positive cultures may be obtained in first week, especially if culture often repeated. Forty per cent positive before fourteenth day and 70–80% in third week; subsequently incidence falls rapidly. *Method*: Triturate portion in broth; stand or incubate. Subculture on fluid enrichment medium and solid selective medium.
>
> *3. From urine*. Bacilli appear in third or fourth week in 25%; often transient. *Method*: Centrifuge urine and culture deposit.

4. Presence of bacilli in other organs. Bacilli have been isolated from numerous sites—rose spots (rarely), lungs in pneumonia, endocarditis, pus from abscesses, etc.

Spleen: Bacilli easily isolated at autopsy. *Method*: Remove spleen entire. Cut with sterile knife and culture.

Peyer's patches and intestinal lymphoid tissue: After a few days.

Gallbladder: Often in large numbers.

Survival of bacillus outside the body

In water. In sterile water cultures of bacilli live many weeks. In natural waters uncultured bacilli, from excreta, die in less than 2 weeks. In aerated water, bacillus lives not more than 2 weeks. Survives in ice.

In milk. Lives and multiplies without changing the milk's appearance.

In soil. Can live several months. Probably does not multiply.

In stools and sewage. Dies in 3–5 days.

On clothes and materials. May live many months.

Antigens and agglutinins in enteric group. All TAB bacilli contain (as do other flagellated bacilli) an antigen in the flagella known as flagellar or 'H' (*Hauch*), and an antigen in the body known as somatic or 'O' (*ohne Hauch*). Agglutinins form independently to these two antigens and can be separately estimated in serum. Agglutinins to part of cell envelope, Vi agglutinins, related to virulence of organism.

Agglutinins rarely detectable in patients until 7th–8th day of disease. Occasionally appearance delayed. Rising titres of great diagnostic significance. H antibodies are IgG and O are IgM.

H Agglutinins (flagellar)

1. Are not present in normal human serum (rarely, up to 1 : 30).

2. Are nearly specific for one organism, e.g. *S. typhi*. Hence, in an uninoculated person their presence is proof of infection with the homologous organism.

3. Titre often higher than O and more persistent, but development less constant.

4. Are produced by inoculation with the vaccine of the organism. After an interval may be present and rise to high titre in various febrile infections, or with slighter causes ('anamnestic reaction'). Hence are not evidence of infection.

O Agglutinins (somatic)

1. Are present in normal serum 1 : 10 or 1 : 20 or rarely 1 : 50.

2. Are not specific for separate members of enteric groups, i.e. are 'group agglutinins'.

3. Are not produced by inoculation with vaccines. Hence presence in appropriate dilutions, especially with 'rising' titre, either in uninoculated or inoculated persons, is evidence of 'enteric group' infection, but cannot identify bacillus.

Note: H *antigens* are destroyed by alcohol but present alone in formolized suspensions of bacilli, and conversely for O *antigens*.

Vi Antigen and Agglutinin (Felix)

Antigen is present in fresh strains from blood cultures, from smooth (S) colonies, rapidly lost on subculture; readily destroyed, e.g. by heat. Indicative of virulence.

Agglutinins highly specific. Titre 1 : 10 is positive. Interfere with O agglutination. Positive in 90% of carriers. Of value in detection of carriers, the carrier state being improbable but not impossible if test negative. Also used for mass screening of suspects, convalescents, and as a test of cure.

Cell-mediated immunity. In addition to humoral immunity cell-mediated immunity is responsible for macrophage activation and granuloma formation in typhoid.

Modes of Infection

Man is sole natural reservoir of enteric organisms, which are excreted in faeces and urine. Contamination of food or fluid from a human source is origin of every epidemic. Transmission may be direct or indirect.

Volunteer experiments showed that ingestion of 10^5 organisms led to disease in 25%, 10^7 organisms in 50% and 10^9 organisms in 90%. As infecting dose increased incubation period decreased but final illness not affected by size of infecting dose.

Water and milk. Drinking water and dairy milk contaminated by sewage are causes of large epidemics. Preliminary increase of diarrhoea usual. Water supply only infective for limited period unless contamination repeated.

Shellfish. Specially liable to infection.

Tinned meat. Has caused epidemic.

Uncooked food. May be infected directly by carrier, e.g. ice-cream.

Direct contagion. From infected clothing, sheets, etc. Rare.

Flies. Have conveyed infection from latrines to cook-house in wartime conditions.

Development in human body. Bacilli after ingestion probably multiply in liver, spleen and mesenteric lymph nodes, during incubation period. Onset of symptoms corresponds with appearance of bacilli in bloodstream. From the circulation, bacilli localize in certain sites, especially lymphoid tissue of intestines.

Morbid Anatomy

1. Intestines. The changes characteristic to typhoid are infiltration of tissues by macrophages containing bacteria. Aggregations of macrophages become typhoid nodules or tubercles. Occur especially in intestine, mesenteric lymph nodes, spleen, liver, bone marrow and less commonly in kidneys, testes and parotids.

In intestine Peyer's patches involved particularly in the last foot of the ileum. Condition is a proliferative inflammation followed by necrosis. Four stages: *Hyperplasia*; *Necrosis and formation of sloughs*; *Ulceration*; *Healing and cicatrization*.

1.1. Hyperplasia. Swelling in Peyer's patches of solitary follicles. Commences with hyperaemia, followed by hyperplasia, viz. increase of lymphoid and macrophage cells. Follicles and patches project above the surface. Blood vessels compressed, hence projections are often greyish. Condition at maximum from eighth to tenth day.

Necrosis is usual result. *Resolution* may occur in mild cases, by degeneration of cells and absorption without ulceration.

1.2. Necrosis and Formation of Sloughs. Necrosis of swollen lymphoid elements, resulting in formation of sloughs. Deepest in patches near ileocaecal valve. Usually involves submucosa; may perforate peritoneum.

1.3. Ulceration. Separation of sloughs. Extent and depth depend on necrosis. Typhoid ulcer results from separation of slough.

Characters: Long axis in line of intestine. *Shape*: usually irregular oval. *Edges*: soft, undermined, swollen, not indurated. *Floor*: smooth; usually formed of muscularis. *Peritoneal surface*: changes slight.

1.4. Healing and Cicatrization. Granulation tissue forms and covers floor.

Epithelium then extends inwards from edge of mucosa.

Healed ulcer is smooth, slightly depressed and pigmented.

Finally, almost no sign of scar remains.

Stricture and intestinal obstruction never result.

Typhoid bacilli are present in tissues in early stages, but diminish or disappear during necrosis.

Large Intestine. Lymphoid elements affected in one-third of cases. Severity diminishes with distance from ileocaecal valve. Occasionally is extensively affected, and then often severe in sigmoid and rectum, with marked changes in ileum.

2. Mesenteric lymph nodes. Hyperaemic and may exhibit changes as in intestinal lymphoid tissue. Suppuration very rare. Rupture of node extremely rare: may cause peritonitis or fatal haemorrhage.

3. Spleen. Invariably enlarged in early stages. *Increase moderate.* Soft consistency. Changes of hyperaemia and, later, hyperplasia, returning to normal about fourth week. Rupture very rare. Typhoid bacilli scattered throughout, often in typhoid nodules.

4. Other organs

Lungs. Bronchitis in early stages. Hypostatic congestion in toxaemic cases. For pneumonia, *see* Complications, p. 113.

Heart. Myocarditis in toxaemic cases. *See also under* Complications, pp. 110–1.

5. Voluntary muscles. Zenker's hyaline degeneration may occur. Affected muscles may rupture. Abdominal muscles, adductors of thigh, and pectorals most common.

6. Blood. Anaemia usual: is mild in most cases but occasionally severe. A haemolytic element present. Probably caused by complement-fixing immunoglobulins on erythrocyte surface.

Symptoms

In untreated patients the course of typhoid, subsequent to the incubation period and days of onset, is commonly considered in three stages. *Antibiotic treatment usually cuts short development of symptoms and nowadays stages seen much less frequently than formerly.* In cases of ordinary severity these stages frequently correspond, reasonably closely, to periods of one week each and are thus referred to. May be summarized as follows:

First stage or week. Bacteriaemia and development of symptoms. Rising temperature.

Second stage or week. Localization of organisms in small intestine. Increasing toxaemia. Fastigium of pyrexia. Results of ulceration of intestine.

Third stage or week

In milder forms: fever remits, healing of intestinal ulcers begins, signs of improvement commence.

In severe forms: period of dangerous complications and advancing toxaemia.

The course may be of any degree of severity, e.g. abortive forms with a few days' pyrexia and malaise and mild forms of normal duration but little severity.

Incubation period. Commonly 10–15 days. Ordinary limits 5–23 days.

Period of onset. Onset insidious. Very rarely abrupt. Increasing malaise until patient takes to bed.

First week. Symptoms varied. *Headache*: rarely absent, persistent and severe. *Tired*, pains in limbs. *Anorexia*: abdominal discomfort, beginning. *Constipation*: diarrhoea less often at onset. *Epistaxis*: early symptom, rarely serious. *Cough*: especially in children. Tongue furred.

> *Physical signs*
>
> *Temperature*: Rises steadily by 'steps'. On evening of fourth day reaches 39·4–40 °C (103–104 °F).
>
> *Pulse*: Slow compared with temperature—in adults rarely exceeds 105. Becomes dicrotic.
>
> *Blood pressure*: Low.
>
> *Facies*: Cheeks flushed; eyes bright.
>
> Gradual advance during week: toxaemia increasing, memory defective, slight mental confusion, deafness, muscular relaxation and inert posture, abdomen beginning to distend.
>
> *End of first week*: between seventh and tenth day, note: (1) spleen becomes palpable; (2) Rose spots appear; (3) Agglutination reaction becomes positive.

Second week. Increasing toxaemia and results of ulceration of intestine.

Mental torpor. Expression dull. *Face* pale, may be malar flush, pupils dilated, lips dry: characteristic appearance. Tongue dry and raw. *Constipation*: may persist obstinately (good prognosis). *Diarrhoea*, if present, 'pea-soup' stools: abdomen distending and tender.

> *Physical Signs*
>
> *Temperature*: Fastigium, remains constant.
>
> *Pulse*: Varies with toxaemia; slow or rapid.
>
> Loss of weight rapid.
>
> Toxaemia advances in severe cases: delirium, may be death.
>
> *End of second week*: serious complications from ulceration of intestine: (1) Haemorrhage; (2) Perforation.

Third week

Mild and Favourable Cases. Temperature remits, falling by steps. Signs of improvement appear.

Severe Cases. Dangerous complications and advancing toxaemia.

Unfavourable Symptoms. (1) *Mental symptoms* pronounced: 'typhoid state' or delirium; (2) *Temperature* remains high or rises; (3) Cardiac weakness: may be fatal failure; (4) Pulmonary complications: pneumonia, hypostatic congestion; (5) Extreme weakness and wasting; (6) Severe diarrhoea.

Fourth week

In Ordinary Cases. Convalescence commences. *Appetite* returns, often ravenous. *Temperature* gradually becomes normal. *Tongue* cleans. Mental and abdominal symptoms subside. General condition is extremely weak.

In Severe Cases. Toxaemia increases. 'Typhoid state" may occur; face cyanosed; clammy perspiration; dry fissured tongue; sordes of lips; lungs congested; rapid, feeble pulse, often irregular.

Coma vigil: Patient lies with open eyes, muttering and oblivious to surroundings. Incontinence of urine and faeces. Tremors of lips, tongue and limbs. Twitching of fingers (subsultus tendinum). Picks at bedclothes (carphologia). Is a sign of extreme toxaemia, and mortality very high.

Fifth and Sixth weeks. In ordinary cases, general progess. In protracted cases, convalescence commences. *Relapses, recrudescences, complications* and *sequelae* may occur.

Special Features and Complications

Modes of onset. Onset usually insidious. *Localization* to one system may occur: extremely deceptive, and diagnosis difficult; onset may be acute.

Commonest localizations are: *Lungs:* lobar and bronchopneumonia. *Nervous system:* meningism and meningitis. Also mental disturbances and rarely mania, other forms rare.

Ambulatory or latent forms: Patient may 'fight the disease' and remain at work until symptoms and signs of the 'second week' are present. Subsequent course often very severe. Delirium common.

Fever

Variations during Acute Stages

1. Temperature often high when first observed: 'steps' in rise having occurred previously.

2. Rapid rise to 39·4–40 °C (103–104 °F) may occur with rare initial rigor, or with lobar pneumonia or localization of symptoms.

3. Sudden fall indicates perforation or intestinal haemorrhage.

4. In severe cases, febrile period may persist for many weeks.

5. Rise during course may occur with: (i) Increasing severity; (ii) Lobar pneumonia or other complications. Hyperpyrexia, above 41 °C (106 °F), of serious prognosis.

Aspirin usually causes sudden fall followed by rapid rise.

Rigors. Not common. In general, a rigor suggests a complication, and repeated rigors an error of diagnosis.

Rash

> *Time of appearance*: Seventh to tenth day; may be later.
> *Frequency*: Rarely absent except in children and old persons.
> *Site*: Abdomen and chest commonest, then back and thighs. Face, hands, and feet very rare.
> *Characters*: Rose-red, slightly raised, flattened papules. Disappear entirely on pressure, and reappear rapidly on release.
> *Size*: Two to four mm.
> *Number*: Usually scanty and widely scattered. Frequently less than a dozen. Appear in successive crops, persist about three days, then fade, leaving slight brownish stain. Number of spots bears no constant relation to severity of attack.

Other Eruptions

Sudamina and miliaria: Not infrequent with sweats.

Skin—various lesions

> *Odour*. Of 'abdominal' character in severe cases.
> *Sweats*. Skin usually dry. Sweats may occur with venous thrombosis, haemorrhage, or perforation.
> *Bedsores*. In severe cases tend to form rapidly.
> *Boils*. Not uncommon, in convalescence.
> *Herpes Labialis*. Very rare.
> *Hair*. Often falls out during convalescence of severe cases. Grows again as before. Permanent baldness very rare.

Blood changes. Mild leucopenia with relative lymphocytosis a classic feature but inconstant.

> *Polynuclear leucocytosis* occurs with peritonitis or septic complications. Repeat white cell count after chloramphenicol treatment if haematological complications suspected.
> *Erythrocytes and Haemoglobin*. Progressive secondary anaemia with a haemolytic element. Rarely severe until third week.
> Changes persist into convalescence, and gradually disappear.

Cardiovascular System

> *The Pulse*
> *First week*: (1) *Rate*: In adults, rarely exceeds 105, even with high fever. Usually 85–95. This relatively slow pulse is very common and of importance in diagnosis. In children more rapid. In severe cases with high temperature, may be rapid throughout: prognosis serious. (2) *Character*: Dicrotic pulse common.
> *Subsequent weeks*: Frequently more rapid, 110–130, but may remain slow throughout. *Not dicrotic*.
> *The Heart*
> Myocarditis in 1–5% cases: may be cardiac failure or arrhythmias. Many cases in S. Africa in 1975 with good response to chloramphenicol. Pericarditis—rare.

During convalescence: Cardiac arrhythmias and bradycardia common.

Blood Pressure. Characteristically low. With haemorrhage may be rapid fall. Following perforation, initial rise common.

Venous Thrombosis. In 2–3%. Usually during 3rd or later week.

Arterial Thrombosis. Very rare. Extremely blue and pulseless. Gangrene unusual.

Alimentary System

Appetite. Lost early. Ravenous in convalescence.

Vomiting. Strikingly rare: suggests complications.

Thirst. Constant. Must be gratified.

Tongue. At onset, thin moist fur, which gradually thickens. In ordinary cases dry in second week. Cleans in fourth week or in convalescence. Saliva diminished. Mouth must be kept clean.

Parotitis. Rare, but mortality formerly high. Frequency 1%. Chiefly in third week of very severe cases.
Very rare when mouth properly treated. Generally suppurates.

Oesophagus. True typhoid ulceration may occur: very rare. Dysphagia. Stricture may follow.

Abdominal features. Abdominal tenderness. From a few days after onset. Pain rarely severe, except with complications: may simulate appendicitis.

Abdominal Distension. Meteorism or tympanites: due to loss of tone of muscular coats of intestine or stomach. Moderate degree common, on palpation feels doughy. *If severe*, prognosis bad: distension impedes heart and lungs and favours perforation: occurs also in peritonitis.

Diarrhoea. *Note*: diarrhoea with 'pea-soup' stools is a characteristic symptom, but occurs in less than 50% of cases, and with modern avoidance of purgatives is considerably less common. Begins in second week. Profuse diarrhoea is serious.

Cause. Inflammation of gut, especially large intestine. No relation between diarrhoea and extent of ulceration.

Character of Stools. Thin, large quantity. Reaction alkaline.

Mucus scanty. Shreds from sloughs are very rarely recognizable. Defaecation painless.

Constipation. Prognosis good. May occur with advanced ulceration.

Local Damage to the Intestine. This is the cause of the two serious complications—haemorrhage and perforation—at the end of the second or during the third week.

Intestinal Haemorrhage. Serious and important complication.

Frequency: In 2–8% of different series before introduction of antibiotic therapy. Much reduced by such therapy. Incidence increases with age, rarer in children.

Time of occurrence: Between end of second and beginning of fourth week, the time of separation of sloughs (*Note*: slight haemorrhage from congestion may occur in first week; unimportant except for diagnosis).

Symptoms: Faintness and collapse. Sudden anaemia. Manifestations as in other forms of shock due to acute haemorrhage. *Temperature*: rapid fall. *Pulse*: rapid and low tension. *Stools*: blood, bright or tarry. Death may occur before passage of blood.

Perforation of Typhoid Ulcer

Frequency: Variable. In reports of different series totalling 40 000 cases between 1909 and 1969 incidence varied from 0·7 to 17·9% (Christie). Causes 25% (at least) of deaths from typhoid. Antibiotic treatment probably does not reduce frequency though it makes it less fatal even if more difficult to recognize.

Age: Rare over 40 years, and in young children.

Time of occurrence: First to third week. In fourth and even fifth week if pyrexia persists. Very rare when temperature normal.

Site: Usually in ileum; commonly within 30 cm of ileocaecal valve. Occasionally in sigmoid and appendix. Rarely in other sites. *May be several perforations*. Mutliple perforations often in an area of paper-thin partially matted gut.

Cause of perforation: Separation of sloughs: slough often adherent to edge of perforation. Perforation may be pin-point, or, less often, extensive from separation of large slough.

Previous course of attack: Usually severe toxaemia: particularly with diarrhoea and meteorism: associated with haemorrhage not uncommonly. *May occur in mild attacks*.

Symptoms: Three stages often recognizable: (*a*) Shock immediately on perforation; (*b*) Latent period or 'period of repose'; (*c*) Symptoms of general peritonitis. Toxic state and existing abdominal distension modifies and obscures usual symptoms of intestinal perforation.

a. Shock on Occurrence of Perforation. Shivering, sudden pain in or near right iliac fossa: signs of shock. Maybe restlessness in a previously apathetic patient. Temperature falls. Pulse rapid. Blood pressure rises.

b. Latent Period. Initial symptoms often subside in one to two hours with temporary period of repose. *May be extremely deceptive*. Not always present, or incomplete, and the preceding and following stages merge.

c. Symptoms of General Peritonitis develop. Temperature rises again. Leucocytosis usually present: important in diagnosis, but may be absent.

Diagnosis: Often difficult. From: (1) *Haemorrhage*: abdominal symptoms slighter, and blanching. May be very difficult, and may coexist; (2) *Appendicitis*: difficult, but differential diagnosis unimportant; (3) *Phlebitis of iliac veins*: very rare; (3)*Peritonitis* from other causes: very rare.

Spleen. Becomes palpable at beginning of second week in 70% of cases. Soft. Size moderate. Red pulp congested and contains typhoid nodules.

Liver. Slight enlargement usual. Typhoid nodules present. Cloudy swelling of hepatocytes and focal necrosis common. Jaundice rarely.

Gallbladder. Occasionally acute cholecystitis during attack. Chronic cholecystitis and gallstones may develop even after long interval due to persistence of *S. typhi* in gall bladder. Their presence in gallstones may induce carrier state.

Respiratory System
1. *Epistaxis*. Frequent early symptom.
2. *Bronchitis*. Presence at onset almost invariable. Physical signs: crepitations at bases. Symptoms slight.
3. *Hypostatic Congestion*. Not uncommon in later periods of severe attacks. Symptoms often absent. *Mortality* high.
4. *Bronchopneumonia*. Serious. Occurs particularly in children.
5. *Lobar Pneumonia*. Less common than bronchopneumonia in children. Rare in adults and when it occurs is then usually in 3rd week. Rusty sputum often absent.

Nervous System. The *mental state* is often affected and frequently for a period subsequent to attack. *In febrile stage* in ordinary forms, there is mental dullness with stupor or mild delirium. Sleep is almost continuous, insomnia being a severer condition. The various changes can, in general, be referred to three stages: (1) At onset; (2) Febrile and toxic period; (3) Convalescence.

Memory. At onset, memory usually deficient. Subsequent to attack, memory of illness is hazy. Memory is impaired during convalescence.

Delirium. Rarely absent in severe cases.
1. *At Onset*. Not common. In rare cases (especially in 'ambulatory' form), confusion, delirium, or mania may be earliest symptom.
2. *In Febrile Period*, during second and third weeks or subsequently. Various types. May be quiet and stuporose or continuously restless. Rarely violent except alcoholics. For Coma Vigil, *see* p. 109. Suicidal tendencies may be present even in mild delirium.

Convulsions. Very rare. Causes various. May occur at onset, in children or may result from meningism or meningitis.

Peripheral neuritis. Guillain-Barré type of syndrome. Occurs late in disease or during convalescence. Severe pain and swelling in affected area; most frequently extensors of lower extremity.

'Tender toes': Cause doubtful: may be due to relative deficiency of B vitamins brought about by the infection. Tips of toes extremely sensitive to weight of bedclothes; no swelling.

Painful cramps: Not uncommon, especially in calves. Possibly a myositis; rarely venous thrombosis.

Hemiplegia: Probably due to thrombosis.

Meningeal symptoms
1. *Meningism*: especially in children and at onset of illness.
2. *Meningitis*: A rare late complication.

Psychoses

1. Delusions arising in febrile period may persist. Dementia may occur but progress is good.

2. Impairment of memory well known but not permanent. May result from typhoid encephalomyelitis.

Eye. Affections very rare. Optic neuritis.

Ear. Temporary deafness common in early stages.

Renal System.   *Retention of Urine*. A frequent early symptom.

Febrile albuminuria: Common. Kidney not permanently affected. May be due to immune complex mediated glomerulonephritis.

Nephritis: Rare. Glomerulonephritis with renal failure or nephrotic syndrome may develop. Occasionally tubular necrosis follows acute haemolysis.

Bacilluria, Cystitis and Pyelitis

Bacilluria from typhoid bacilli occurs frequently: about 20%. Rarely before third week. Pus or albumin usually present. Cystitis usually caused by *E. coli*; occasionally by typhoid bacillus.

Periostitis and Bone Abscess. May develop during convalescence or at interval after attack, even many years. Are particularly likely to occur in sicklaemic persons. Ribs, tibia, femur commonest sites. Onset as painful node. May subside or abscess slowly forms; recovery tedious; recurrence frequent. Pus usually contains typhoid bacillus, either in pure culture or with pyogenic organisms.

Arthritis. Monarticular or polyarticular. Hip most common. 'Typhoid dislocation of hip' may occur spontaneously.

'Typhoid Spine.' Characterized by severe pain in lumbar and sacral regions. Very rare. Usually adult males during convalescence. No radiographic changes or physical signs. Prolonged complete rest always cures. Aetiology uncertain. Often confused with tuberculosis and brucellosis of spine.

Varieties

Typhoid fever in children. Usually more acute than in adults. After 10 years of age disease approximates to adult type.

In Infants under 2. Rare. Congenital infection known. Diagnosis usually suggested by possibility of infection (as in epidemics) rather than by symptoms. Mortality high in cases diagnosed. Often an acute respiratory presentation.

In Childhood. Most frequent variations from adult type:

Morbid anatomy: Intestinal lesions are not so marked. Ulceration may be absent. In undoubted typhoid, changes may not exceed those of simple diarrhoea.

Mortality: In the developing world may be up to 30%.

Onset: Often sudden. Vomiting is common initial symptom.

Temperature: Initial rise frequently more rapid, curve less typical, duration shorter. Usually higher than in adult cases of same severity.

Pulse: More rapid, but comparatively slow for febrile disease in children. Dicrotism rare.

Rash: Less frequent, and is scanty.

Spleen: Nearly always palpable.

Meningitis: Typhoid meningitis mostly a disease of children under 5.

General progress: Symptoms usually milder but in developing countries often a severe disease. Marked delirium and 'typhoid state', rare. Meningism, like meningitis relatively common. Anaemia and respiratory symptoms commoner than in adults.

Complications and sequelae: Haemorrhage and perforation rare. So also otitis media. Temporary aphasia, without apparent cause, is peculiar sequel: recovery in a few weeks.

Typhoid fever in the aged. Incidence low. Fever not high and course usually atypical. Pneumonia and heart failure common. Mortality high.

Typhoid fever in pregnancy. Pregnancy gives no immunity. Abortion in 70%.

Relapses
Occur in about 10% of cases in absence of antibiotic treatment. Frequency varies in different epidemics.

1. *Ordinary or true relapse*. Occurs after temperature has become normal. Average interval 5 days; rarely exceeds 2 weeks. Diagnosed by presence of two of the triad; (1) Steplike temperature; (2) Rash; (3) Enlarged spleen. Relapse usually shorter and milder than original attack, but in rare instances is more severe. May be several relapses, becoming progressively milder. Duration 7–21 days; occasionally longer.

2. *Intercurrent relapse*. Occurs before temperature has become normal. Often very severe. Complications not uncommon.

3. *Spurious relapse, recrudescence*. Transient rise of temperature of a few hours' to one or two days' duration are not uncommon during convalescence.

No satisfactory explanation for relapses is known, the blood at the time being strongly bactericidal to typhoid bacilli. Possibly due to reinfection of bloodstream by bacilli protected by lying latent in gallbladder or elsewhere.

Diagnosis
Methods of diagnosis. Typhoid fever (or enteric group) should be suspected in temperate climates if a fever lasts a week without falling to normal and without manifestations of another disease. Suspect it particularly in persons recently returned from tropics or subtropics. It may be simulated by many febrile conditions, especially with splenomegaly. There are three groups of data for diagnosis, depending on: (1) Symptoms and signs; (2) Bacteriological examinations (*see* p. 104); Beware of misdiagnosis resulting from pyrexia due to intercurrent illness in a typhoid carrier; and (3) Agglutination reactions (*see* p. 105). Repetition is important in all pathological examinations if inconclusive.

> *Symptoms and Signs*. Variable. No one symptom or sign is characteristic in early stages until end of first week. Most suggestive are: (1) Insidious onset; (2) Temperature curve; (3) Relatively slow pulse; (4) Headache. The typical triad of typhoid is: *rash, enlarged spleen* and *the temperature curve*.
>
> *Blood*. Leucopenia with relative lymphocytosis.

Differential diagnosis. *Difficulties in diagnosis* arise from: (1) Localization of symptoms in special organs at onset; (2) The general symptoms and course.

1. *Localization of symptoms*
a. *Pneumonia: Pneumonia at onset* may mask other symptoms.
b. *Meningeal Symptoms*: Lumbar puncture may decide.
c. *Appendicitis.*
2. *General Symptoms and Course*
a. *Tuberculosis*. The usual error is diagnosing tuberculosis as typhoid: the reverse is less frequent.

Acute Miliary Tuberculosis. May simulate typhoid, with insidious onset and indefinite malaise. *Temperature* generally more irregular. *Pulse* more rapid. Sweats, dyspnoea and cough (if pulmonary).

Tuberculosis Peritonitis. This may simulate typhoid fever when occurring with acute onset.

Tuberculous Meningitis. Vomiting is frequent early, the abdomen is retracted, there are convulsions, and the temperature is irregular. Inequality of pupils and squint are common. *Lumbar puncture* decides the diagnosis.

b. Septicaemia and pyaemic conditions: Note in general: (1) Onset more abrupt; (2) Temperature less regular; (3) Pulse rapid from onset. (4) Sweats and rigors frequent; (5) Leucocytosis common; (6) Aetiological factor may be present, e.g. septic foci; (7) Progress often rapid.

Bacterial endocarditis, osteomyelitis, appendicitis and intraperitoneal abscesses are special difficulties.

c. Influenza: Onset more acute, and respiratory and upper air-passages more affected.

d. Malaria. Difficult in continuous febrile *Plasmodium falciparum* infections. Diagnosis by specific tests. May coexist.

e. Typhus fever: Sudden onset: high fever without remissions: rash on fourth day: delirium: crisis. Weil–Felix reaction positive. Agglutination test for typhoid H agglutinins may be positive in inoculated persons.

f. Undulant fever: Shorter course with relapses. Agglutination with *Brucella*.

g. Various conditions: Psittacosis, amoebiasis, febrile glandular fevers.

Prognosis

Antibiotics. Can eliminate toxaemia at all stages and hence greatly reduce mortality.

Mortality. Debilitating conditions are adverse factors, e.g. obesity, fatigue, alcoholism. Death rate lowest at 6–10 years.

Adverse features. Evidences of severe toxaemia—especially severe delirium or coma; profuse diarrhoea, incontinence and meteorism; failing heart and circulatory failure.

Serious complications. Haemorrhage, perforation, pneumonia.

Of little value in prognosis are: profuse rash, initial bronchitis, dicrotic pulse.

Prophylaxis

Prophylactic measures involve: (1) Prevention and control of epidemics; (2) Investigation of typhoid carriers, especially among cooks and dairy employees; (3) Prevention of direct infection from a patient or carrier; (4) Antityphoid inoculation.

1. *Prevention and control of epidemics.* All water and milk should be boiled during epidemics.

Water supply. Contamination by sewage causes large

epidemics. Usually explosive, many cases infected simultaneously. Water supply only remains infective for limited period unless contamination repeated.

Milk and milk products. Contamination usually by carriers: includes cream and ice-creams. Often a stream of cases.

Food.

See Modes of Infection, p. 106.

2. *Typhoid carriers.* Excreta usually free of bacilli in 2–3 weeks after convalescence: may persist indefinitely as carriers.

Classification. (*a*) Convalescent carriers: within few months (say 3–6) of convalescence: in 5% of cases. (*b*) Chronic carriers: in 2%. (*c*) Healthy carriers: no known attack: more commonly in children.

Site of Infection. (*a*) Intestinal carrier: focus usually in gallbladder. (*b*) Urinary carrier; rarely chronic.

Presence of bacilli in excreta often intermittent.

Agglutination Reaction. Titre usually high, but may be intermittent or absent. Chronic carriers stated in 90% to have permanently high Vi titres (1:10 is positive): needs confirmation. Infecting organism should be typed by Vi-bacteriophage method.

Treatment. Chloramphenicol unreliable. Ampicillin or amoxycillin 100 mg/kg/day orally for 12 weeks. Probenecid to block excretion given in doses of 2 g daily throughout this course. Co-trimoxazole in doses of 480 mg orally twice daily for 12 weeks is an alternative. Cholecystectomy often successful if chemotherapy fails.

3. *Prevention of direct infection from patient.* Patient must be isolated or barrier nursed.

Attendants. Wear protective clothing. Wash hands carefully after attending patient and rinse in disinfectant such as 1% cetrimide solution. Must not prepare food.

Duration of Isolation. No patient should be regarded as non-infective until the stools and urine are negative at least at three examinations at daily intervals.

4. *Antityphoid inoculation.*

Monovalent vaccine containing only *S. typhi* is now generally used as it causes fewer side effects than TAB and trials with a TAB vaccine suggest that little protection against paratyphoid is obtained.

Acetone-inactivated vaccine preserves Vi antigen and is superior to older phenolised vaccine. Two subcutaneous injections given, preferably separated by 3–6 weeks. First contains 500 million organisms in 0·5 ml, second double this dosage. Intradermal injections of double strength vaccine contain 1/10 of subcutaneous amounts give equal protection and less marked side effects. Children less than 10 years old given half doses in otherwise unchanged schedule. *Orally administered vaccine* is under development.

Local reaction and constitutional symptoms commence in 4–6 h and last 1–3 days. Usually slight but occasionally marked local reaction, or in others constitutional symptoms with little local change. The local reaction is swelling, pain and redness. The reaction is usually considerably less after the second injection. Relieved by aspirin and codeine.

Results: The value of antityphoid vaccination has been questioned, but WHO studies confirmed its value.

Protection is high for one year. After this it varies in different individuals, but is often considerable for two years.

Case Mortality. The course of the disease if infection takes place is not modified by inoculation and case mortality is not reduced.

Treatment

Specific chemotherapy now rapidly alleviates toxaemia and pyrexia. Attention is still necessary to the general and dietetic management since haemorrhage or perforation may occur after the temperature is normal if intestinal ulceration has developed.

General management. Nursing in bed essential with blanket bathing and attention to pressure points; posture frequently to be changed and mouth cleansed after food. Aperients not to be given, even if constipated.

Diet. Antibiotic treatment has obviated need for strict diet. Any light food suitable. Attention to fluid balance and electrolytes important. In tropics parenteral administration of saline and glucose often necessary and of potassium chloride in oral doses of 0·5–1 g daily.

Chemotherapy

Chloramphenicol. Generally agreed the most effective antibiotic for typhoid and revolutionized its treatment. It is bacteriostatic, not bactericidal. Resistance to it an increasing problem since 1972, particularly in Brazil and Mexico.

Dosage: 30–50 mg/kg patient's body weight daily until temperature dropped to 100 °F, then reduced by one-third until patient afebrile when reduced by further third of original and there maintained 10 days to prevent relapses. Total daily dose divided into 4 individual doses. In very ill patients give initial doses of 0·5 g i.v.

Precautions and results

Relapses: Respond to further dosage and are prevented by continuing treatment for 10–14 days.

Haemorrhage and perforation: May occur after temperature normal and all toxaemia relieved, and hence general care and management must be continued. If perforation occurs continue chloramphenicol administration parenterally.

Reactions of Herxheimer type, sometimes with haemolytic anaemia, may occur if large initial doses used; loading doses therefore not advised. Reactions may be controlled by corticosteroids.

Carriers:

Urinary carriers usually relatively easy to cure by doses of chloramphenicol approximately double those used for treatment of uncomplicated typhoid fever.

Intestinal carriers — See p. 117.

Ampicillin. Inferior to chloramphenicol except for carriers. Given orally, in doses of 20–25 mg/kg q.d.s. till 10 days after defervescence of fever.

Amoxycillin. As effective as ampicillin. Given orally in doses of 25–33 mg/kg t.d.s. till 10 days after defervescence of fever.

Co-trimoxazole. Tablets contain 80 mg trimethoprim and 400 mg sulphamethoxazole; 2 given orally b.d. 10–14 days. Children 2–5 years ¼ and 6–12 years ½ this daily dosage. Seems almost as good as chloramphenicol and less toxic, although neutropenia has followed its use and there have been treatment failures and few cases of *S. typhi* resistance to the drug. The injectable preparation is available.

Corticosteroids reduce toxaemia and mortality in patients with mental changes and/or severe toxaemia. After starting antimicrobial therapy give 3 mg/kg dexamethasone or equivalent of other corticosteroid by intravenous infusion over 30 min then 1 mg/kg at same rate 6-hourly for 8 doses. Do not administer corticosteroids in 3rd or later week as they may then increase risk of intestinal perforation or haemorrhage.

Paratyphoid Fever

Paratyphoid A and B infections resemble *S. typhi* infection, but tend to be milder and often atypical. Under Morbid Anatomy and Symptoms the common differences from typhoid fever are noted. No sharp clinical distinction can be drawn between para A and B infection, but para C tends to be septicaemic and is also serologically distinct.

Types
Now recognized: (1) *S. paratyphi A*; (2) *S. paratyphi B* (*S. schott-mülleri*); (3) *S. paratyphi C* (*S. hirschfeldii*). There is only one serotype of *S. paratyphi A* but there are many of *S. paratyphi B* and C.

Epidemiology
Spread commonly by milk, milk products and meat (due to carriers); by water less often than *S. typhi*. Para B has approximately the same geographical distribution as *S. typhi*, but is less common in tropical than subtropical countries. Para A is rare in Europe and America, but not uncommon in India. Para C is rare, occurs mainly in Balkans and Guyana.

Bacteriology
Morphology and methods of isolation. As for *S. typhi*. Septicaemic stage is short, and blood cultures must be taken early.
Culture characteristics
1. No change in: lactose, saccharose, inulin.
2. Produce acid and gas in: dextrose, mannitol, dulcitol, maltose.
3. No formation of indole.
4. Action on milk: *S. paratyphi A*—permanent acidity: *S. paratyphi B* and C—slight initial acidity, permanent alkalinity commencing on third day.
Paratyphoid C.   *S. paratyphi C* may be isolated from almost typical enteric, but

has a tendency to atypical forms; has also been isolated from diarrhoeal, pulmonary, and various septic conditions without enteric symptoms. Thus differs from other enteric bacilli in its clinical manifestations. Also differs serologically. In infections or inoculations with *S. paratyphi C*, serum contains no group agglutinins, i.e. does not agglutinate T, A, or B (last occasionally slightly); agglutinins to *S. paratyphi C* itself may be absent, and diagnosis may depend on isolation of bacillus. *S. paratyphi C* is also not agglutinated by T, A, or B antisera (last occasionally slightly). Typical strains of *S. paratyphi C* and of *S. suipestifer* (*S. choleraesuis*, hog cholera, var. *kunzendorf*) may be indistinguishable even by absorption, but differ biologically.

Morbid Anatomy
The colon is more frequently and lymphoid tissue less frequently affected than with *S. typhi* infection. Catarrh of the intestine without actual ulceration may be present.

Symptoms
Clinical course may be identical with ordinary or even severe forms of *S. typhi* infection, i.e. it may cause a septicaemic illness with marked toxicity but usually is more limited to the bowel and tends to produce diarrhoea without marked toxicity, and sometimes may cause symptomless infections. All gradations between these extremes occur. Incubation period shorter, about 10 days. Case mortality, in civilian hospitals, about 2%, but may be severer in epidemics. Toxaemia, complications and fatal results are unusual.

Differences from 'typhoid fever'. The following refer to paratyphoid fever of moderate severity, occurring in persons not inoculated with paratyphoid vaccine.

　1.　*Onset*. Often more rapid.

　2.　*Rash*. Occasionally very profuse, very large spots (or small areas) of irregular outline, of deeper colour than typhoid, or sometimes a bluish tinge, not entirely fading on pressure, and leaving a slight stain: may almost resemble measles.

　3.　*Temperature*. Rise more rapid: often 40–40·5 °C (104–105 °F) in a few days. Course more irregular, and sustained fastigium unusual. Fall more rapid. Duration about 2 weeks.

　4.　*Pulse*. Frequently very slow throughout.

　5.　*Spleen*. Enlargement may be marked. May be tender.

　6.　*Sweating* and *Shivering* more common.

　7.　*Toxaemia* rare. Patients with temperature of 40 °C (104 °F) and a profuse rash often exhibit no toxic symptoms or psychical disturbance, and feel well after first few days.

Diarrhoeal and dysenteric onset. Slight diarrhoea not uncommon at onset. Instances occur with acute onset and diarrhoea of dysenteric or food-poisoning type. These only occur in sporadic cases, paratyphoid never producing an outbreak of such type, alleged occurrence being due to confusion of paratyphoid and food-poisoning bacilli.

Complications
As in typhoid fever, but of far greater rarity.

　Salmonella bacteraemia and salmonella osteitis are common in sicklaemics, possibly because their macrophage function is impaired by excessive erythrophagocytosis. Similar salmonella bacteraemia may occur in persons with schistosomiasis and in *S. haematobium* infections salmonellosis may lead to chronic urinary infections with the organism and to increased calculus formation and urinary tract fibrosis.

Diagnosis
General diagnosis as in typhoid fever. Differentiation from typhoid A and B rests entirely on bacteriological and serological tests.

Treatment
Gastroenteritic forms of paratyphoid are best treated with supportive therapy only. Antibiotics appear to prolong excretion of bacilli. Severe forms with toxicity are treated as typhoid.

Chapter 32   # BACTERIAL FOOD POISONING

Diseases of many kinds may be conveyed by or arise from ingestion of food, but the term 'food poisoning', though not clearly defined, is usually applied to certain acute conditions, due to bacterial infection or ingestion of bacterial toxins and characterized mainly by gastroenteritis, often occurring in so-called epidemics or outbreaks, attacking a number of persons within a short space of time. *Salmonellae, Staphylococci, Clostridia, Campylobacter foetus, Yersinia enterocolitica* and *Vibrio parahaemolyticus* commonest causative organisms.

Note: Bacilli of enteric group, dysentery, diphtheria, scarlet fever and certain other organisms may be spread by food and milk fluids, and may cause epidemics, but these are not usually included as 'food poisoning'.

'Food Poisoning' caused by Infection with Salmonellae

N.B. Salmonella 'food poisoning' may occasionally be caused by consumption of cooked food in which cultures of salmonellae have been killed and their enterotoxins remain. In such cases illness is usually acute and self-limiting. The following section applies to infection with living organisms.

Modes of Contamination with Bacteria
(1) Animal infected when slaughtered; (2) Food, during preparation for consumption, contaminated by human 'carrier' or by excreta of rats and other rodents.

Substances Affected
Commonest today is battery-reared poultry among which *S. gallinarum* and *S. pullorum* infections are common. Dried egg similarly affected. Pork commonly, mutton rarely; often pies, sausages, etc. Also milk.

Bacteriology
Bacterial food poisoning is usually due to organisms of the salmonella group; *S. typhimurium* (*aertrycke*) most commonly. Other salmonellae commonly involved

are *S. brandenburg* usually in ham and sausages, *S. dublin* in beef products, *S. choleraesuis* in pork preparations, *S. gallinarum* and *S. pullorum* in poultry and *S. oranienburg* in spray-dried eggs. *S. enteritidis*, identified by Gaertner in 1888, has been isolated from many animals and their products. There are many other members of this group.

Cultural properties. In investigating outbreaks remember that most of these organisms ferment glucose and other sugars with production of gas and hence 'blow' tins containing food infected with them. *S. typhi* and *S. gallinarum* are exceptions in this respect. The organisms are mostly culturally identical. *Agglutination reactions* and *antigen typing* enable these organisms to be distinguished.

Note: Bacilli of enteric group and other organisms may be spread by milk and food, and have thus caused large epidemics, but these are not usually included as 'food poisoning'. Botulism caused by toxins from *Clostridium botulinum*, though also not usually classed as a food-poisoning disease, is a specific form of food poisoning causing bulbar paralysis; gastrointestinal symptoms are usually either slight or absent.

Morbid Anatomy

Acute gastroenteritis; Peyer's patches unaffected, no ulceration. Bacilli often recoverable from bile and spleen. In non-fatal cases, affection is mainly of small intestine.

Symptoms

Outbreak of food poisoning usually possesses following features: (1) Symptoms commence almost simultaneously amongst a number of those consuming the food; (2) Illness limited to those eating the food, *but not all necessarily become ill*; (3) In large outbreaks, every degree of severity is usually present; (4) In bacillary infections as distinct from ingestion of bacillary toxins, excreta of patients are infective, and condition may spread subsequently as an epidemic, e.g. in institutions and camps, constituting 'secondary infections'.

Incubation period. Variable 8–48 h.

Onset. Sudden gastroenteritis. Abdominal pain and tenesmus, diarrhoea, nausea and usually vomiting. Commonly: headache, cold sweats; often shivering and syncope when severe. Cramp in muscles.

Physical signs. No characteristic. Abdomen tender but usually not rigid. Spleen not enlarged. No rash. Temperature: in severe cases often 37·2–38·9 °C (99–102 °F), but may be apyrexial. Character of stools: blood and mucus rare, mucus never in masses as in dysentery. Blood occasionally while motions very frequent. Acetonuria if vomiting severe.

Progress. Initial symptoms usually the severest. Diarrhoea often continues for few hours; rarely severe more than 2–5 days. Improvement usually rapid and recovery in 6–8 days. Continued vomiting is most serious symptom, and present in most fatal cases.

Carriers

Rare.

Mortality

Low. Vomiting usually persistent in fatal cases.

Diagnosis
Numerous simultaneous cases in household or assembly of individuals. Diagnosis from: (1) *Dysentery*: by absence of mucus from stools and by specific organisms; (2) *Enteric fever*: by sudden onset and rapid maximum severity. (3) *Appendicitis*.
Specific diagnosis. Bacteriological examination of stools and vomit. Agglutination reactions with recognized strains. In an outbreak of any extent, many cases may give negative results, but few positive examinations are sufficient to establish the cause.

Treatment
Fluid in plenty.
Diet. For 24 h fluids only. As diarrhoea ceases, diet can be rapidly increased. Combat dehydration and electrolyte loss.
Chemotherapy. Usually unnecessary and may prolong disability and infectivity. Otherwise as for bacillary dysentery (*see* p. 132): short course and smaller dose usually sufficient.

Further Management
Ensure stools culture negative before considered free from infection. Especially important for food handlers.

Investigation of an Outbreak
Note: (1) Clinical symptoms; (2) Bacteriological examination of excreta and agglutination reactions; (3) Epidemiology: (*a*) date, time, and number of persons attacked; (*b*) relations to any common meal, or consumption of same article of food, or food prepared by same person or persons; (4) Examination of residue of food consumed, especially bacteriologically; (5) Mode of preparation of food, cleanliness of kitchen, cooking and apparatus employed; (6) Examination of cooks; (*a*) previous or present attack of diarrhoea; (*b*) bacteriological examination of excreta and agglutination tests, for identification of 'carriers'.

Staphylococcal Food Poisoning

Frequency of staphylococcal food poisoning only recently recognized: accounts for many mild outbreaks.

Mode of Contamination
Often unelucidated: certain outbreaks definitely traced to staphylococcal infections on hands of cooks, etc. Milk and cream cake fillings often infected, but 7 h at 30–37 °C usually required for sufficient concentration of staphylococci to build up. Enterotoxin withstands boiling for 30 min. Contaminated meats, soups and stockpots allowed to stand and then reheated are common sources of toxin.

Bacteriology
Only coagulase-positive strains of staphylococci produce enterotoxin. It is not haemolytic.
   Gel-diffusion tests and injection into isolated loops animal bowel used to recognize toxins. Kittens easily affected by intraperitoneal injection of filtrate.

In outbreaks, suspected food should be examined.

Symptoms
Incubation period. Short: 2–4 h, may be 30 min.
Onset. Nausea, vomiting. Diarrhoea variable, acute and rarely associated with fever.
Progress. Usually lasts 6–8 h. Recovery rapid: about 24 h. Death very rare.

Treatment
Simple measures usually sufficient. Codeine or Lomotil as for travellers' diarrhoea (*see* p. 133).
(*See also Clostridium difficile.*)

Clostridial Food Poisoning and Enteritis Necroticans

Aetiology
Clostridium perfringens (*Clostridium welchii*) present in faeces of many humans, animals and blow-flies and bluebottles and especially pig faeces. Common in dust and sewage. Food readily infected if hygiene poor.

Enteritis necroticans
C. perfringens type C ingested in pork. Toxin produced by organismal growth in intestine is not inactivated because malnutrition or dietary factors reduce proteases in intestinal contents. Toxin destroyed by proteases. Sweet potatoes contain trypsin inhibitors which reduce protease destruction of toxin. Sweet potatoes are the main staple diet in New Guinea areas where enteritis necroticans occurs.

  Ascaris lumbricoides may further predispose by secreting trypsin inhibitors.

Bacteriology
Many strains of *C. perfringens*. Type A causes gas gangrene. Several strains cause food poisoning. All are anaerobes and spore-bearing.

  Type C causes enteritis necroticans, the most important clostridial 'food poisoning' syndrome.

Pathology
Enteritis necroticans affects small intestine from a few cm to almost the whole. Mucosa necrotic, intestinal wall thinned and dilated.

Symptoms
Incubation period usually 48 h, varies from 1 to 7 days. Abdominal pain, distension, diarrhoea with blood in stools. Vomiting.

Treatment
1. Reduce distension with nasogastric tube.
2. Restore fluid and electrolytes.
3. In New Guinea 50% patients needed resection of affected part of small bowel.

4. Full course penicillin or chloramphenicol, initially administered intravenously.

Prognosis
Mortality 15–40% in enteritis necroticans.

Clostridium Difficile
Recently found to cause most cases of colitis following antibiotic administration for sterilizing gut contents. These cases were formerly thought to result from staphylococcal overgrowth. The organism is found in soil, animal faeces and in 30–60% of stools in newborn infants and 3% of normal adults.

Aetiology
After antibiotic administration for attempted sterilization of gut contents, e.g. for surgery or liver failure, the organism colonizes the gut contents in the absence of normal competitors. Has been recovered especially by endoscopic studies. It produces toxins designated A and B. Type A produces fluid accumulation and haemorrhagic inflammation of gut and type B is cytopathic.

Clinical features
Profuse watery diarrhoea containing mucus during antibiotic administration or for up to 4 weeks after its cessation. There is abdominal pain and tenderness with fever and leucocytosis, and dehydration, hypotension, anasarca and toxic megacolon may follow.

Diagnosis
1. *Endoscopy* reveals plaques of pseudomembranous colitis with inflammation, haemorrhage and oedema of bowel wall. The pseudomembranous plaques overlie an intact mucosa with inflammatory exudate in the lamina propria.
2. *C. difficile toxins* are demonstrated by assay of cytopathic changes in tissue culture. The toxins are neutralized by *C. difficile* antitoxins and other toxins that cross react with them. Counter-immunoelectrophoretic and ELISA techniques have also been developed.
3. As the organism's name suggests, its culture requires specialized techniques and laboratories.

Treatment
Orally administered vancomycin, 125–500 mg q.d.s. for 7–14 days, or metronidazole 1500 mg/day orally or intravenously, or bacitracin orally, 500 mg q.d.s.
    Cholestyramine orally in doses of 4 g t.d.s. for 5 days binds *C. difficile*. Fewer patients respond than with antibiotics but those who do are less likely to relapse. Patients should be isolated.

Prognosis
Without specific treatment mortality 20%.

Other 'Food Poisoning' Organisms

Vibrio parahaemolyticus grows in salty waters, especially the sewage-containing coastal Pacific. Transmitted to man in crabs and raw fish especially as eaten in Far East. No man-to-man transmission.

Symptoms
Abdominal pain, diarrhoea, headache, fever.

Treatment
Symptomatic. In serious cases dehydration may need correction, *see* Chapter 42, pp. 189–190.

Bacillus cereus. Produces spores which contaminate dust. Grows on vegetables, especially cooked rice and potatoes left in warm kitchen and then reheated. Severe outbreaks traced to meals in Chinese restaurants in Britain recently.

Symptoms
Abdominal pain, diarrhoea, vomiting.

Treatment
Symptomatic.

Campylobacter Infections

Aetiology
Campylobacter are curved rod or comma-like organisms that principally infect animals, particularly cattle, sheep and poultry. Recent developments in cultural techniques have shown that they not uncommonly infect man. Milk, water and man-to-man transmission by the faecal-oral route are the main modes of infection.

Pathology
Jejunitis and colitis may be produced. Colonic appearances may be indistinguishable from those of acute ulcerative colitis.

Symptoms
Abdominal pain and diarrhoea associated with fever, malaise, headache, myalgia and nausea with little or no vomiting. When colitis is present blood and leucocytes may be found in the stools. The illness usually lasts less than 7 days.

Diagnosis
A presumptive diagnosis may be made by using the phase contrast technique to identify in faeces comma-shaped organisms that have a typically darting type of motility.
    Culture of the organism is with selective media incorporating bacitracin, vancomycin, polymyxin B sulphate, trimethoprim or other agents.

Treatment
Only symptomatic treatment is usually required. In severe cases erythromycin or tetracycline may be administered orally.

Yersinia Enterocolitica Infection

Aetiology
Y. enterocolitica is a gram-negative, facultatively anaerobic rod-like organism. It

is difficult to isolate from faeces as it grows more slowly than the common faecal organisms and hence its importance as a cause of diarrhoea in man has only recently been recognized.

Many isolates have been made from domestic and wild animals and the organism has been found in milk, meat, cheese, ice cream, sea food, poultry and surface water in wells, lakes and streams. Infection is by consuming contaminated food or drink, and man-to-man spread by the faecal-oral route has been reported.

Pathology
Organism appears to invade the bowel wall and may reach regional lymph nodes, producing granuloma-like lesions. Colitis has been demonstrated as has ileitis and mesenteric adenitis.

Symptoms
Diarrhoea with fever and abdominal pain that may mimic appendicitis. The diarrhoea may continue for up to 14 days and the stools may contain blood. However, many infections are asymptomatic.

Extra-intestinal Complications
Non-suppurative arthritis, erythema nodosum, uveitis, Reiter's syndrome, carditis, thyroiditis, acute glomerulonephritis, hepatitis, pancreatitis and haemolytic anaemia have been described.

In patients, particularly those with cirrhosis of the liver, in whom *Y. enterocolitica* occurs as an intercurrent infection septicaemia may develop. Metastatic foci of the infection have then been found in intra-abdominal abscesses, osteomyelitis, meningitis and the lungs. Erysipelas-like skin lesions have also been reported.

Diagnosis
Y. enterocolitica is best isolated from faeces by culture at low temperatures to inhibit overgrowth by other oganisms contained in the stool. Various selective media, particularly incorporating novobiocin or carbenicillin, may also be used.

Treatment
Most infections require symptomatic treatment only. In severe infections gentamicin, chloramphenicol, tetracycline or co-trimoxazole may be tried. The organisms are resistant to penicillin and cephalothin and their sensitivity to erythromycin is variable. Infected persons should be isolated.

Chapter 33   **DYSENTERY**

Dysentery is characterized clinically by: (1) Passage of frequent small stools; (2) Presence of mucus and blood; (3) Abdominal pain and tenesmus. These symptoms constitute dysentery when due to certain specific causes. The intestinal symptoms are the result of an *inflammatory* or *ulcerative colitis*, a condition which may also arise from causes other than dysentery.

Types
Dysentery is of two main types: (1) *Bacillary*, due to certain specific bacilli; (2)

Amoebic, due to protozoon *Entamoeba histolytica* (considered here for convenience).

The term 'dysentery' is used now to imply the presence of one of these two groups of organisms, however mild the symptoms may be, and its definition is aetiological rather than clinical. Either may cause a simple diarrhoea without the characteristic symptoms. Extensive epidemics are usually bacillary dysentery, and, when the death rate is high, are generally due to Shiga's bacillus.

Schistosomal infection may cause diarrhoea but symptoms follow a subacute or chronic course.

1. Bacillary Dysentery

Bacteriology

Two principal groups of bacilli of genus *Shigella*: (1) *Sh. dysenteriae* (formerly *Sh. shiga*). This is a specific organism without strains, constant in its bacteriology: it excretes a powerful exotoxin. (2) *Sh. flexneri/boydii* group. This represents a group with numerous strains differing serologically. Five strains were early identified and titled, V, W, X, Y, Z; of these, V, W and Z are now accepted as separate strains and X and Y regarded as products of subcultures. Other strains have now been identified and are represented by numerals. The group forms endotoxins and recently recognized exotoxin.

Sh. boydii are recognized by their distinctive type antigens and lack of group antigens whereas *Sh. flexneri* contain one or more group antigens as well as type antigens.

Sh. sonnei differs from the *Sh. flexneri/boydii* group in being a late lactose fermenter instead of a non-lactose fermenter. It is also antigenically distinct and homogeneous. It also has recently been recognized to produce exotoxin.

Morphology. Non-motile, non-sporing, gram-negative bacilli resembling colityphoid group. Grow on ordinary media. *Selective media*: sodium desoxycholate citrate and tellurite, citrate and rosolic acid.

Cultural characters

> *Carbohydrates*. Except as noted under *Sh. sonnei*, lactose is not fermented by any of the group. No gas formed by any strain.
>
> *Mannitol*. Enables initial separation of *Sh. dysenteriae* from *Sh. flexneri/boydii*. Former produces neither acid nor gas in it, latter forms acid without gas. Further separation largely by characterization of antigens or phage typing.

Bacteriophage

Most gastrointestinal gram-negative bacteria susceptible to bacteriophage. Specific phages known for most *Shigellae*. Phages are bacterial viruses which will kill or alter the bacteria.

Modes of Infection

Resemble enteric, viz. by water, food, flies and contamination by excreta of infected persons. Epidemics in tropics specially spread by: (1) Faecal pollution of water; (2) Contamination of food by faecal-feeding flies or by carriers.

Carriers. More common than formerly believed. Discovered by careful culture of stools in which *Shigellae* quickly die. Culture therefore necessary almost immediately stool passed.

Morbid Anatomy

The large intestine is mainly affected. The entire colon may be equally involved, but frequently the maximal change is in the sigmoid, extending above and below with diminishing severity. The terminal ileum is frequently hyperaemic for a varying distance.

In acute, rapidly fatal cases, the mucous membrane is hyperaemic, dark red and thickened: there is superficial necrosis, but usually no ulceration: may be bile stained.

In less acute forms of longer duration, ulceration commences in the lymphoid follicles, numerous small superficial ulcers forming on transverse folds of mucous membrane. The edges may be thickened and infiltrated, but are never undermined (as occurs in amoebic dysentery). Destroyed mucous membrane is characteristically green.

In chronic forms, thickening of the mucous membrane: may be nearly 1·5 cm thick: most marked on summits of folds. In severe chronic cases the thickening causes uniform rigidity of bowel wall and decrease in size of lumen.

Peritoneal adhesions may form.

Symptoms

Incubation period. May be a few hours only, and probably rarely exceeds 3 days. Occasionally up to 8 days.

Onset. Onset and development of characteristic symptoms always rapid. Often sudden and abrupt. Occasionally insidious for 1 or 2 days.

Symptoms at onset. Vary greatly in severity.

> *Frequent small stools.* May be almost continuous.
>
> *Abdominal pain.* Colicky pain and tenesmus. Between stools there may be little pain.
>
> *Vomiting.* Common at onset: may be for 1–2 days.
>
> *Headache.* Usual.
>
> *Character of stools.* Each motion of small quantity. A few initial stools may empty the intestine of faecal matter. Subsequently: In mild cases may remain faeculent but in severer forms red-blood-tinged mucus ('red-currant jelly'), or clear mucus and blood. Alkaline. *Microscopic*: numerous pus cells; red cells; large macrophage cells (to be distinguished from amoebae): bacilli scanty. *Entamoeba coli* common.
>
> *Temperature.* Variable: high, low, or moderate.
>
> *Pulse.* Rapid.
>
> *Blood count.* No change.

Clinical Forms

Dysentery may be of any grade of severity with differences in clinical manifestations and great differences in mortality. Forms range from fulminating through severe and moderate to mild.

Fulminating forms. Usually caused by *Sh. dysenteriae* infections. Abrupt onset. Watery diarrhoea, vomiting, subnormal temperature. Rapid dehydration, collapse, toxaemia and death if untreated. Often no typical dysentery stools and may suggest cholera or food poisoning.

Severe forms. Complaints of: (1) Abdominal pain; (2) Thirst. On examination, dryness and coldness are marked.

> *Onset*. Usually abrupt and severe: but not so invariably, for 1 or 2 days may suggest moderate attack. Severe forms are always *dehydrated*.
>
> *Stools*. Very numerous. Almost pure blood, with varying amounts of mucus. Desire for stool almost continuous.
>
> *Skin*. Dry and inelastic. A bluish flush on cheeks, of limited area, is common. *Extremities cold*. These features are due to dehydration and increase in blood viscosity.
>
> *Abdomen. Retracted. Rigidity is unusual. Tenderness* often extreme, especially on left side, but on palpation contraction usually does not occur. Pain preceding and accompanying stools, but may be only slight between motions.
>
> *Anus*. Excoriated and painful. Rectal prolapse common. Haemorrhoids aggravated.
>
> *Tongue* dry. Fur variable, may be absent.
>
> *Temperature*. Not characteristic: usually high, 39·4 °C (103 °F) or subnormal. *Pulse* rapid and small.
>
> *Vomiting* not infrequent, and a very serious symptom when occurring at this stage. Also *hiccup*.
>
> *Muscular pains and cramps* not uncommon: especially anterior thigh and calves.
>
> *Subsequent progress*. (1) Symptoms more severe. Prostration increases. Discomfort extreme. Incontinence of urine and faeces. Mental wandering common, but mind may remain clear. Progressive failure. Death usually from: (*a*) Peripheral circulatory failure, or (*b*) Anuria, uraemic coma. (2) Slow gradual improvement. Convalescence prolonged. Rapid recovery does not occur.
>
> *Mortality* varies with availability and quality of treatment. High in malnourished persons and in times of national or regional disasters, war, famine, earthquakes, etc.

Moderate forms. All above features modified to a varying extent. Stools usually faeculent, may contain some visible blood and/or mucus.

Mild forms. Symptoms of any degree of mildness may result from infections with dysentery bacilli.

Chronic forms. Persistence of symptoms following acute attacks rare with modern treatment but relapses sometimes occur and stools may or may not then be culturally positive. The irritable bowel syndrome occasionally persists for months after an attack.

Notes on symptoms

> *Serious symptoms*. High fever. Passage of offensive sloughs. Hiccup.
>
> *Temperature*. Not of great prognostic significance. (*a*) *Severe forms*: commonly high at onset, but usually subnormal when condition has developed. (*b*) *Moderate forms*: temperature is some measure of severity. High temperature is a sign of severe infection, especially when persistent. Fall of temperature is a sign of improvement. Milder cases have slight pyrexia.

Vomiting. Occasional vomiting at onset is common and of little importance. Persistence or onset of vomiting later is serious symptom.

Sweating. A sweating patient is rarely in immediate danger.

Complications and Sequelae

Arthritis. Onset usually during convalescence. Large joints, especially knees, affected. May occur in mild cases. Considerable effusion: fluid contains polynuclear leucocytes. *Complete recovery is almost invariable and suppuration never occurs*, but duration may be months.

Heart unaffected.

Reiter's syndrome. This, manifested by arthritis, iritis and mucus membrane lesions, a classical complication. Now known to occur only in those with tissue type HLA-B27. The rarity of the syndrome in endemic areas reflects the rarity there of this tissue type.

Haemolytic uraemic syndrome. In severe dysentery caused by *Sh. dysenteriae* type 1. Disseminated intravascular coagulation with anaemia, thrombocytopenia, haematuria and/or renal failure. Infecting organisms often difficult to isolate and antibiotic resistant. In the kidneys tubular and cortical necrosis may occur. Haemodialysis is usually needed in management.

Stenosis. Healing ulcer encircles gut. May cause intestinal obstruction. Rare.

Peripheral neuritis. Rare. Commonest after toxic *Sh. dysenteriae* infections.

Boils. Occasionally troublesome.

Haemorrhoids. Common, may cause blood in stools during convalescence.

Peritonitis. Perforation rare. In later stages and after severe attacks only. Peritonitis may be general or localized by adhesions. Perforations often multiple. Death rate high.

Diagnosis

Diarrhoea of any form, mildness, or severity, may result from infection with dysentery bacilli; but in epidemics characteristic cases will occur. The ultimate diagnosis depends on specific methods.

Diagnosis from non-dysenteric conditions

> 1. *Enteric.* Onset rarely acute. Mucus in stools unusual. Agglutination reactions and bacteriology.
> 2. *Bacterial food-poisoning.* Characterized by simultaneous affection of many individuals. Condition is mainly ileitis or enteritis, and blood is unusual after initial severe motions, and mucus not prominent. Short duration.
> 3. *Ulcerative colitis.* By history and negative bacteriology.
> 4. *Diverticulitis.* Polyposis.

Diagnosis from amoebic dysentery

	Bacillary	Amoebic
Onset	Acute	Often more gradual: initial diarrhoea not uncommon
Symptoms	Toxaemia. Tenesmus. General tenderness	Toxaemia slight. Tenesmus unusual. Tenderness localized.
Progress	Most severe at onset	Irregular. Tends to be chronic

[cont. over]

	Bacillary	Amoebic
Stools. Often indistinguishable but characteristically:	Small, numerous, odourless, alkaline. Mass of glairy tinged mucus. Pus cells and clotted blood. Motions when formed are coated with mucus.	Large, offensive, acid. Mucus, blood, and faecal matter more intimately mixed. Small masses of blood-tinged mucus. Motions when formed are mixed with mucus.
Complications	Arthritis	Hepatic abscess. Amoeboma.
Morbid Anatomy	Sigmoid most affected. Ileum often hyperaemic. Ulcerations superficial. Mucus membrane thickened	Caecum and ascending colon mainly. Ileum rarely affected. Ulcers with undermined edges in long axis

Special methods of diagnosis

1. *Examination of stools*. Examine for bacilli and also for amoebae and amoebic cysts (*see* p. 137). Culture from rectal swab or, in later stages, sigmoidoscope scrapings. Microscopic examination for polymorphonuclear exudate an important procedure. Addition of methylene blue helps identification of polymorphs.

2. *Agglutination*. Agglutinins usually appear early, by second day, and usually maximum by sixth day but are transient and those to *Sh. flexner* and *Sh. boydii* are complicated by multiplicity of strains. Now little used.

3. *Sigmoidoscopy*. After 10 days. Presence of diffuse inflammatory changes typical.

Prognosis

In severest forms, mortality high unless treatment given early, *in moderate forms*, usually low. The relative frequency of these two forms varies greatly with the causal bacillus. (*a*) *Shiga infections*: Severe forms common and convalescence prolonged even in milder forms; but simple diarrhoea may result from them. (*b*) *Flexner group*: Mortality low.

Treatment

Principles are: bed-rest; prevention of, or correction of, dehydration; in severe cases treatment with sulphonamides or antibiotics.

1. *Fluids and electrolytes*. Dehydration major cause of death in children; important at all ages. In infants and young children correct dehydration with half-strength physiological saline made isotonic with glucose (NaCl 0·9%, glucose 2·5%). Daily fluid requirements: 20 ml kg body weight. Ensure this amount given plus any needed to make good abnormal loss. Give also 0·5–1 g potassium chloride orally daily to adults and proportionally less to children. Intravenously never exceed 13 mEq (0·5 g)/potassium/h for adults and half this amount over 24 h. Fantus test useful guide to salt depletion where laboratories not available. Under 2 g chloride per litre urine as indicated by Fantus test means sodium depletion and consequent extracellular dehydration.

For further information, *see* Chapter 42.

In severe cases only fluids given in first 24 h.

2. *Diet*. Semi-fluids until stools fewer than 5/day, then light diet given as condition improves.

3. *Specific therapy*. Resistance of *Shigellae* to sulphonamides and antibiotics is

now widespread. The situation differs from outbreak to outbreak and from the beginning to the end of a given outbreak for transference of resistance takes place speedily. In outbreaks therefore reserve specific drugs for seriously ill patients. More liberality with drugs is permissible for individual patients not part of an epidemic. Ideally sensitivities of causative organism should first be determined but this causes delay in treatment of an ill patient.

Co-trimoxazole (BNF) in a single adult dose of 4–6 tablets with 2·5 g tetracycline often gives good results irrespective of the sensitivities of the causal organism in severe cases.

Drugs reducing intestinal motility e.g. diphenoxylate (Lomotil) prolong the illness and excretion of organisms.

Sonne Dysentery

Sonne Bacillus differs from shiga-flexner groups in:
1. Late lactose-fermenter.
2. Ferments mannitol. Clots milk.
3. Not agglutinated by *Sh. dysenteriae* and *Sh. flexner* sera.

Symptoms
Usually mild diarrhoea: rarely acute, with vomiting and collapse. May present with fever and meningeal signs in children. Often causes outbreaks among children in institutions or day-nurseries.

Treatment
Vide supra. Particular attention needed to fluid and electrolytes in young children.

Traveller's Diarrhoea

Synonyms
Many and bizarre, e.g. Hong Kong dog, Montezuma's revenge, Delhi belly and gippy tummy.

Causes
Mild shigella infections in some cases but British Army/MRC research teams showed pathogenic *Escherichia coli* often responsible, especially *E. coli* 0148. Some cases from which no organisms isolated almost certainly caused by toxins in food especially from killed staphylococcal cultures in meats, soups, milk products and synthetic creams. Campylobacter (q.v.) causes some cases as do viruses, including the Norwalk agent and related viruses. Diarrhoea lasting more than a few days usually caused by giardiasis or other organisms.

Epidemiology
Affects travellers within few days of arriving in fresh location. Particularly associated with consumption of water and food prepared in poor hygienic conditions; however, carriers can work even in kitchens of best hotels. Greatest incidence in group travelling from developed to developing countries. Also affects those proceeding from one locality in tropics to another. In first locality they may

have acquired some immunity to local organisms and do not have immunity to organisms in the fresh location.

Symptoms
Diarrhoea, abdominal pains, anorexia, nausea, vomiting, fever, myalgia, headache, weakness, dizziness and faintness. Symptoms abrupt in onset and persist only for 24–72 h.

Treatment
Self-limiting but codeine phosphate 30 mg, once or twice daily, codeine compound tablets (BP) 2 three or four times daily, or diphenoxylate hydrochloride 2·5 mg and atropine sulphate 25 mg (Lomotil) 4 tablets initially and 2 every 6 h may bring relief. Correction of dehydration important.

Prevention
Hygiene!—Avoidance of: (1) Uncooked foods especially cream and cake fillings; (2) Foods such as cold meats which since cooking have been handled or exposed to flies; (3) Soups cooked, then allowed to stand and reheated. These are a common cause of staphylococcal toxin-induced enterocolitis.
Drug prophylaxis. Most favourable reports from use of 1 tablet Streptotriad b.d. or t.d.s. Streptotriad tablets each contain sulphadiazine 100 mg, sulphadimidine 100 mg, sulphathiazole 100 mg and streptomycin 65 mg.

Infantile Gastroenteritis
A gastroenteritis of gradual or abrupt onset and of varying severity though usually mild. Dehydration is an important complication. The cause is usually *E. coli* infection, especially with types 0111, 026, 055, 0119 and 0125–8 or rotavirus infection. Particularly occurs in outbreaks in nursery schools and similar establishments. Fluid and electrolyte replacement, orally, or in severe cases intravenously, is the most important aspect of treatment.

2. Amoebic Dysentery

Amoebic dysentery is caused by infection with the protozoon *Entamoeba histolytica*. Characterized by afebrile diarrhoea: typically has insidious onset and chronic course, with tendency to latency and relapses. Metastatic amoebiasis is due to penetration of amoebae into tissues of intestine and spread by bloodstream: liver usually affected.

The Amoeba
Entamoeba histolytica. The only pathogenic intestinal amoeba. General characteristics:
1. Size: 25–50 μm diameter, commonly about 35 μm.
2. Clear refractile ectoplasm with a granular vacuolated endoplasm.
3. Amoeboid movements active. Clear pseudopodia are thrown out and retracted.
4. Often contains erythrocytes.
5. Nucleus indistinct and eccentric.
Cysts
1. *Size*: 10–14 μm diameter. Round.

2. *Nuclei*: 2 or 4 in number.
3. Chromidial body present.
4. Cyst wall thin and indistinct.

E. hartmanni morphologically similar to *E. histolytica* except that it is smaller (15–35 μm in diameter) and its cysts are less than 10 μm in diameter. Almost certainly non-pathogenic. Has caused much confusion in past.

Entamoeba coli. Non-pathogenic. Size rather larger than *E. histolytica*. Distinction often extremely difficult, depending on: (1) absence of ectoplasm, (2) amoeboid movements sluggish, (3) erythrocytes rare and never numerous, (4) nucleus central and more distinct.

Cysts: Distinction from *E. histolytica* depends upon:
1. *Size*: diameter 15–29 μm: sometimes 30 μm. (Smaller cysts may occur; also *E. histolytica* are occasionally larger than 14 μm.)
2. *Nuclei*: 6 or 8, sometimes more. Simplest and most reliable mode of distinction.
3. No chromidial body.
4. Cyst wall more distinct.

Endolimax nana (*Entamoeba nana*). A small (6–12 μm), non-pathogenic amoeba. The cysts are same size as *E. histolytica*, and contain 1, 2, or 4 nuclei, but are of oval shape.

Iodamoeba bütschlii. No evidence of pathogenicity.

Presence of Entamoeba histolytica *in stools*. *Vegetative forms* in acute stages only. Fresh stool must be examined, as amoebae rapidly disintegrate. Examine unstained or with a little weak neutral red, preferably on a warm stage. *Cysts*: Pick out portion of mucus: place on slide with Lugol's iodine solution; this renders nuclei more distinct and also stains glycogen granules. Examine slide with a 5 mm lens and confirm with oil-immersion lens. *Faust's flotation method*: Addition of $ZnSO_4$ brings cysts to the surface. Method: Solution of $ZnSO_4$, 33%, is poured onto centrifuged deposit from stool suspension, shaken, and centrifuged again: cysts concentrate on surface.

Modes of Infection

Active forms of amoebae die very rapidly even in faeces. *Cysts* have long endurance in moisture, faeces and water, but are rapidly killed by drying. Spread of disease entirely by cysts, from presence in stools and frequency of 'carriers'. Epidemics may be water-borne. Cooks, if 'carriers', infect food. Flies and cockroaches may transmit by feeding on faeces and subsequently defaecating on food.

Development of cysts. On ingestion pass unchanged through stomach; wall dissolved by pancreatic juice; amoebulae escape and develop into vegetative forms.

Morbid Anatomy

Caecum and ascending colon are usually most affected. The entire large intestine may be involved: less often sigmoid and rectum. The ileum escapes.

Path of amoebae. Amoebae enter mucous membrane through crypts of Lieberkühn, multiply, and mainly spread in the submucosa.

Infiltration of submucosa. Earliest stage of oedema, multiplication of fixed cells, and round-cell infiltration. Polynuclear leucocytes are scanty at all stages.

Prominences due to small abscesses appear on gut, size of pea.

Ulceration. Mucous membrane over prominences necroses and sloughs, forming *ulcers* with irregular outline, ragged and characteristically *undermined edges*. Floor often has black tenacious slough. In submucosa undermining of the mucous membrane is prominent feature. Ulcers may coalesce, forming large ulcerated areas, base covered with sloughs. Intervening mucous membrane almost normal. Amoebae are in the spreading edge.

Healing results by formation of fibrous tissue. Local contractions may result, but not a stricture, since ulcers tend to spread in long axis of gut.

All stages of ulceration and repair may be present simultaneously in the same specimen.

In chronic cases. Wall thick in some parts, in others thin, scarred and pigmented.

Amoeboma (amoebic granuloma). Tumour formed in chronic cases by granulation tissue, fibrous tissue and products of ulceration. Forms in any part of colon, especially sigmoid and at flexures; may cause colonic obstruction. In rectum may form large mass and protrude at anus. Dangerous to operate without previous treatment.

Adhesions. Not uncommon.

Symptoms
Incubation period. Probably 3 weeks to 3 months.

Insidious onset. Bowels loose. Typically an afebrile diarrhoea. Local and general disturbances slight. Caecum or sigmoid may be tender.

Stools. Number 3 or 4 daily. Flecked with mucus; streaks of degenerated blood.

Chronic form. Recurrent diarrhoea and constipation. Vague ill health and loss of weight. Colon sometimes palpable and tender.

Acute form. Not common. Onset sudden, but often previous diarrhoea. Symptoms in general resemble bacillary dysentery but less tenesmus and toxaemia, and usually afebrile.

Latent forms. Cysts in stools but often no history of dysentery. Irregular gastric and dyspeptic symptoms. May be complications.

Fulminating forms. Rare.

Progress
Chronic course usual: improvement and relapses. Uncomplicated almost invariably recover, most permanently.

Complications and Sequelae
Important.

Liver abscess. See Amoebic Hepatitis and Amoebic Abscess (p. 138).

Localized peritonitis and adhesions. Not uncommon in chronic cases, especially over thickened intestine, e.g. caecum. May be confused with appendicitis, but operation useless.

Perforation and peritonitis. Rare except in later stage of severe attacks. Mortality high owing to extensive lesions of intestine. *Haemorrhage* rare but may be fatal.

Colon. Never stricture. May be dilated.

Appendicitis. Not uncommon.

Skin. May become infected around anus. With spreading ulceration.

Other complications as in bacillary type, but no arthritis.

'Carriers'
Attack of dysentery often leaves a chronic carrier. Other carriers may have no

history of attack but develop complications. Many carriers found on routine test have no symptoms but are potential source of infection. Incidence of symptomless carriers very high in many tropical countries: approximately 0·5% in Britain.

Diagnosis
By examination of stools and sigmoidoscope scrapings for vegetative and amoebic cysts. *See* Bacillary dysentery (pp. 128–134) and *Balantidium coli* (p. 140). also from intestinal neoplasm, cholecystitis and chronic intestinal lesions. Beware of combination of bleeding piles with non-infective diarrhoea. *Sigmoidoscopy*: Ulcers often visible in sigmoid. *Radiographs*: Little assistance in routine cases but may be valuable for complications, e.g. amoeboma.

Treatment
No one drug adequately eradicates both vegetative and cystic forms.
Specific therapy

> **A. In acute cases with trophozoites in the stool**
> 1. *Metronidazole* (Flagyl): Has largely replaced emetine, being less toxic and possessing amoebicidal activity in the liver. May, however, cause T wave flattening in ECG and usually causes nausea, anorexia, giddiness, lassitude and dark coloration of urine. *Dose* 800 mg t.d.s for 5 days. Best followed by course of diloxanide.
> 2. *Tinidazole* acts similarly to metronidazole and may be used instead of it. Dose 2 g (or for children 50 mg/kg) orally daily for 2–3 days.
> 3. *Diloxanide furoate* (Furamide): Non-toxic and alone cures 95% chronic cases and 75% acute dysenteric cases when given in doses of 20 mg/kg body weight daily for 10 days. Best used after 3–5 days course of metronidazole or emetine to ensure any amoebae in liver are killed.
> 4. *Antibiotics*: Oxytetracycline probably most satisfactory antibiotic to use but has no direct action on amoebae. Acts by killing bacteria with which amoebae live in symbiosis. Cures 80–90% cases intestinal amoebiasis, no effect on hepatic forms of the disease. Dosage 30 mg/kg body weight daily for 10 days. As in case of diloxanide, antibiotics are best given after short course of metronidazole or emetine. Especially valuable if peritonitis threatens/or is present.
> 5. *Emetine or dehydroemetine hydrochloride*: Much less used than formerly but popular in some countries. *Dosage*: Subcutaneous or intramuscular injection, 60 mg in 1 ml distilled water daily for 3–5 injections. Is lethal to vegetative tissue-invading forms. Produces cessation of diarrhoea and absence of blood and mucus; also acts on metastatic vegetative forms, e.g. amoebic hepatitis. No effect on cysts and chronic stages. Repeated courses within 2 or 3 weeks are dangerous, ineffective and may result in emetine-fast

forms. Dehydroemetine less toxic and as effective as emetine.

B. In carriers and chronic cases with cysts only in stool. Recommended course is 3 days metronidazole followed by 10 days diloxanide in dosage given above. Metronidazole omitted by many physicians. Metronidazole alone less effective in eradicating such infections than diloxanide. Di-iodohydroxyquinoline an alternative in doses of 250–500 mg q.d.s. for 20 days. Its side effects include gastrointestinal irritation, headache and very occasionally optic neuritis.

3. Amoebiasis of the Liver (Amoebic Hepatitis and Liver Abscess)

In metastatic amoebiasis, amoebae enter the bloodstream of the intestine, and reach the liver through the portal vein. From the liver they may rarely reach the brain and other organs.

Aetiology
Previous dysentery. History in high percentage of cases. May have been mild. Occasionally no record: in some of these sigmoidoscopy reveals small ulcers with cysts present.
Interval since dysentery. May be acute within few weeks. May be 5–10 years or longer.
Alcohol. Epidemiological evidence hints at alcohol as a predisposing factor.
Mode of onset. May be: (1) Acute or subacute: symptoms develop rapidly: may be shortly after dysentery. (2) Chronic: slow development.

Amoebic Hepatitis
A slight degree of tender hepatomegaly often accompanies acute amoebic dysentery. Its origin is contested but probably caused by metastatic foci of amoebae with surrounding inflammation. One or more of these foci may develop into abscesses. The hepatitis may be due to bacterial invasion of the liver. Almost all observers now agree that chronic amoebic hepatitis does not exist. Where chronic hepatic symptoms persist, cause likely to be one or more small abscesses or hepatitis caused by alcohol or other agent.

Amoebic Abscess

Symptoms
Progress rapidly.
1. Constitutional symptoms (less marked in chronic forms). (1) *Fever*: irregular, rising to 103°. (2) *Rigors*. (3) *Profuse sweats*. (4) From septic absorption: sallow complexion, wasting, anorexia, furred tongue.
2. Pain. (1) Over liver; (2) Back and *right shoulder*.
3. Liver enlarged and tender. Abdominal muscles rigid. If abscess, dullness, usually increased upwards in mid-axillary line, from common position of abscess (top of right lobe); if in the left lobe, tender tumour in epigastrium.

4. Icterus. Very rare.
5. Pulmonary symptoms at right base. Cough and pleurisy. Liver dullness raised. Diminished movements and breath sounds.
Chronic forms. Slow development. Symptoms slighter.
Leucocytosis. 10 000–25 000; mainly polynuclears. May be absent. No ascites, nor enlargement of spleen.

Morbid Anatomy of Abscess
Commonly single, in right lobe and on diaphragmatic surface. Occasionally two or more or a loculated abscess present. Early abscess: contents grey yellow. Larger abscess: necrotic walls, contents reddish mass of blood and liver tissue.

Contents are sterile (in absence of secondary infection), are not purulent, and consist of detritus. Amoebae only present in recent abscess: in old abscesses only found in walls.

Diagnosis
Difficult in early stages. History of amoebiasis important. Diagnosis from: (1) *Malaria*. Often simulated by recurrent pyrexia and rigors. Malaria parasites in blood; (2) Gallstones, cholecystitis and complications; (3) Pneumonia and pleurisy, right base; (4) Subphrenic abscess; (5) Fever associated with carcinoma in liver.
Special examinations. (1) Leucocyte count; (2) Stools for cysts but note their absence does not exclude hepatic amoebiasis; (3) Radiography of liver and chest. Diaphragm over affected lobe of liver raised and relatively immobile; (4) Aspiration of the liver (with due precautions and preparation for operation if necessary); (5) Radioactive scintillography shows area of diminished radioactivity corresponding to abscess; (6) Ultrasonic scanning of liver very valuable in demonstrating abscesses and their position. Very helpful as a preliminary to aspiration. Amoebic fluorescent antibody test positive in this and other parenteral forms of amoebiasis.

Perforation
Occurs into:
1. Lungs. Most common. Either direct into lung or via pleural cavity. Symptoms: (1) Cough; (2) Signs at right base; (3) 'Anchovy sauce' sputum when lung perforated—contains amoebae, liver tissue, pus scanty.
2. Other sites. Externally. Stomach. Peritoneum (local or general infection). Pericardium.

Treatment
Metronidazole or tinidazole. Now the drug of choice. Dosage as for dysentery. Unless abscess small aspiration also needed.
Emetine injections. As for dysentery. Rapidly successful with small abscesses and in stage of hepatitis.
Chloroquine. Is amoebicidal: concentrates in liver: good results. Initial doses of 600 mg base daily for 5 days followed by 300 mg base daily for 14–21 days.
Aspiration. If evidence of much pus. Aspirate up to 1200 ml: repeat if necessary. Puncture in eighth or ninth intercostal space in anterior axillary line or at a tender spot if present. Give preliminary 1–2 days' treatment with metronidazole or 1–2 subcutaneous injections of 60 mg emetine hydrochloride. Complete course of metronidazole or emetine followed by diloxanide as for dysentery.

Secondary infections. Treat with antibiotics. Note antibiotics useless for primary amoebic infection of liver. Open operation rarely justified.

Prognosis
Good. Mortality low with modern treatment.

Intestinal and Urogenital Protozoa other than Entamoeba

Giardiasis

Aetiology
Giardia lamblia (syn. Giardia intestinalis). A flagellate protozoon, which inhabits the duodenum and jejunum. Pyriform in shape, with a characteristic saucer-shaped depression and four pairs of flagella: length about 20 μm. Encysted non-flagellated form also occur.

Commonly associated with diarrhoea, often with features of malabsorption of fats and sugars. Never invades mucosa but partial villous atrophy and extensive infiltration of lamina propria with lymphocytes, plasma cells and polymorphs occur.

Diagnosis: Giardia cysts demonstrable in formed stools and trophozoites in unformed stools. *The string test*. Very effective. A brushed nylon thread is swallowed by attaching it to a gelatine capsule. Microscopic examination of absorbed duodenal juice often reveals trophozoites when string recovered. May be found in bile by duodenal tube suction, especially in achlorhydria, but no evidence of invasion of gallbladder or ducts.

Treatment
Mepacrine hydrochloride (atebrin) 0·1 g t.d.s for 7 days is specific as is metronidazole in doses of 400 mg t.d.s. for 5 days or 200 mg t.d.s. for 8 days.

Balantidium Coli
A ciliated protozoon: oval shape: size 50–80 μm by 30–60 μm. Encysted forms occur. Infection from pigs. Produces ulcers indistinguishable from amoebic dysentery. Symptoms as in chronic dysentery. May invade lymph glands but never liver. May be latent. Diagnosis from amoebiasis by demonstrating balantidium in scrapings from ulcers or in excreta: number scanty.

Treatment
Tetracycline 2 g daily for 10 days.

Trichomonas Vaginalis
A flagellate protozoon: pear-shaped: size 10–15 μm by 7–10 μm: reproduces by fission. No encysted form known. About 10% women infected: produces vaginitis. In males rare, may cause prostatitis. Diagnosis from gonorrhea needs care. Metronidazole in doses of 400 mg b.d. or t.d.s. for 7 days is usually effective. For vaginitis metronidazole can also be given in pessaries containing 500 mg; one is inserted daily for 10–20 days.

Trichomonas Intestinalis. Tetramitus Mesnili. Paramecium Coli
No proof of pathogenicity.

Isospora Belli
A coccidian parasite exclusively found in man in the epithelial cells of whose small intestine the life-cycle is completed. It is rare in temperate regions but not uncommon in the tropics. It usually causes self-limiting diarrhoea and sometimes fever. Malabsorption has also been described. Co-trimoxazole (BNF) in doses of 2 tablets twice daily for 5–8 days may be used if treatment is required.

Chapter 34   # STREPTOCOCCAL INFECTIONS

Conditions in which a group of constitutional symptoms occurs, with or without local manifestations or suppuration, as the result of invasion of the bloodstream by bacteria.

Bacteriaemia without resulting manifestations is not regarded as septicaemia: probably not uncommon temporarily, as after minor operations, e.g. tonsillectomy.

Streptococcus
Streptococci include numerous strains, pathogenic and non-pathogenic. Essential proof of pathogenicity is production of haemolysis.

Primary Division
Certain strains cause haemolysis, i.e. lysis of red cells, when grown on blood agar plates, resulting in area of blanching around the colonies. Hence primary division into:
1. *β-haemolytic streptococci* (*S. haemolyticus, S. pyogenes* and many others). Produce complete haemolysis around colonies: known as β haemolysis. Includes nearly all strains pathogenic to man—viz. Group A. But all haemolytic streptococci are not pathogenic: they are present in nasopharynx in 20% of persons, but only one-third are potential pathogens.
2. *α-haemolytic streptococci* (*S. pneumoniae* formerly known as pneumococci, *S. mitis* and *S. faecalis*). Produces green discoloration and partial lysis.
3. *Non-haemolytic*. Also known as γ-haemolytic. Many strains. Non-pathogenic.

Grouping of Streptococci
Lancefield differentiated by antigenic qualities of carbohydrates in the organism's cell wall. Serogroups A to H and K to O known. Groups A, B, C, D and G most important to man.

Group A streptococci have in cell walls protein M which induces type-specific immunity. It may also be an anti-phagocytic and virulence factor.
Value of tests. The main value of grouping today is that different groups vary in antimicrobial susceptibility. Group A (*S. pyogenes*) and also *S. viridans* are very sensitive to penicillin G. Group B are susceptible but less so. Group D enterococci (*S. faecalis*) are resistant to penicillin G; non-enterococcal Group D streptococci (*S. bovis, S. equinus*) are, however, penicillin sensitive.

Strain Typing

Proves that infection with one type does not protect against infection with another: thus cross-infection in hospital wards is cause of so-called 'relapse' in scarlet fever. Typing facilitates investigation of origin of local epidemics of haemolytic streptococcal infection.

Streptococcal Toxins

Haemolytic streptococci produce several toxins which are enzymes or other extracellular products. These include: (1) *Streptolysin O (haemolysin)*. Antistreptolysin O titres are of diagnostic value in rheumatic fever. (2) *Streptokinase*: liquefies fibrin. These two, i.e. (1) and (2) are produced by groups A, C and G. (3) *Erythrogenic toxin*. Produced by toxigenic Group A strains. Scarlet fever strains produce most. Used in Dick test for scarlet fever. (4) *Diphosphopyridine nucleotidase*. Produced by Group A and particularly by type 12, nephritogenic strains. (5) Hyaluronidases. Group A. Hyaluronidase probably helps these streptococci to spread rapidly through tissues.
Virulence of haemolytic streptococcus. Apparently much less than 50 to 100 years ago—e.g. case mortality of scarlet fever now very low.

Disease Specificity of Types

The former designation of certain strains as *S. scarlatinae, S. erysipelatis, S. puerperalis* etc. now outmoded. Difference in strains attributed to variation in amount produced of the different toxins. (The tendency of scarlet fever, erysipelas, etc. to pass from one person to another predominantly, though not exclusively, in the same clinical form remains true).

Anaerobic Streptococci

Puerperal septicaemia is frequently due to anaerobic strains.

Clinical Syndromes produced by Streptococcal Infection

The main syndromes are of 3 groups: (1) Suppurative; (2) Immunologically mediated complications of clinical or subclinical infection, e.g. rheumatic fever; (3) Toxin-mediated disease, e.g. scarlet fever.

Suppurative Streptococcal Syndromes

Streptococcal Pharyngitis

Aetiology

Usually Group A streptococci. Occurs particularly in childhood and early adult life.

Clinical Features

Causes: (1) Fever more than viral pharyngitis; (2) Painful cervical lymphadenitis; (3) Absence of influenza-like symptoms. Pharyngeal exudates and peripheral leucocytosis usual but may be equally present in viral pharyngitis.

Complications

Peritonsillar abscess, i.e. quinsy—usually requires surgical incision. Rheumatic fever, glomerulonephritis, erythema nodosum.

Diagnosis
Throat culture most reliable means. Antibody responses often equivocal.

Treatment
One intramuscular dose 0·6 g benzathine penicillin; phenoxymethyl penicillin or erythromycin orally 250 mg q.d.s. for 10 days. Antibiotics do not usually shorten course of acute illness but prevent rheumatic fever and other streptococcal complications.

Streptococcal Pneumonia
Now uncommon.

Aetiology
Usually Group A streptococci. Pneumonia caused by pneumococci, i.e. *S. pneumoniae* is a separate clinical entity. May follow measles, influenza or aspiration of exudate from streptococcal throat infection.

Clinical Features
Illness often severe.

Complications
Empyema not uncommon and organizes rapidly into fibrous coating to lungs which then require surgical decortication.

Diagnosis
Culture and typing of organism in sputum or blood. Pneumococcal polysaccharide antigens detected by CIE (countercurrent immunoelectrophoresis), useful if infection partially treated when cultures may be negative.

Treatment
Daily intramuscular benzathine penicillin 0·6 g till fever resolves then dose is tailed off.

Streptococcal Meningitis

Aetiology
Group A streptococci: Almost always in young persons. Infection usually has spread from middle ear or mastoid. Group D and *S. viridans* rare causes of meningitis and in such cases organism usually reaches meningi from infective endocarditis. Group B streptococci important cause in neonates.

Treatment
Penicillin intravenously at least 0·6 g daily. Gentamicin is also often added for Group D infections, 2–4 mg/kg daily i.m. and/or 1 mg daily intrathecally.

Streptococcal Septicaemia

Morbid Anatomy (fatal cases)
Blood often fluid from presence of streptokinase produced by the streptococci. *Spleen* large and soft. *Petechial haemorrhages* common; especially on serous

membranes. *Arterial walls* stained. *Kidneys* and other organs show cloudy swelling.

Source of Infection
Often obvious and local, e.g. finger-prick, tonsillitis. Septic abortion or pelvic inflammation. Site may be trivial and overlooked.

General Characteristics
Variations in intensity of symptoms depend on virulence of organisms and resistance of tissues: (1) *Rigors* and *sweats*; (2) *Pyrexia*: May be daily remissions or intermissions, or steady rise; (3) *Pulse*: Small, soft and rapid; (4) *Gastrointestinal disturbances*: Diarrhoea in severe forms; (5) *Prostration* marked; (6) *Mental symptoms*: Delirium if debilitated; may remain mentally clear; (7) *Anaemia*: Develops rapidly, hypochromic type. Spleen may be palpable; (8) *Pain* not marked; joints may be tender and swollen; (9) *Haemorrhages*, petechial or purpuric. Transient erythemata, etc. may occur; (10) *Leucocytosis*: (*a*) Total leucocytes increased ($10\,000–100\,000/mm^3$); (*b*) Polynuclear cells relatively increased (up to 90% or higher); (11) *Urine*: Albuminuria rarely absent. Abscesses may form.

Prognosis
Especially serious if: (1) No localization of infection; (2) Absence of absolute polynucleosis; (3) Severe rigors; (4) Apyrexial.

Treatment
Penicillin intravenously at least 1 megaunit daily plus gentamicin 2–5 mg/kg daily i.m.

Erysipelas
A spreading inflammation of the deeper layers of the skin, with local and constitutional symptoms, due to a haemolytic streptococcus; may invade subcutaneous tissues, producing cellulitis.

Aetiology
Group A streptococci. No special strain responsible and tonsillitis, scarlet fever and erysipelas may result from common source. Erysipelas once established, however, tends to transmit as erysipelas. Is contagious, conveyable by third person or by bedding, etc. of a patient, but infectivity is low. Probably invariably starts from an abrasion. Commoner in women, especially in puerperium. Also after surgical operations.

Alcoholism, nephritis, diabetes and debility are predisposing factors.

Recurrence, especially on the face. Sometimes a longstanding break in the skin may be responsible.

Morbid Anatomy
Streptococci are present in the spreading edge, in the lymphatics of the skin and subcutaneous tissues.

Symptoms (facial erysipelas)
Incubation period. 1–7 days.

Onset. Malaise, rigor, pyrexia. Initial focus over nose and cheeks or at local abrasion.

Local symptoms. (1) Skin red, hot, smooth, tense and oedematous; (2) Blebs common; (3) Definite spreading red edge develops; (4) Advances at the edge, while centre fades. Face and features swell enormously, especially eyes, lips and scalp. Neck swollen and glands enlarged. Pus may form under scalp. Mouth, throat and larynx may be involved.

Constitutional symptoms. Temperature high: usually no remissions. Headache may be severe and suggests meningitis. Symptoms severe in old, alcoholic, or debilitated subjects. *Delirium*, especially in alcoholics or when scalp is involved. Albuminuria usual.

Complications
Oedema of glottis serious. Meningitis rare. Rarely: pneumonia, pyaemia, septicaemia, nephritis. If it affects the leg in an elderly person longstanding oedema may result.

Course and Prognosis
Self-limited. Spreading edge dies out. Temperature often falls about fourth to fifth day. Mortality very low if previous health good.

Treatment
Isolation advisable or good barrier nursing
Chemotherapy. Penicillin, 0·6 g i.m. initially followed by 0·25 g phenoxy-methyl penicillin orally 4-hourly for 7 days. If there is a history or symptoms suggesting penicillin hypersensitivity erythromycin 250 mg 6-hourly for 4–6 days may be used.

Local Treatment
If pus collects delay incision till erysipelas is under control.

Other Streptococcal Syndromes of the Suppurative Class
These include bacterial endocarditis which is commonly caused by group D streptococci (*S. faecalis* and *S. bovis*) and viridans streptococci. Group B streptococci may also be causes especially after parturition and in diabetes mellitus. Some forms of impetigo and myositis also fall into this group of infections.

Immunologically Mediated Complications of Clinical or Subclinical Streptococcal Infection

Rheumatic Fever
Disease characterized by fever and migratory arthritis, and a tendency to affect the heart causing carditis which may result in permanent heart valve lesions. It is a late sequela of pharyngitis caused by Lancefield group A streptococci.

Note: Attacks vary greatly in severity of general symptoms and extent of joint lesions. Manifestations may be slight, but risk of cardiac lesions still exists. In the nineteenth century, rhuematic fever was a very severe illness with extreme tenderness of joints, sour sweats and high temperature. The change is not due to introduction of salicylates, since this type is not now met with at onset, but is comparable with the fall in virulence of scarlet fever.

Aetiology
Primary factor. Probably a tissue response of allergic or autoimmune nature, which may be determined by inherited factors, associated with pharyngitis caused by Group A beta-haemolytic streptococci.
Climate
Universal. Now uncommon in the developed world.
Season. In England, maximum in October and November, minimum in February and March. Varies greatly in different countries. In America, maximum in March.
Age. Most frequent from 5 to 15 years; first attacks very rare in adult life; never under 2 years.
Sex. Males more common than females, except between 10 and 15 years.
Hereditary influence. Generally accepted: most marked in children.
Predisposing causes. Environment important, e.g. bad hygienic surroundings; 20–30 times more common in slums than in good environments. May be related to increased person-to-person spread.
Immunity. One attack definitely predisposes to others.

Morbid Anatomy
Aschoff's nodes are the primary lesion: present characteristically in myocardium. Are spindle-shaped 'submiliary' bodies, i.e. smaller than miliary tubercles. *Histology*: (1) General fibroblastic proliferation; (2) Aschoff's large endothelioid cells, one or more nuclei, scattered; (3) Lymphocytes and plasma cells—varying numbers, may be numerous; (4) Necrotic tissue often in centre. May be present as above several years after acute attack, but in old cases replaced by fibrous tissue.
Changes in valves. As in 'endocarditis', *see* p. 148.
Joint changes. Slight. Synovial membrane may show hyperaemia. Non-erosive. Fibrinous exudate. Sterile effusion.

Modes of Onset
1. Insidious. Vague pains in limbs. *Note*: 'Growing pains' are not rheumatic.
2. Sudden onset. Typical acute articular rheumatism.
    An attack of tonsillitis without joint symptoms may result in similar cardiac lesions.

Symptoms
Preliminary symptoms. Sometimes none remembered, but streptococcal tonsillitis or pharyngitis precedes acute rheumatism by 1–6 weeks.
Major manifestations. Carditis, polyarthritis, chorea, subcutaneous nodules and erythema marginatum.
Minor manifestations. Arthralgia, fever, history of previous rheumatic fever or evidence of pre-existing rheumatic heart disease, and certain laboratory findings (discussed below).
(*Note*: Presence of 2 major or 1 major and 2 minor criteria plus evidence of recent group A infection indicates a high probability of rheumatic fever.)
Onset. Abrupt. Chill but no rigor. Condition fully developed in 24 h.

Characteristic symptoms are: (1) *Joints* swollen and painful; (2) *Face flushed*; (3) *Sweats*; even in absence of sweats the skin is moist, and in spite of pyrexia is never dry: (4) *Temperature*, 38·3–39·4°C (101–103°F); (5) *Pulse* soft and rapid, 100–120. Ordinary febrile symptoms present. Pain may cause sleeplessness.

Joint affection (Arthritis). Characteristics are:

Multiple Joints affected: especially larger joints, often symmetrically. In severe attacks, many attacked simultaneously.

Frequency of Involvement: Order: (1) Knee; (2) Ankle; (3) Wrist; (4) Elbow; (5) Shoulder. Vertebral, sternoclavicular, jaw and phalangeal joints very rare.

Joints: Swollen, red, hot to the hand, exquisitely tender and extremely painful on movement. Changes are mainly inflammation of periarticular tissues. Tissues are infiltrated with serum, but oedema and pitting of the skin on pressure is absent even in severe cases. Tendon sheaths involved. *Extensive effusion into joint rare*. In some cases no discernible change.

Course: Wanders from joint to joint, e.g. as knee recovers, wrists swell. Change may occur in 24 h. In space of 3 or 4 days many joints may have been affected. Lasts up to 4 weeks. Resolves without residual damage.

Joint Fluid: Turbid. Contains numerous polynuclear leucocytes, but never has appearance of pus. *Suppuration never occurs*.

Directly acute symptoms subside, joint usually appears normal.

Temperature. Rise rapid, 38·3–39·4 or 40°C (101–103 or 104°F): rarely higher. Irregular. Falls gradually. First recorded temperature usually the highest, owing to subsequent administration of salicylates. Pyrexia after 5 days' treatment with salicylates suggests endocarditis or pericarditis, or error of diagnosis.

Heart. Systolic murmur frequent at apex.

Pulse. At onset 100–120. Soft. Tracings often show slight irregularity. Falls with temperature. With salicylates may become very slow, 40–50, but this is of no importance.

Laboratory Findings

Sedimentation rate raised. C-reactive protein in blood.

Throat swab. Shows group A streptococci in only a minority of cases.

Serology. Shows raised anti-O streptolysin titre in 80% of cases. With additional serological tests for recent group A infection the frequency of positivity rises to 95%.

Urine. May contain protein, red cells and white cells.

Blood. Polynuclear leucocytosis. Normochromic, normocytic anaemia.

Progress

In absence of complications and without drugs, fever and acute symptoms subside in about 10 days. With salicylates fever rarely exceeds 4 days. Occasional deaths from acute rheumatic carditis. More marked carditis is associated with increasing risk of residual rheumatic heart disease. Chorea, which is often not associated with acute carditis, is commonly associated with chronic rheumatic heart disease.

Complications

Cardiac lesions. Though described here as a complication, cardiac changes are truly a part of the disease as much as arthritis.

Endocarditis: Most serious feature of rheumatism. Special features. *Frequency* about 50% of cases. No direct relation to severity of arthritis. Increases with number of attacks, diminishes with age. Children rarely escape.

Valves commonly affected, in order of frequency: (1) Mitral alone; (2) Mitral and aortic; (3) Aortic alone—rare.

Mitral stenosis only develops slowly, and hence is not recognizable during acute stages of a first attack.

Pathological changes are of simple endocarditis: verrucose and infective form rare during attack of rheumatism.

Subsequent progress: Signs and symptoms of endocarditis slight in first attack, but pathological changes tend to advance after attack of rheumatism has passed.

Mortality low during the acute attack.

Pericarditis: Especially in children. Special features: (1) Commonest in socially under-privileged groups; sexes equal; (2) Slightly more frequent in first attacks, but mortality in first attack is 40% and in second 10%; (3) May occur at any time during attack, with or without endocarditis; (4) Effusion may occur (20% of cases), *but is never purulent*; (5) Arthritis usually severe.

In fatal cases, endocarditis also nearly always present.

Myocarditis: Probably frequent, leading to dilatation. Abnormalities of heart rhythm: more often first-degree heart block, second- and third-degree less often.

Hyperpyrexia. Formerly common, now extremely rare.

Pulmonary complications. Rare. Pleurisy may occur with pericarditis, usually dry, but may be effusion. No true pneumonia, but occasionally collapse and congestion.

Skin. *Erythema marginatum* begins as red macule or papule. Extends outwards, centre becomes normal. Coalescence of adjacent lesions to cause serpiginous or circinate appearances.

Rheumatic nodules. Evidence of serious attack. Occur on fibrous tissue and periosteum of bones lying close under the skin, e.g. olecranon, tendons and fasciae especially about elbows and wrists, also on occiput, scapulae and vertebrae. Number usually 3 or 4, rarely 20–30, occasionally very numerous. Best recognized by drawing skin tight and palpating gently. Almost confined to children. Incidence is still greater in chorea. Pericarditis has been observed subsequently in many cases.

Chorea (Sydenham's Chorea; St Vitus' Dance). Often occurs without any other manifestations of rheumatic fever. Characterized by jerky, erratic, inco-ordinated flailing movements of arms and legs. May recur unilaterally. Facial grimacing, tics and protrusion of tongue. Generalized muscle weakness. Grip waxes and wanes on examiner's finger ('milkmaid's grip'). Pendular knee jerks. Emotional lability causes personality change. May alternate with attacks of acute rheumatism. Special tendency to affect heart.

Diagnosis

Usually simple. A high rise of anti-O streptolysin titres, with each episode of streptococcal infection is noted in those who develop rheumatic fever. Temperature always subsides within 5 days of efficient salicylate treament, unless endocarditis or pericarditis present. Diagnosis from:

Osteomyelitis. Point of tenderness of bone always present. Rheumatic fever is not monoarticular.

Acute rheumatoid arthritis. Tends to attack smaller joints. Does not wander from joint to joint. Chronic articular changes.

Secondary arthritis. Septic arthritis in pyaemia and septicaemia. Gonorrhoeal arthritis (q.v.).

Congenital heart disease. In cases of cardiac lesions without history of rheumatic attacks.

Gout. Age of patient; aetiology; previous attacks; small joints usually affected, especially great toe and thumb.

Chronic meningococcal septicaemia and staphylococcal septicaemia may both closely simulate rheumatic fever.

Prognosis
Immediate. Fever and joint symptoms subside rapidly under salicylates. Evidence of endocarditis may persist. Death in first attack very rare, usually pericarditis.

Remote. Depends on: (1) Cardiac lesions; (2) Liability to recurrence.

Treatment
Indication is to protect heart specially.

Antibiotics. Do not modify the course of the disease but should be given. Penicillin either orally or i.m. for 10 days. Erythromycin in penicillin-allergic patients.

Rest in bed. At least 4 weeks. Longer if there is active carditis and heart failure.

Local treatment. Cradle to support weight of bedclothes.

Salicylates. Sodium salicylate recommended for routine use in patients with polyarthritis who have no carditis or mild carditis.

Adults: Initially up to 90–100 mg/kg of sodium salicylate/day to obtain a blood level of 30–40 mg %. Once symptoms are relieved the dose is lowered to a level adequate to prevent pain and fever.

If salicylate is not well tolerated soluble aspirin must be tried up to 80 mg/kg body weight/day in 4 divided doses.

Action of salicylates: Usually rapid. Ease the articular pains, and cause fall of temperature. It is doubtful whether they lower the incidence of endocarditis.

Cortisone. Severe carditis with heart failure, those who cannot tolerate high dose aspirin, or those whose symptoms and signs are not sufficiently controlled by aspirin. Prednisolone 40–60 mg/day in divided doses reducing the dosage after 2–3 weeks.

Convalescence
Progress slow, especially if evidence of carditis.

Rheumatic Fever in Children
Differs from clinical condition in adults by more insidious character. Does not occur under 2 years of age.

Articular lesions. Often slight and overlooked; and endocarditis often progresses to mitral stenosis and incompetence without any illness being observed.

Recurrent tonsillitis or sore throat may be the only manifestation, or possibly endocarditis may occur without other symptoms.

Complications are more common in childhood: chorea, pericarditis, rapid anaemia and also subcutaneous nodules.

Differential diagnosis. From:

Acute osteomyelitis: *monarticular*. Constitutional symptoms very severe. Pain is not in joint.

Acute poliomyelitis: May be associated with hyperaesthesia.

Infantile scurvy: Age under 2 years.

Congenital syphilis: Occurs as (1) *Syphilitic epiphysitis*: age under 2 years, affects epiphyses and not joints; (2) *Symmetrical synovitis*: painless, at age of puberty.

Still's disease: Rare. Chronic. Spleen and glands often enlarged. Heart unaffected.

Prophylaxis

1. Social improvement. This is an important aspect of community care. Better housing, less over-crowding, better general nutrition all tend to reduce incidence of rheumatic fever.

2. Treatment of streptococcal infections. Early diagnosis and effective doses of penicillin are essential.

3. Chemoprophylaxis. Those who have had one attack may be saved further damage to the heart by the use of long-acting penicillins, e.g. phenoxymethyl-penicillin 125 mg b.d. given orally, or benzathine penicillin 0·6 megaunits by i.m. injection once a month. *Note*: This is painful and blood levels variable.

Erythromycin is an alternative to penicillin. Chemoprophylaxis may be required for 5 years, or longer if environmental conditions predispose to streptococcal infections.

4. Tonsillectomy is indicated only where strong evidence of chronic or recurrent tonsillitis, not responding adequately to antibiotic therapy.

Erythema Nodosum

Characterized by tender erythematous swellings usually confined to extensor aspects of lower limbs.

Aetiology

Mainly in children and young adults. Females commoner.

Pathogenesis

Now considered to be a non-specific cutaneous response to bacterial allergens. Common primary infections: (1) Tuberculosis—eruption forming manifestation of a primary tuberculous infection, Mantoux test having been observed to change from negative to positive; (2) Streptococcus; (3) Meningococcus—occurs typically in meningococcal septicaemia. (4) Sarcoidosis; (5) Leprosy: Erythema nodosum leprosum (ENL) is common in patients suffering from lepromatous or dimorphous leprosy when treatment is started; (6) Drug hypersensitivity. *Note*: (1) cardiac lesions are; (2) salicylates occasionally helpful if there is associated arthropathy; (3) joint pains not greater than in urticaria.

Symptoms

1. *Local eruption.* (1) Round or oval swellings; (2) Usually on extensor aspects of lower limbs, rare above knees: occasionally on arms; (3) Bilateral; (4) Size: up to 5 cm in diameter; (5) Number very variable; (6) Colour: red deepening to

purple; (7) Very tender. Swelling involves subcutaneous tissues: may be oedema around. *Duration*: 10–20 days.
2. *Constitutional*. Slight pyrexia and malaise. May be sore throat and joint pains.

Diagnosis
Simple.

Treatment
Symptomatic. Rest in bed. The indications from the causal factor must be considered.

Acute Poststreptococcal Glomerulonephritis
Group A streptococci especially M type 49 causing cutaneous lesions may be followed in 2–3 weeks or more by glomerulonephritis and those causing pharyngitis especially type 12 by this complication in about 10 days. Recovery is usual though renal failure sometimes ensues.

Acute Anaphylactoid Purpura

Occasionally results, particularly after scarlet fever.

Toxin-mediated Streptococcal Disease

Scarlet Fever (Scarlatina)
Acute infectious disease due to various strains of haemolytic streptococci producing erythrogenic toxin, characterized by inflammation of the fauces and a punctate erythematous rash followed by desquamation and by a tendency to complications. The disease is less common and less serious than formerly.

Epidemiology
Geographical distribution. In all temperate climates. Endemic and frequently epidemic. Uncommon in tropics. Epidemic prevalence is irregular and no periodicity is distinguishable.
Season. Marked seasonal prevalence. Increases during summer to maximum in October, rapid fall in December, minimum in March. Slight fall in August due to closure of schools.
Age. Most frequent about 5 years of age. Over 80% under 10 years. Frequency diminishes in each subsequent decade.
Virulence. Varies considerably in different epidemics and years. Present mortality under 0·1%, highest about 5 years of age. *Susceptibility* not so universal as in measles. One attack usually protects for life.
Susceptibility of animals. No occurrence in nature and no experimental transmission.

Aetiology
Usually caused by streptococci of group A but sometimes by groups C or G. (Haemolytic *Staphylococcus aureus* may produce erythrogenic toxin and clinical scarlet fever.) Prevalent type in an area may vary from year to year. In scarlet fever, the organisms remain localized in the fauces. However, scarlet fever sometimes results from infection elsewhere than the throat, e.g. a wound or in

puerperal sepsis. The essential cause is a streptococcal or other infection in which enough erythrogenic toxin is produced. If the infection does not produce enough then immunity to scarlet fever does not develop. Some infections, especially of the throat, acquired from a patient with scarlet fever are of this type.

Conveyance of infection. (1) *Droplet infection* from infected persons. (2) *Infected articles*: may be conveyed by clothes, books, etc. for long distances and time; (3) *Third persons*; (4) *Carriers*: these may be apparently healthy in which case specific treatment usually clears up their infection readily or they may have infected discharging foci in the middle ear or elsewhere. (5) *Milk-borne epidemics*: have resulted from milk infected in transit by individual with scarlet fever.

Infective material from patient. (1) *Secretion of throat, nose and ear* containing virulent organisms main cause of infection. Infectivity highest in prodromal and eruptive periods: (2) *From skin.* Scales probably only secondarily infected, and therefore not infectious when nasopharynx is clear.

Cross-infection; relapses; complications. Immunity developed to one strain, does not protect against infection with another type. Cross-infection consequently occurs in hospital wards: accounts for 'relapses', and many complications and 'return cases'.

'Return cases'. Using penicillin therapy it is possible to eliminate the organism so that the carrier problem is not so serious, and return cases, that is patients from the household of the original sufferer, are now rare.

Pathology
Nothing characteristic apart from kidneys. Rash due to damage to capillaries with perivascular infiltration with monocytes. It is not visible post mortem unless haemorrhagic. Fauces: acute inflammation. *Cervical lymph nodes* may be enlarged. Pulmonary complications frequent in fatal cases.

Renal changes. Nephritis not uncommon; changes usually not characteristic, but occasionally a pure 'glomerular nephritis'.

Clinical Varieties
Five types: (1) Simple ordinary form, scarlatina benigna; (2) Malignant or toxic; (3) Haemorrhagic; (4) Septic or anginose; Intermediate types occur. *All severe forms are rare.* (5) Surgical and puerperal.

Scarlatina sine eruptione. Modern conception is infection in an individual who is immune to erythrogenic toxin.

Symptoms
Incubation period. Generally 2–4 days, most commonly 3 days. Limits ½–6 days.

1. Simple scarlet fever (scarlatina benigna). Three stages: (1.1) Invasion; (1.2) Eruption; (1.3) Desquamation.

> *1.1 Stage of invasion*
> *Onset*: Sudden. Chilly sensations; definite rigors infrequent. Convulsions not uncommon in children: also epistaxis.
> *Initial symptoms*: (*a*) *Sore throat*, with some tenderness on swallowing or in submaxillary region; (*b*) *Vomiting*, early and constant. Sore throat is commoner in adults, and vomiting in children; (*c*) *Temperature* rises rapidly, often 39·4–40 °C (103–104 °F) when first taken; (*d*) *Pulse* very

rapid, especially in children. *Skin dry* and very pungent. *Face* flushed. *Tongue* furred. General malaise and constipation.

No definite diagnosis until rash appears. If early signs mild, attack mild; if severe, attack may still be mild.

1.2 Stage of eruption. Rash commences 24–36 h after onset, i.e. on second or third day; occasionally more rapid: rarely delayed for 4 days. General *exacerbation of symptoms*: throat more swollen and painful, tongue more furred, temperature higher, and pulse more rapid. Symptoms increase for 2–3 days; then, simultaneously, rash fades, defervescence occurs, and symptoms abate.

Convalescence usually on sixth to eighth day.

1.3 Stage of desquamation. As rash subsides, skin is stained and rough. Desquamation or peeling commences on the neck, follows order of rash, *and occurs last on palms and soles*. May commence before rash faded on limbs. Extent proportional to rash. On the face it begins at numerous foci and separates as powder; on abdomen as scales; on soles of feet as large flakes. Most marked in second week, usually complete in 4 weeks except soles. May be many weeks. Usually slight in infants. Slight secondary desquamation is common. Nails subsequently have transverse ridges not infrequently. Desquamation occasionally absent in infants.

Mild forms. All symptoms may be very mild.

Special features

Rash. Onset on second or third day.

Distribution: Commences on neck, behind ears, and upper part of chest; spreads over body, usually in a few hours; may take 2 or 3 days.

Chest and neck, flexor surface of elbows and knees, and inner aspect of thighs most affected.

Face, scalp, palms and soles very rarely affected.

Character: A vivid, scarlet eruption, composed of two factors: (*a*) scattered red spots, on (*b*) basis of general erythema. Disappears on pressure, unless petechial. Traditionally described as 'punctate erythema', better represented by 'small spots of red ink on red blotting paper'. When erythema is intense no puncta may be observed.

Skin smooth at first, then rough. Swelling and inflammatory oedema not infrequent, especially on hands. *Miliary sudamina* or even vesicles may be present. *Petechiae* not uncommon, especially in folds and creases of skin and on neck. Itching varies: rarely excessive. *Rash on extremities* sometimes blotchy and macular.

Duration: Usually 2–3 days: darkens in colour and fades roughly in order of appearance, last from sites where thickest. Generally absent by seventh to eighth day. Petechiae may persist longer. When rash subsides, may be transverse, brown staining with tiny petechiae at flexures, especially elbow and popliteal space (Pastia's sign).

Facial Aspect. Cheeks flushed, while mouth and nose are pale, so-called 'circumoral pallor'—Filatow's sign—often very suggestive. Bluish, peach-blossom tinge of cheeks, as if rouged.

Tongue. In stage of invasion is furred in centre, with red papillae projecting, and red at edges, the 'strawberry tongue'. Fur clears on third or fourth day, leaving surface red and raw, 'raspberry tongue'.

Fauces. The changes may be: (*a*) Slight redness and swelling; (*b*) Follicular tonsillitis; (*c*) Membranous angina—great tenderness and induration in neck and swelling of glands.

Cervical Lymphatic Glands. Palpable.

Skin. Hot and extremely pungent.

These symptoms, with the early occurrence of vomiting, and the subsequent desquamation, are the characteristics of scarlet fever.

Rhinorrhoea. Mucous discharge common.

Blood. Polymorphonuclear leucocytosis present.

Urine. Febrile changes with early albuminuria.

Gastric disturbance. Uncommon after initial vomiting.

Spleen. Rarely palpable.

2. Malignant or toxic scarlet fever. Characterized by slightness of throat lesions with severe constitutional symptoms. *Onset* severe—serious vomiting, high temperature and delirium. Fauces little changed. *Rash dusky*, or may be absent.

Subsequently: dyspnoea, rapid pulse, hyperpyrexia, coma and cardiac failure. Is a toxaemia.

While mortality used to be high in this form of the disease, all the severe forms are now uncommon, and more effective therapy has reduced mortality.

3. Haemorrhagic scarlet fever. Very rare. Haemorrhages into skin and from mucous membranes, including epistaxis and haematuria. Prognosis very serious.

4. Septic or anginose scarlet fever. Characterized by ulceration and necrosis, commencing in fauces and spreading widely.

5. Surgical and puerperal scarlet fever. Infection with relevant organisms at puerperium and in surgical conditions, especially burns and scalds.

Important Complications

1. Otitis media. Rare after age 15 years. Due to extension of inflammation from fauces. In septic forms and angina common, but also in mild attacks. May be no pain until otorrhoea occurs. In two-thirds of cases is due to primary infection and develops at the end of first week; in remainder is due to cross-infection and develops in third or fourth week.

Progress. Usually good, with *efficient treatment*, discharge ceasing in 2–4 weeks, and in these cases hearing not greatly affected. Complete deafness from labyrinthitis rare. *Mastoid abscess* develops occasionally: Under treatment with antibiotics discharge may cease in few days.

2. Renal (see also Pathology, p. 152).

Initial albuminuria. Of febrile origin not uncommon while temperature high, disappears when temperature falls: unconnected with subsequent nephritis. No subsequent symptoms.

Nephritis. Onset usually towards end of third week: may be later, usually in cross-infections. No age exempt, but commoner in children. May occur even in mild cases, but especially in septic forms.

Symptoms: All grades of severity, from simple albuminuria to acute diffuse glomerular nephritis with definite symptoms, and blood, casts and much albumin in urine.

3. *Rhinitis.* Frequent. Nasal discharge at first thin and irritant, later mucopurulent; often obstinate; undoubtedly infective.

4. *Adenitis.* Almost constant. (i) In simple and mild types, submaxillary glands tender and swollen; (ii) in anginose and septic types, extreme, swelling of glands, with cellulitis or subsequent sloughing. An adenitis may occur in third week, especially with nephritis. Rarely a suppurative adenitis develops in the fourth week. *Retropharyngeal abscess* occasionally occurs during convalescence.

5. *Arthritis* (*see also* Rheumatic fever, p. 147). (i) *Multiple arthritis* (rheumatism): very frequent in adults, uncommon in children. Commences at end of first week. Small joints mainly affected. Changes in joints slight or absent. Usually, but not invariably, reacts to salicylates. Prognosis good. Chorea and cardiac affections rare; (ii) *Pyaemic suppuration* of joints: rare.

6. *Cardiac complications.* (i) Sudden death during convalescence, usually no previous warning, very rare; (ii) Endocarditis, rare; (iii) Malignant endocarditis or purulent pericarditis in septic type.

7. *Bronchitis.* Common in children; usually present in fatal cases.

Relapses. True relapses occur in about 1%.

Association with other diseases. Not uncommon: with diphtheria in 2%, chickenpox 2%, measles 1–2% of cases.

Diagnosis

Often simple, especially in cases of moderate severity: in mild forms, may be difficult: in the rare very acute forms, diagnosis may depend on existence of an epidemic, or knowledge of exposure to infection or a previous attack. Diagnosis never certain previous to eruption. Cultures from fauces may show relative streptococci.

Differential Diagnosis

Difficulties in diagnosis arise from: (1) Inflammations of the fauces: (*a*) follicular and catarrhal tonsillitis; (*b*) diphtheria; (2) Various eruptions: measles; rubella; smallpox; initial rashes; erythemata of various types.

Lassa fever. Rash more localized and blotchy. Unusual in childhood. Clinical condition more severe than usual for degree of pyrexia present. N.B. Scarlet fever uncommon in tropics.

Erythemata. The rash in erythemata of various origins may resemble scarlet fever more or less closely. Desquamation may follow any erythema. The history and other symptoms usually indicate the diagnosis. The most important are:

1. *Drug rashes.* Especially belladonna, quinine and salicylates. Iodide and bromide rashes are usually pustular.

2. *Allergic rashes*

3. *Septic rashes*

4. *Enema rash.* Generally within few hours of enema, and usually confined to trunk.

Diagnosis in post-febrile stage. Rash may linger on outer surface of legs. Peeling latest on palms and soles. Transverse lines at elbows, and cervical glands, may assist.

Prognosis
Age. Highest mortality in infants under 1 year. Greatest number of deaths occur at about 5 years. Mortality subsequently very low, and diminishes with increasing age.
General mortality. Usually less than 0·2% but varies in different epidemics.
Clinical types. Malignant and anginose types have highest mortality: usually cardiac failure either in first few days or later stages. *Ordinary types*: deaths very uncommon with modern therapy.
Serious symptoms. Bronchitis in children. Severe vomiting. Hyperpyrexia, very rapid pulse, delirium. Excessive oedema or exudation on fauces. Rapid emaciation in later stages.

Treatment and Management
Chemotherapy. In mild case phenoxymethylpenicillin. Adult dose 0·25 g 6-hourly for 5 days but duration of treatment increased if progress not rapid. If oral treatment cannot be used one i.m. injection of 0·6 g benzathine penicillin will usually be adequate. More serious and complicated cases require 0·3 g 6-hourly for 5 days. If there is circulatory failure 40 mg prednisolone i.m. and 10 mg 6-hourly for 24 h, 10 mg 4-hourly during the next 24 h, then tailed off.
Otitis media. Treat immediately with antibiotics.
Hyperpyrexia and delirium. Especially occurs in septic type. Treat by hydrotherapy. Above 39·4 °C (103 °F) tepid sponge. If still rises, warm bath, commencing at 32·2 °C (90 °F) cooling to 26·6 °C (80 °F). If delirium present, cold packs preferable. Antipyretic drugs useless.
Duration of infectivity. With specific therapy in uncomplicated cases 8 days from onset. Patients may return to school or work 14 days from onset. It is now customary to obtain one negative throat swab before discharge. This will not reveal all convalescent carriers but will detect heavy excretors who can then be given further specific (penicillin) treatment (*see* p. 145). Desquamation may be disregarded.
Quarantine for contacts. School, work and family contacts are not now quarantined but should remain at home if they develop any suspicious symptoms. Any handling milk should cease to do so if they are contacts.

Chapter 35   STAPHYLOCOCCAL INFECTIONS

Recognition of pathogenic groups and identification of individual strains is difficult. Earliest classification was based on pigmentation of colonies, viz. aureus, albus and citreus: citreus is rarely pathogenic. Now main pathogens *Staph. aureus, Staph. epidermidis* and *Staph. saprophyticus.*

Relation of Biological Properties to Pathogenicity
Coagulase production, i.e. power to coagulate plasma, is best test of pathogenicity. Fermentation of mannitol and liquefaction of gelatin less reliable.

Staphylococcal Toxins
Production of haemolytic toxin (α toxin) is related to pathogenicity. Leucocidin also produced, but variable. An enterotoxin in some strains produces 'food poisoning'. Some elaborate an exotoxin which causes necrosis of the subepidermal skin. Others produce an erythrogenic toxin which can cause clinical 'scarlet fever'.

Identification of Particular Strains
All coagulase-producing strains are now classified as *Staph. aureus* and the others are *Staph. epidermidis* or *Staph. saprophyticus*. Strains of *Staph. aureus* are currently classified by antibiotic sensitivity, some by antigenic structure, and most by phage typing of which there are 4 major groups. Group 1 found particularly in hospitals. Group 2 (phage type 71) causes vesicular skin eruptions in infants—bullous impetigo and staphylococcal scalded skin syndrome. Group 3 are mostly antibiotic resistant. Group 4 contains enterotoxin-producing strains; some such strains are also in group 3.

   Staph. saprophyticus differs from *Staph. epidermidis* in being resistant to novobiocin and in producing acid in aerobic growth in mannitol. There are other cultural and antigenic differences. Its identity as a separate species is disputed by some authorities.

Staphylococcal Infections
Can be divided into superficial, affecting skin and adnexa, and deep causing septicaemia and infection of deeper organs and tissues. *Staph. aureus* tends to produce cutaneous lesions, i.e. boils, carbuncles; metastases may follow (pyaemia) either multiple or single foci, e.g. osteomyelitis, perirenal abscess, otitis media. Also causes food poisoning.

   Staph. epidermidis was considered of little pathological importance till the era of heart valve replacement came in. It was then found to be a common cause of infections on prosthetic valves and of endocarditis on natural valves following cardiotomy. It also infects hip and other joint prostheses and vascular prostheses, particularly those in the inguinal region. The organism is normally abundant in the groin and anal region, in the nose and axillae.

   Staph. saprophyticus causes some urinary infections in young women.

Staphylococcal Septicaemia

Source of Infection
Skin infection e.g. boils, currently particularly after transurethral prostatectomy, after prolonged use of intravenous indwelling catheters and in steroid therapy. It may originate from bed-sores.

General Characteristics
Rigors and sweats; pulse often rather slow: pyrexia: moderate polynucleosis. Often there is profound malaise and weakness. It is prone to occur in childhood or late in life. In almost a quarter of patients it is a complication of an already fatal disease such as acute leukaemia.

   Pyrexia of unknown origin. Often a presenting manifestation, especially in a patient with or who recently has had an indwelling catheter or scalp needle. The longer a catheter remains in situ the greater the chance of septicaemia. Frequent after 72 hours.

Metastatic abscesses. May appear at many sites, e.g. pleura, pericardium, lungs, perinephric (especially in adults), osteomyelitis (especially in children) hip joint.

Anaemia. Almost invariable in established cases.

Albuminuria. Present in one-third of patients, half of whom will also have haematuria.

Diagnosis
Special methods.

(1) *Blood culture*; In more than 90% of patients not on antibiotics it will be positive. Three specimens should be taken at 2-hourly intervals.

(2) *Culture from anterior nares, skin lesions or suspected site of infection.* May reveal causative organism and enable sensitivities to be determined.

(3) *Counter immunoelectrophoresis.* Enables detection of serum antibody to staphylococcal cell wall, teichoic, acid even before blood culture positive. Ouchterlony method also used. Diagnosis may be simple, if primary focus obvious.

Differential Diagnosis
(1) *Enteric fever*; (2) *Infective endocarditis*; (3) *Malaria*; (4) *Acute miliary tuberculosis; (5) Brucella abortus; (6) Rheumatic fever* (in staphylococcal septicaemia). Other causes of obscure pyrexia.

Remember staphylococcal septicaemia often complicates other serious illness for which indwelling catheters or prolonged steroid therapy have been used.

Treatment
Chemotherapy. Every effort should be made to culture the organism and determine its sensitivities. Urgent initial treatment before the culture report may be with Methicillin 1g i.m. or slowly i.v. every 4–6 h or cephaloridine given i.m. or i.v. in a dose from 2 to 6 g daily in severe infections, and also with gentamicin given i.m. in a dose of 80 mg every 12 h.

Important to keep careful watch for renal failure, and not to prolong the high dose of gentamicin because of VIIIth nerve damage.

Flucloxacillin is an alternative and may be given i.m. or orally in doses of 500 mg 6-hourly or i.v. 0·5–1 g every 4–6 hours. Children are given ¼–½ the adult dose.

Length of antibiotic treatment. If there is an easily treatable or removable focus of the infection, 2 weeks if not at least 4 weeks. Endocarditis requires 6 weeks and if a prosthetic valve is present treatment should be for at least 12 weeks. The valve may have to be replaced in order to obtain a cure.

Prevention
Topical antibiotic ointments, but not quarternary ammonium antiseptics, at site of indwelling catheters reduce incidence of secondary sepsis. Infusion of hypertonic glucose, or other fluid containing substances that predispose to phlebitis (e.g. some antibiotics) increase the risk of septicaemia. Special care is needed in the use of these substances and where possible an alternative route should be employed.

Prognosis
Invariably fatal if not treated but with treatment approximately 40%. Mortality greater in those over 50.

Other Deep-seated Staphylococcal Infections
Staphylococci may give rise to meningitis and brain abscess, to pneumonia, empyema and lung abscess. In this category it is now recognized as the initial bacterial pathogen in the lungs of children with cystic fibrosis. Staphylococci are important causes of endocarditis and have been recognized as such particularly in heroin addicts. The organisms are the commonest infecting agent in acute osteomyelitis and are second only to gonococci as causes of septic arthritis.

Staphylococcal Enterocolitis
See section on food-poisoning organisms.

Chapter 36   **DIPHTHERIA**

Specific infectious disease due to *Corynebacterium diphtheriae*, and characterized by local symptoms due to a fibrinous exudate, usually on mucous membranes of fauces or larynx, and by constitutional symptoms due to the bacilli at the site of exudate.

Aetiology and Epidemiology
Geographical distribution. Almost universal, but most prevalent in temperate and cold climates; however, over the past 25 years there has been a progressive decline in incidence and mortality related to effective immunization of children and the early use of antitoxin in therapy.
Season. Especially in winter months. Highest in dry years. In England, slight fall in August and maximum in October and November.
Age. Frequency and mortality are greatest between 1 and 5 years: Rare under 6 months (inherited immunity) and over 50.
Individual susceptibility important (*see* Schick Test, p. 161).

Modes of Infection
Very contagious. Transmission usually occurs almost directly from one person to another, e.g. from kissing, by interchanging of pencils, etc. at schools. Sources of infection:
1. *Directly from individual* with typical active diphtheria, by droplet infection.
2. *Fomites.* Bacilli may live for months but indirect infection rare and of theoretical importance.
3. *Diphtheria carriers.* Immunization programmes have led almost to their disappearance in developed countries.
4. *Subjects of atypical diphtheria,* e.g. mild tonsillitis. Severe attack may occur in infected individual.

In the following the human contact is not so direct:

5. *Epidemics due to milk* of historical interest. Now very rare.
6. *Accidental infection from cultures*

No transmission takes place by water or by air. No infection from domestic animals.

One attack does not confer immunity.

Bacteriology

Corynebacterium diphtheriae was discovered by Klebbs in 1883, and isolated by Loeffler in 1884. Commonly known as Klebs–Loeffler bacillus.

Morphological characters. A non-motile, non-sporing bacillus. Length and appearance very variable: varies from a short bacillus with rounded ends, to irregular forms with swollen 'clubbed' extremities; the latter 'involution' forms are common in cultures of more than 48 h growth. May stain uniformly, but more commonly shows 'beaded' appearance or irregular staining: due to granules (especially in *mitis* strains, often absent in *gravis*), often 'bipolar' but may be scattered through bacillus. Arrangement of bacilli in films from cultures often characteristic, groups resembling 'Chinese letters', due to the organism bending lengthways before division. From tissues, bacilli are often separate, unless numerous.

Stains. *Gram-positive*, but fairly easily decolorized. Better stained as routine by Loeffler's alkaline methylene blue, or by toluidine blue. Neisser's stains, the original Bismarck-brown or the cresoidin method, exhibit the granules better.

Special characteristics. (1) Irregular staining; (2) Arrangement.

Cultural characters. Grows well on all ordinary media in subcultures. Initial cultures from tissues to be made on Loeffler's blood serum or blood-tellurite-agar medium (claimed to be more reliable). *Growth is rapid* at 37 °C. Colonies may be visible in 12 h: colonies on tellurite media become greyish-black in colour as do streptococci and staphylococci. On Tinsdale's agar *C. diphtheriae* develops a brown-grey halo and produces a garlic-like odour: bacilli may be found in films after 6–8 h. Very resistant to drying. Carbohydrate fermentation: Forms acid without gas in glucose, never ferments saccharose.

Distribution of the bacillus in the tissues

1. *In the membrane.* Mainly in superficial portions and on surface. Bacilli do not penetrate below membrane.

2. In *other sites*, especially mucous membranes. Occasionally present in *rhinitis, conjunctivitis*, and, less commonly, otitis media; also in vulva. Very rarely in ulcerative endocarditis.

3. *In skin lesions* (e.g. desert sores) *and wounds.* As secondary invaders.

Inoculation into animals. Subcutaneous inoculation into leg of guinea-pig with 48-h broth culture in suspension is used to test virulence of bacilli. *Result.* Death in 36–72 h, with rapid loss of weight; great oedema at site of inoculation; *haemorrhages into adrenals* and serous membranes; bacilli at site of inoculation only.

Toxin and antitoxin. Toxins from cultures of the bacillus on inoculation cause symptoms of the disease except for absence of membrane. Death in diphtheria is due to action of toxin and not to extension of bacilli. Animals can be immunized to a high degree by injections of the toxin, and horses are thus used for production of diphtheria antitoxin serum.

Toxicity of strains. *Gravis, intermedius* and *mitis* strains can be distinguished by cultural characters on rabbit-blood-tellurite medium. *Gravis* strain, but not others, ferments starch and glycogen; *mitis* strain alone is haemolytic. Strain toxicity can be changed *in vitro* by treatment with bacteriophage but this has not been demonstrated in the field. It could account for the sudden appearance of diphtheria in communities. All strains produce same toxin but in *gravis* infections serum therapy often little effect. Cause of different severity is uncertain.

Diphtheroid Bacilli

Many diphtheroid bacilli are morphologically similar to *C. diphtheriae* and are distinguished by differential fermentation of glycogen, starch, glucose, sucrose and maltose. In managing patients, however, the diagnosis of diphtheria must be made on clinical criteria and treatment instituted while awaiting bacteriological results.

Schick Test

Distinguishes between those susceptible and those not susceptible to an attack of clinical diphtheria.

Theory of Test. (1) Presence of $\frac{1}{30}$ unit of antitoxin per ml of blood gives immunity to diphtheria; often present in normal persons; (2) Such amount prevents any reaction after injection of MLD of diphtheria toxin (minimal lethal dose kills a 250-g guinea-pig at end of 4 days).

Technique. Inject *intradermally*, not subcutaneously, $0 \cdot 1$ ml of a saline solution containing $\frac{1}{50}$ MLD (obtainable fresh from Wellcome and others) into flexor surface of the forearm. In opposite arm inject, as control, toxin heated to 75 °C for 10 min.

Reactions. Read after 24 h, 48 h and between 4 and 7 days.

1. *Positive.* Circumscribed area of redness, diameter more than 10 mm by 4th day. If control is negative a positive result can be read at 48 h.

2. *Negative.*

3. *Non-specific or pseudo-reaction.* Appears early and disappears within 2–3 days.

4. *Combined pseudo- and positive reactions.* Positive persists after pseudo-fades.

5. *Schick test* is not affected by antitoxin given 6 h or more after test injections.

Interpretation of results

1. *Negative and Pseudo-reactions.* Indicates immunity.

2. *Positive and Combined Reactions.* Indicates susceptibility.

Active Immunization

In infancy. Best begun at 6–16 weeks of age with triple vaccine of diphtheria, pertussis and tetanus (DPT). Three injections of $0 \cdot 5$ ml given i.m. at monthly intervals and a booster just before starting school.

Older infants and young children. Paediatric diphtheria-tetanus vaccine (DT) available and given in two doses of $0 \cdot 5$ ml separated by 6 weeks followed by a booster in 6–12 months.

Older children and adults. Use adult diphtheria-tetanus vaccine (DT) in same spacing as young children plus booster dose at 10-year intervals.

For diphtheria immunization *per se* similar doses ($0 \cdot 5$ ml) of alum precipitated toxoid (APT), purified toxoid aluminium phosphate (PTAP) or toxoid antitoxin floccules (TAF) may be used.

During epidemics of poliomyelitis the giving of a prophylactic inoculation against diphtheria may result in paralysis of the injected limb, and the risk is greater if the injected material contains aluminium. Therefore it is then advisable to use TAF for diphtheria immunization.

TAF contains a small amount of horse serum so should be avoided in any subject of allergy.

Carriers

Presence of diphtheria bacilli usually in nose or fauces without clinical symptoms occurs in:

1. *'Convalescent Carriers'*, subsequent to an attack. Isolation necessary; usually becomes negative in 6–8 weeks. *Gravis* infections are most persistent, *intermedius* transient.

2. 'Contacts'.

Only those with virulent bacilli constitute carriers.

Disposal of chronic carriers. Often causes difficulty. No legal necessity apparently (in Great Britain) for notification of healthy carriers, or removal to hospital. But practitioners incur responsibility if treating such carriers lightly.

Treatment of chronic carriers. Erythromycin 250–500 mg, (children 125–250 mg) orally 6-hourly for 7 days clears most. If it fails tonsillectomy may be effective as may correction of other nasopharyngeal disease, if present. Ordinary active and passive immunization and antiseptics useless.

Carriers normally discharged form hospital after 3 negative swab cultures. A further culture should be made 1–3 weeks later.

Contacts

When an outbreak of diphtheria occurs, all contacts (*but not others*) must be examined. Those with clinical symptoms or faucial changes are immediately separated and isolated. Disposal and treatment of all depends on: (1) Examination of throat swabs; (2) Schick test; (3) Virulence or avirulence of bacilli.

Swab positive. Isolate. Divide into:

1. *Schick-positive. Give antitoxin.* Subsequent division into:
      1.1 Bacilli virulent: This group are frequently incubating diphtheria and develop symptoms. Treat as diphtheria.
      1.2 Bacilli avirulent: Further isolation unnecessary. Active immunization advisable.
2. *Schick-negative.* Divide into:
      2.1 Bacilli virulent: Are 'chronic carriers'. Treat as above.
      2.2 Bacilli avirulent: No isolation or immunization necessary.

Swab negative. No isolation. Divide into:

1. *Schick-positive.* Active immunization.
2. *Schick-negative.* Immunization unnecessary.

Quarantine Period

Till dealt with as under 'Contacts' or, if infected, till 3 successive cultures taken at 24-h intervals are negative.

Pathology

C. diphtheriae elaborates a toxin which is a pro-enzyme. It crosses cell membranes

and inactivates a factor needed for the translocation step of protein synthesis.
Diphtheritic membrane. Is termed 'false' as it consists of invaded necrotic mucosal layers and is not an exudate overlying an intact surface.
Common sites: *Tonsils and neighbourhood*, and *larynx.* Also occurs on pharynx, trachea, epiglottis, nares. In fatal cases, often in accessory sinuses. Rarely, on conjunctiva.
Macroscopic characters
    1. *Colour of membrane* greyish-white; later may darken.
    2. *Adherent, and leaves bleeding surface on separation.* In later stages separates easily.
    3· *Is superficial*: only in rare cases extends deeply.
    Disappears by disintegration.
    Histology. Membrane is formed by coagulative necrosis of epithelial cells, with exudation of fibrin and, in deepest layers, of polynuclear cells. Frequently the epithelial cells are shed early. Tissues below membrane are but little affected. Diphtheria bacilli present mainly on surface and at edge of membrane.
    Faucial diphtheria. Initial slight catarrh of fauces. Membrane formation commences usually at one spot, either on tonsils or at junction of uvula and tonsil, and spreads over tonsil, pillar of fauces, uvula, over soft palate and often over pharynx; *is not confined to tonsil.*
    Laryngeal diphtheria. Membrane may include rima. Spreads upwards to epiglottis; downwards may extend even to bronchioles. Faucial membrane usually present.
Lymph nodes. *Enlarged in neck and under jaw*; in severe cases extreme. Mainly due to secondary streptococcal infection and not rapidly affected by antitoxin.
Heart. In fatal cases cloudy swelling, fatty change, oedema and multiple foci of plasma cells and lymphocytes.
Pulmonary lesions. *Bronchitis and bronchopneumonia* may occur and be fatal, especially in laryngeal type. Pneumococcus is commonest organism: *Membrane may extend down trachea to bronchi; rarely to bronchioles.*
Nervous system. May be fatty degeneration of myelin sheaths.
Other changes, not characteristic
    Blood. Definite leucocytosis and relative increase of polynuclear cells.
    Kidney. Fatty degeneration and tubular epithelium may be damaged.
    Liver and spleen. Toxic changes.
    Adrenals. Haemorrhages are rare.

Duration of Infectivity
Isolate until: (1) Three consecutive negative swabs at intervals of 4 days; (2) No local lesion or discharge.

Severity of Infection
Usually related to strain: *gravis, intermedius*, or *mitis.*

Symptoms
Incubation period. Usually 2–5 days, most commonly 2.
Early symptoms. Insidious: not characteristic. General malaise. Temperature about 38·4 °C (101 °F); rarely exceeds 39·4 °C (103 °F). Slight hoarseness: sore

throat often unnoticed in children. Face grey. May be convulsions in infants. Trace of proteinuria very frequent.

Clinical types. (1) Faucial; (2) Laryngeal; (3) Anterior nasal; (4) Nasopharyngeal; (5) Cutaneous; (6) Various. Membrane may affect more than one site.

1. *Faucial Diphtheria.* In children is a silent disease—little pain, complaint, or crying—symptoms being toxaemic.

> *Early symptoms.* As above. Some difficulty in swallowing. Tonsils: general catarrh; membrane often commencing on first day. Glands in neck and under jaw tender and slightly enlarged on affected side.
>
> *Third day. Membrane (see* Morbid Anatomy, *above)* on tonsils, palate and uvula: may fill aperture. Glands larger. Temperature is variable. General malaise and toxaemia. Pain as a rule only on swallowing.
>
> *Fourth to fifth day.* Membrane extensive, Glands large. Breath has characteristic foetor. Tongue furred. Urine reduced. Albumin almost constant.
>
> *Mild forms (Mitis).* Toxaemia slight. Subsequently membrane disintegrates. Signs disappear. Convalescence in 7–10 days. Constitutional symptoms generally defervesce in proportion to extent of membrane.
>
> *Malignant forms (Gravis* and *Intermedius):* Toxaemia severe. Ashy face. *Pulse* feeble, rapid. Bradycardia or marked variations in pulse rate are of serious significance. Membrane varies, slight or extensive. Oedema of fauces often intense. Periadenitis of cervical glands and cellulitis producing '*bullneck*'. Nasal discharge common. Vomiting. Albumin increases. Prostration marked. *Death* from cardiac failure: often sudden: usually in 3–8 days. *Larynx* often involved.
>
> *Haemorrhagic symptoms* rare but very serious.
>
> *Tonsils* may show following variations : (1) Punctate exudate as in follicular tonsillitis; (2) General pultaceous exudate; (3) Miliary membrane at several points; (4) Catarrh. In severe cases with little membrane, virulent bacilli often numerous in nares.

2. *Laryngeal Diphtheria.* Commonest about 3 years of age. Nearly always secondary to faucial diphtheria, and faucial membrane, cervical nodes and symptoms present.

> *Early stage:* An acute laryngitis producing 'croup', viz.: (1) Hoarseness; (2) Harsh cough; (3) Inspiratory stridor; (4) Inspiratory recession above clavicle.
>
> *Clinical varieties:*
>
> 1.   Onset sudden, but symptoms not severe. *Paroxysms of dyspnoea* for a few hours, due to spasm of glottis. Membrane slight. Prognosis good.
>
> 2. Onset less sudden. Dyspnoea becomes continuously worse, without spasms. Colour livid. Cyanosis and 'croup' increase. Restlessness, vomiting and coma. Condition

associated with spread of membrane down trachea. Pulmonary complications. Prognosis very bad.
Temperature rarely high unless faucial symptoms marked.
In adults, laryngeal diphtheria is rare, but is often overlooked; width of larynx prevents blockage and hence there is no croup. Membrane spreads to fine bronchi, with severe symptoms and high mortality.

3. *Anterior Nasal Diphtheria.* Constitutional symptoms slight. Thin sanious discharge. Membrane extensive or slight. Liable to spread infection.

4. *Tonsillopharyngeal Diphtheria.* (*Gravis* and *intermedius* infections.) Extends from faucial diphtheria. Membrane may extend to anterior nares, but variable. Thin sanious discharge. Cervical adenitis, cellulitis and oedema ('bullneck'). Toxaemia extreme. Reaction to antitoxin often slight: high mortality: sequelae severe in survivors.

5. *Cutaneous Diphtheria.* (*a*) Acute forms, e.g. local ulcers, whitlows, or, rarely, gangrene. Always in association with throat lesions; (*b*) Chronic form. Common in hot climates. Superimposed on a skin lesion, e.g. desert sore, impetigo, scratches. Sores are deep, circular, with bluish rolled edges and leathery, black membrane on base. Paralyses not uncommon, usually late after sore healed, tend to affect symmetrical muscles and especially lower limbs.

6. *Various.* Any tissue may be infected, progress indolent to malignant, e.g.: (*a*) Wounds: as in cutaneous type; (*b*) Conjunctiva: mild conjunctivitis or membrane on lids, usually direct inoculation, rarely rapid sloughing; (*c*) Vulva and vagina: primary or secondary to fauces; insidious, slough forms, inguinal glands enlarged, toxaemia severe, diagnosis difficult; (*d*) Prepuce: following circumcision; (*e*) Middle ear: rare; extension from nasopharynx.

Complications
1. *Cardiac.* Acute circulatory failure in acute stages is serious risk of *gravis* forms, rare in *mitis* forms. Vomiting suggestive onset of failure. Pulse rapid, feeble, often irregular: may be gallop rhythm. Blood pressure falls very low, must be carefully watched. E.C.G. shows changes in most cases of faucial diphtheria.
2. *Vomiting.* Dangerous sign.
3. *Albuminuria. Almost constant*, and *very early*, not uncommon on first day. Amount large in severe cases. Anuria serious. Subsequent nephritis very rare.
4. *Pulmonary. Bronchitis and bronchopneumonia* nearly always present in severe cases.
5. *Rashes.* Diffuse erythema occasionally even in absence of antitoxin.
6. *Lymph nodes.* Periadenitis and cellulitis of neck may develop; occasionally suppuration; due to streptococci.
7. *Relapses.* Rare.

Sequelae
Of extreme importance: (A) Paralysis; (B) Cardiac failure.
A. *Post-diphtheritic paralysis.* Strict sequel: occurs in second or third week of convalescence: of toxic origin.
   Frequency. 10–15%: higher in adults. Most common in *faucial type. Usually following severe cases*, but also in mild forms. Heart usually also affected.

Progress. From onset of paralysis takes 2–7 weeks to become complete. Progress may be arrested at any stage.

Order of Progression. (1) Palate; (2) Eye; (3) Limbs; occasionally (4) Trunk; (5) Diaphragm; (6) Intercostals. *Special senses never affected*. Facial paralysis rare. Involvement of sphincters very rare.

1. *Palate: Nearly always affected first*, usually from fourteenth to twenty-first day of illness. Earliest signs: *Nasal voice*; *regurgitation of food through the nose*. On examination: *Palate relaxed, motionless, insensitive, and reflex absent*: changes often incomplete in milder degrees. *Constrictor of pharynx* affected in severe cases, whence difficulty in deglutition, and choking. *Larynx* affected in late stages with widespread paralysis: paralysis of adductors, causing hoarseness and weak cough: may simulate relapse of laryngeal diphtheria. Anaesthesia of larynx may lead to aspiration of food.

2. *Eye*: Frequency of affection next to palate commonly occurring some time between twenty-eighth and thirty-fifth day. Most common is *loss of power of accommodation* from paralysis of ciliary muscles, revealed by difficulty in reading. *External rectus* most commonly affected of extrinsic muscles. Diplopia and squint of every grade to complete ophthalmoplegia externa (very rare). *Pupils* often sluggish: may react to light and not to accommodation (very rare apart from diphtheria and encephalitis lethargica). Argyll Robertson pupil very rarely.

3. *Limbs*: *Legs* more frequently affected than arms; commences with weakness in walking and occurring from the forty-second to the seventieth day of illness. *Knee jerk* and deep reflexes abolished. With complete paralysis, *wasting* of muscles is often extreme. *Sensation* is usually affected, but marked loss is unusual. Reaction of degeneration very rare.

4. *Trunk muscles* May be inability to move head.

5. *Diaphragm*: Special danger to lungs from accumulation of mucus.

6. *Intercostals*: Respiration seriously affected.

A generalized type of paralysis occurs in which the last three groups of muscles are specially affected: otherwise their involvement is uncommon.

Cause of Death in Paralysis. (1) *Respiratory failure* from paralysis of muscles; aspiration pneumonia; massive collapse of lungs; (2) *Cardiac failure*.

Prognosis in Paralysis. When mild, recovery complete in a few weeks. Severe cases, prolonged. *Paralysis never persists with life* except from hemiplegia of vascular origin. Mortality in adults very low.

B. *Cardiac failure.* Apart from acute stage, failure most common in third week. Cardiac symptoms may occur thus:

1. Patient with paralysis of any degree allowed to get up: may be suddenly fatal.

2. Patient without paralysis allowed up under 3 weeks after severe attack.

3. Rarely occurs in bed, after severe attack, on slight exertion.

Slight symptom is tachycardia.

Serious symptoms are precordial pain, vomiting, ventricular arrhythmias and dilatations; may be cardiac arrest; mortality very high.

Differential Diagnosis

1. *Faucial diphtheria*. Diagnosis necessary from: (i) Streptococcal tonsillitis; (ii) Scarlet fever. Less commonly from glandular fever, lassa fever, agranulocytosis, leukaemia, secondary syphilis, thrush, quinsy, Vincent's angina and herpes of palate. Scalds of pharynx and curds of milk have caused mistakes.

Streptococcal tonsillitis: Onset rapid. *Temperature* high, 40 °C (104 °F). Face flushed. Any membrane present limited to tonsils and leaves no bleeding surface on separation.

Scarlet fever: Sudden onset with vomiting. *Temperature* high, 39·5 °C (103 °F). *Pulse* rapid. Face flushed: circumoral pallor. *Tongue* strawberry. *Rash*.

Glandular fever: Not uncommon mistake in anginose type: mononucleosis present.

Lassa fever: So far only occurs in West Africa; rash usually present and the patient is more ill than the degree of fever would suggest. Virus isolation and immune studies performed in special laboratories will confirm or exclude Lassa fever.

Quinsy: Tonsillar abscess, diphtheria never suppurates.

2. *Laryngeal diphtheria*. Diagnosis from: (i) Acute laryngitis; (ii) Measles; (iii) Retropharyngeal abscess; (iv) Bronchopneumonia. Less commonly from laryngismus stridulus, foreign body and papilloma of larynx.

Acute laryngitis: Often difficult. Constitutional symptoms slight. Bacteriology. Primary acute laryngitis in infants is nearly always diphtheria.

Measles: Catarrhal symptoms. Koplik's spots. No membrane present. Later, typical rash.

Retropharyngeal abscess: In infants. Recognized by position of head and by palpation.

Bronchopneumonia: Expiratory stridor. Retraction of lower ribs.

Laryngismus stridulus: Recurrent nocturnal attacks of dyspnoea. Sudden onset. No membrane. Slight general symptoms. Spasm relieved by warm bath.

Papilloma of larynx: Haemorrhage occurs.

Association with other Specific Fevers
Frequent with measles and scarlet fever (q.v.); prognosis serious.

Prognosis
Case mortality. Greatest in infants, in malignant diphtheria and when administration of antitoxin delayed.

Dangerous symptoms. Very irregular *pulse*, especially if slow. Low temperature with symptoms of prostration. Repeated vomiting. Marked albuminuria. Convulsions. Haemorrhages. Severe oedema with 'bullneck' (*see* Gravis Type). Myocarditis most likely to be fatal in 3rd week and respiratory failure later than that time.

In *faucial diphtheria*. Extensive membrane. Great enlargement of glands.

In *laryngeal diphtheria*. Deaths due to asphyxia or bronchopneumonia, absorption of toxin slight.

In *paralysis*. Extensive paralysis. Involvement of respiratory muscles. Signs of cardiac weakness. Vomiting.

Treatment
Methods of primary importance are: (1) Injection of antitoxin; (2) Treatment of laryngeal obstruction when necessary; (3) Rest. *Note*: In presence of symptoms, commence treatment without waiting for bacteriological report. Only in mildest cases is it justifiable to await 6 h after doing Schick test.

1. *Injection of antitoxin*
   Test dose. If history of previous dose of serum always give test dose of 0·1 ml of

serum by subcutaneous injection. If no reaction in 30 min, give full dose. If reaction (shivering, general rash etc.) repeat very small but gradually increasing doses every 30 min subcutaneously. Hydrocortisone is of value during desensitization. With initial injections 0·5 ml of 1 in 1000 adrenalin solution is also given subcutaneously.

Dosage. Depends on duration of disease, extent of membrane, and degree of toxaemia, and but little on age. Aim is to give all the antitoxin in one dose.

If mild with membrane on one tonsil give 20 000 u i.m.   *With membrane on both tonsils and moderate toxaemia*: 40–80 000 u of which half is given i.m. and half i.v.

Severe: give 100 000–200 000 u i.v. The larger doses are given when there has been delay in treatment.

Anterior nasal diphtheria: 10 000 u usually sufficient.

Concentrated serum: Highly refined globulin-modified (protein-digested) sera contain 6000 u or more per ml: are almost protein-free and reactions are rare.

Hypersensitiveness: Occurs in those who have had previous serum injection more than 10 days previously: may be many years. Symptoms may develop with great rapidity, especially with intravenous injections; if intramuscular, more commonly in ½ h to 3 h: occasionally in one or more days. In acute cases, rapid onset of collapse. When less severe, shivering or rigor, dyspnoea, cyanosis, vomiting, varying degree of cardiac weakness and prostration, rash. Very rarely fatal except in asthmatics. Administer corticosteroids. *The possibility of a reaction is never a contra-indication to intramuscular injections for curative purposes.*

2. *Chemotherapy*. Penicillin and erythromycin are effective in vitro against *C. diphtheriae* but in patients their value is problematic. Most physicians, however, recommend in addition to antitoxin 0·6 g benzyl penicillin 8-hourly till the patient can swallow with ease and then phenoxymethyl penicillin orally in doses of 250–500 mg 6-hourly. Duration of penicillin treatment 7–10 days. Erythromycin 100 mg every 4–8 h then 250–500 mg orally every 6 h is an alternative and is preferred if there is penicillin sensitivity. Children are given ¼–½ the adult dose.

3. *Corticosteroids*. For those severely ill, in shock, or with laryngeal diphtheria 5 mg/kg prednisone daily may be helpful.

4. *Rest in bed. Must be absolute, lying flat.*

Duration. In mild cases, for 2 weeks after membrane disappears.

When severe, for at least 2 weeks after disappearance of symptoms and period increased at slightest indication.

Each stage in getting up and convalescence should be gradual and pulse watched. Risk of cardiac failure is present from onset and persists into convalescence.

Treatment of special symptoms

Laryngeal Obstruction. Indications for tracheostomy: increasing dyspnoea, inspiratory recession above clavicles and restlessness. *Intubation* only in hospitals. Aspiration of membrane under endoscopy may be valuable.

'*Diphtheria Carriers'. See* p. 162.

Desert Sore

Widespread in desert areas, in tropics and subtropics: associated with excessive dryness of skin.

Aetiology
Infection with *C. diphtheriae* present in majority. Positive culture obtained in acute stage: later overgrown by other bacteria.

Symptoms
Acute stage. Onset with clear vesicle: bursts, leaving shallow ulcer with grey base. May spread peripherally. Very painful.
Chronic ulcer. After 2–3 weeks: circular, thick margins, undermined edges. Base formed of debris lying on adherent membrane. Pus absent or slight.
Course. Intractable. May last 2 years. Leaves thin tissue-paper scar.

Diphtheritic Paralyses
Not uncommon. About 3 weeks after onset. Accommodation, palate, arms, legs. Polyneuritis and absent knee jerks. Paresis may commence near site of ulcer.

Treatment
Anti-diphtheritic serum: 20 000 u; inject near ulcer. Also penicillin or erythromycin (*see* p. 168). Apply locally bland oily dressing.

Chapter 37   **WHOOPING-COUGH (PERTUSSIS)**

Specific infectious disease characterized by catarrh of the respiratory tract and paroxysms of coughing terminating in a 'whoop', caused by *Bordetella pertussis*.

Incidence
Sporadic cases common. Epidemics frequent. Temperate climates especially affected.
Season. Most prevalent in winter and spring. Maximum in March, minimum in September.
Age. Usually under 6 years, but no age immune. Not uncommon in infants. In old people usually severe.
   Females in excess of males. *One attack usually protects.* Association with measles very common. *Susceptibility* great but not universal.

Bacteriology
Bordet and Gengou, in 1906, described the causative organism now designated *Bordetella pertussis*. Isolated on special blood-agar media from tenacious mucus voided at end of paroxysms. Absent or difficult to isolate in later stages. A small, gram-negative, non-sporing bacillus resembling *H. influenzae. Complement-deviation* occurs with the serum of convalescents and agglutinins may also be present, but of no help in diagnosis. In all 14 strains have been identified but of these 3 are common and the others unusual. Outbreaks of whooping-cough may differ in the proportion of serotypes present.
   B. parapertussis isolated in 1937 and *B. bronchisepticus* have been associated with the pertussis syndrome. The latter organism is commonly found in the respiratory tract of small animals including rabbits, dogs and guinea pigs and its relationship to pertussis problematic.

Morbid Anatomy

No specific changes. Bacilli localized to respiratory tract: causes inflammation of mucous membrane and interstitial tissue with secretion of thick mucus. Lesions post mortem usually those of some fatal complications.

Mode of Infection

Direct contagion from the sputum. A very short exposure may be sufficient. The cough can probably project particles to some distance, but with precautions the tendency to spread, e.g. in a ward, is considerably less than with measles. Transmission by fomites, infected clothes, etc., is proved, but probably rare. No proof of existence of carriers.

Duration of Infectivity

Infectivity usually ceases within a few days of erythromycin therapy. In untreated cases 3 weeks from onset of 'whoop'. After cessation of 'whoop', cough may remain paroxysmal; it is unnecessary to regard this stage as infectious. One attack usually produces life-long immunity.

Symptoms

Divided into catarrhal and paroxysmal stages.
Incubation period. Six to 18, often 10–14 days.
1. Catarrhal stage. Onset insidious yet disease is at its most infectious at this stage. Commences with slight malaise, coryza and cough: not severe, but cough out of proportion to physical signs of bronchitis. *Pyrexia* slight and intermittent. Some gastric disturbance.

Cough. Becomes more frequent and paroxysmal, especially at night: inspiratory spasms develop; finally characteristic whoop starts. In some cases, whooping occurs almost at once: in others greatly delayed, or not at all.
2. Paroxysmal stage. Dated from first whoop. Coryza has previously subsided. Pyrexia slight or absent.

Cough. Course of events in typical paroxysm: (i) *Long inspiration* (often absent), followed at once by (ii) *Series of short expiratory barks*. Thorax fixed, no air enters, face becomes congested. When apparently suffocating, (iii) *Inspiratory whoop*. Congested appearance rapidly passes, but child is exhausted. *Vomiting frequently follows* even in catarrhal stage, and suggests diagnosis. Cycle may recur several times in succession. May be small amount of tenacious mucus at end of paroxysm. Number of *paroxysms* up to 40 a day: *distinctly more frequent at night*. Child becomes aware of oncoming paroxysm. After attack sleeps, or older children complain of headache. Violent sneezing may precede or follow paroxysm.

Face. Lids swollen, conjunctivae congested. Face bloated and miserable.
Sublingual Ulcer. Occasionally present: confined to infants with only two lower central incisors erupted. Never before paroxysmal stage.
Paroxysms. May be brought on by vigorous movement as in playing and also by large meals, infants whoop usually absent: in aged, an occasional whoop.

Physical Signs

In lungs: very slight. During expiratory coughs, resonance may be defective and a few crackles at bases. Pulse becomes very rapid.

Blood Changes
Absolute lymphocytosis. Rise commences early, maximum in 3rd or 4th week, persists into convalescence:
1. Leucocytes 30 000–80 000 or more but initially often a leucopenia.
2. Lymphocytes 60–85%.
Sedimentation rate. Little affected.

Duration
Catarrhal stage very variable. About 1 week, from 3 days to 2 weeks. *Paroxysmal stage*, 4 weeks and upwards. *Adenoids* may cause prolongation.

Complications
Important.
1. *Pulmonary complications*. Cause nearly all fatalities.
   Capillary Bronchitis and Bronchopneumonia. Child remains ill between the paroxysms. Whoop may disappear. Lobar pneumonia rare.
   Lobar collapse. Due to blockage of air spaces by tenacious secretion, most commonly of the right upper lobe. Infants and young children the most vulnerable. Before the antibiotic era this sometimes led on to bronchiectasis but this is now very rare.
   Interstitial Emphysema. May develop. Rarely pneumothorax.
   Tuberculous Lesions. If present activity is stimulated.
2. *Vomiting and emaciation*. The usual vomiting may become excessive.
3. *Enlargement of bronchial glands*. Very frequent.
4. *Convulsions*. Common in infants. Often fatal if persistent. Probably results from anoxia due to severe paroxysms.
5. *Traumatic*. From venous congestion and high pressure. During paroxysms, may cause various complications: (1) Hernia; (2) Prolapse of rectum; (3) Haemorrhages, e.g. *conjunctival ecchymosis*, epistaxis, petechial rashes, membrana tympani. Rarely meningeal haemorrhage, fatal.
Albuminuria occasionally, but nephritis very rare.
Paralyses and peripheral neuritis. Very rare.

Diagnosis
Catarrhal stage. Often very difficult. *Note*: (1) Cough out of proportion to signs in lungs; (2) Cough becoming paroxysmal, especially at night; (3) Cough accompanied by vomiting.
Paroxysmal stage. Typical cases easy, but in young infants whoop may be absent throughout.

Radiology
Cardiac outline may be 'shaggy' from paroxysmal stage onwards. Due to peribronchial thickening and infiltration adjacent to the heart.
Specific. (1) *Culture of perinasal swab*: preferably held in nares while patient coughs. Has replaced older technique of coughing onto a plate. Swab is immediately applied to two plates containing Bordet–Gengou medium one with 2·5 µg methicillin/ml to diminish growth of other organisms. Small silvery colonies of *B. pertussis* appear in 4 days. (2) Fluorescent antibodies: demonstrable in sputum and droplets but false negative and false negative results occur.

Cause of the Whoop
Uncertain. Has been ascribed to laryngeal spasm from local irritation of larynx by mucus (doubtful). Possibly specific irritation of vagus.

Prognosis
Seriousness often overlooked. Continues to be a very serious disease in infants under 6 months. Though rare in the aged it is then a serious infection with significant mortality. Convulsions: high mortality.

Prophylaxis.
Vaccine Inoculation. Protection of infants under 3 months important in view of their susceptibility and the consequent mortality amongst them. Diphtheria, pertussis and tetanus vaccine (DPT) recommended. After primary dose at 4–8 weeks 2 additional doses given at 4–8 week intervals. Booster doses are recommended 12–15 months later and on entry into school.

Treatment
1. *Specific.* Erythromycin, but not ampicillin, penetrates bronchial mucosa and secretions. For infants and young children 125 mg 6-hourly orally.
2. *Corticosteroids.* Reduce severity and duration of illness but should be used only in severely ill where benefits may outweigh risks. Betamethasone has been given orally in doses of 0·075 mg/kg/24 h or hydrocortisone i.m. 30 mg/kg/24 h.
3. *General treatment.* Confine to bed only during catarrhal stage or pyrexia. Support child during paroxysm.
4. *Diet.* Large meals may precipitate paroxysms so meals should be small, frequent and light.
5. *Paroxysmal stage.* A sedative may be needed. For children Paediatric Chloral Elixir (BNF). Dose up to 1 year: 5 ml (200 mg Chloral) diluted with water. For older children Chloral Mixture (BNF) contains 500 mg Chloral/5 ml. Dose 1–5 years 2·5–5 ml, 6–12 years 5–10 ml.

Chapter 38   # HAEMOPHILUS INFLUENZAE INFECTIONS

Haemophilus influenzae infections are distinct from 'influenza' as commonly known.

Haemophilus influenzae. Discovered by Pfeiffer in 1892 in patients with 'influenza' and presumed to be its cause. It was, however, either growing symbiotically with influenza virus or was a secondary invader, but organism is actively pathogenic in certain circumstances. A strain is present in the nasopharynx of 80% of normal people and 50% infants have an *H. influenzae* infection. Asymptomatic nasopharyngeal infection with it may last months and is not always eradicated by antibiotic sufficient to cure haemophilus meningitis. Its importance has increased in recent years by recognition: (i) of its increasing importance as a pathogen in children aged 3 months to 5 years; (ii) of its increasing resistance to ampicillin; (iii) that antibodies to it may be produced by infection with certain non-pathogenic strains of *Escherichia coli* thus raising an intriguing possible approach to production of immunity to it and some other pathogens. Strains become pathogenic when tissue resistance is lowered—haemophilus bronchopneumonia commonly follows influenza, measles, whooping-cough, etc.

Haemophilus infections have high mortality.

Bacteriology
Minute non-motile bacillus or coccobacillus: very pleomorphous. Stains with all ordinary stains, but not readily. Gram-negative. Of the six Haemophilus species *H. influenzae* is the most important. Others include *H. ducreyi*, the causative organism of chancroid, and *H. aegyptius* (Koch–Weeks bacillus), an important cause of purulent conjunctivitis.

There are six serotypes of *H. influenzae* of which type G is responsible for 95% of human infections.

It grows well on chocolate agar (agar containing heated blood) as it requires factors X (haematin) and Y (nicotinamide adenine dinucleotide).

Clinical Manifestations
Meningitis. H. influenzae type G is the commonest cause of meningitis between the ages of 6 months and 3 years. Rare in neonates because of presence of maternal antibodies. Subdural effusions and ventriculitis tend to complicate it with persistent mental and neuropsychiatric sequelae. Otherwise clinical manifestations as in purulent meningitis due to other agents.
Pneumonia. Often in children follows influenza, measles, whooping-cough, etc. Insidious onset with atypical and slight physical signs: early cyanosis. Increasingly being recognized in adults, especially those already debilitated. May cause bronchopneumonia or multiple partial lobar involvement.
Cellulitis. Particularly affects the face in children causing distinctive reddish-blue hue.
Epiglottitis causes very acute illness in children with fever, dysphagia and airway obstruction. Head retraction reduces airway obstruction and meningitis may be suggested but airway obstruction should suggest the diagnosis.
Pyarthrosis. H. influenzae type G is the commonest cause of septic arthrosis in children under 2 years. Large weight-bearing joints most usually involved without osteomyelitis. May be a cause of pyrexia of unknown origin.
Septicaemia. Causes pyrexia of obscure causation, especially in young children and in adults after chemotherapy for malignant disease.
Other sites. Otitis media, empyema, endocarditis, brain abscess, pericarditis, etc.

Diagnosis
Culture, radioimmune assay.

Treatment
Mortality very high before introduction of chemotherapy. Chloramphenicol, streptomycin and sulphadiazine all good.
Chloramphenicol. Diffuses well into joint and cerebrospinal fluid. Use especially in meningitis, arthritis, pericarditis, 250–500 mg 6-hourly. If necessary 1 g may be given i.v. every 6–12 h to adults. To children give 50 mg/kg body weight initially by i.m. injection and 25 mg/kg 6-hourly by injection thereafter. If able to

swallow give these doses orally. In the neonate give 25 mg/kg/day, as the dose regime. Continue 3–6 weeks.

Amoxycillin. Good for chest and ear infections. Dosage 12 mg/kg 6-hourly orally.

Ampicillin. Widespread resistance of *H. influenzae* to ampicillin has been recorded but if the organism has been proved sensitive to it use in place of chloramphenicol in meningitis, septicamia etc. in doses of 30–50 mg/kg 4-hourly i.v. Ampicillin and chloramphenicol should be given until sensitivities of organism determined.

Co-trimoxazole (BNF). Good reports received. Dose, orally, 960 mg every 8–12 h. Children 120–480 mg every 12 h; by i.m. or i.v. injection.

Chapter 39   *MENINGOCOCCAL MENINGITIS (Cerebrospinal Fever; Cerebrospinal Meningitis; Spotted Fever; (In infants) Posterior Basal Meningitis)*

Acute infectious disease, occurring sporadically and in epidemics, caused by the meningococcus, *Neisseria meningitidis*, and characterized pathologically by purulent inflammation of the meninges of the brain and cord.

Note: The clinical course of the disease, as commonly seen, has been radically modified by chemotherapy.

Aetiology and Epidemiology

Age. Commonest cause of meningitis between 3 years and 15 years. Also classically affects young persons living in crowded conditions, as in military camps (*see also* p. 175).

Season. Highest in first half of year: attributed to confinement in dwellings and prevalence of colds and coughs. Transmission facilitated by low absolute humidity. Epidemics around Southern Sahara are usually in the dry December–March period.

Geographic region. In sub-Saharan Africa from Mali in the West to Ethiopia in the East, 'the African meningitis belt', major epidemics occur every 5–10 years, the last in 1982, 1983 and 1984. Epidemics also occur in semi-arid regions of Zambia and Brazil. In Africa the organism is usually *Neisseria meningitidis* type A but in Europe and America it is types B and C. Epidemics immunize the majority of the population and a new epidemic occurs when a non-immune population has built up.

Mode of Infection

Animals are not susceptible (except monkeys experimentally): hence infection is solely from man to man; *spreads by droplet infection*; fomites are not infectious. Infection is from 'carriers', direct infection from a patient being very rare. Epidemics thus spread irregularly, cases apparently being unconnected, but recent work indicates a considerable incidence among siblings and family contacts.

'Carriers'. May be: (1) Convalescent carriers rare: subsequent to an attack: cultures (from nasopharyngeal swabs) usually negative in a few weeks: (2) Chronic carriers: few only have had symptoms, or develop them; unhealthy nasopharyngeal mucosa common. Antibodies to meningococcus develop within 2 weeks of becoming a carrier. In a healthy population, 5% may be carriers: cases may begin to be frequent when carrier rate is 20%; but a high carrier rate in a community, even 50%, is not necessarily associated with increase of cases, the virulence of the strain being also a factor. The 'carrier rate' among soldiers increases as distance between bunks is decreased. Cubic space is a lesser factor.

Treatment. Oral administration of sulphonamides is effective.

Path of invasion. Nasopharynx is infected initially. Next stage is meningococcal septicaemia (onset of symptoms) followed by stage of localization in meninges. Direct spread to meninges by lymphatics from infected sphenoidal sinus is improbable path.

Bacteriology

Neisseria meningitidis discovered by Weichselbaum in 1887. Dies rapidly outside body. Must be distinguished from gonococcus.

Morphology. Mainly in pairs. In CSF and pus most but not all the organisms are within the leucocytes (intracellular). Shape either round or flattened. Gram-negative. Thus closely resembles gonococcus. Possesses a polysaccharide capsule.

Cultures. Grow readily on Gordon's 'trypagar'; large colonies, somewhat opaque. Less readily on ascitic agar. On ordinary agar growth more delicate and often fails. Cultures die readily, and subcultures are necessary every few days. *Involution forms* are common in cultures, cocci being swollen and staining badly. Identify cultures by agglutination.

Serogroups. Nine now recognized on basis of antibodies to capsular polysaccharides; A, B, C, D, X, Z, (Z'), W-135 and 29-E. Serogrouping of mainly epidemiological importance as there are antibiotics effective against all groups.

Presence and isolation of meningococcus
1. Nasopharynx and accessory sinuses in 'carriers'.
2. Blood in early stage of disease. Isolated in about 25%.
3. CSF during disease.
Rarely isolated from nasopharynx during disease.

Agglutinins. Appear in blood about fourth day: to infecting strain only.

Antisera. Produced in horses and monkeys: only effective against homologous strain.

Morbid Anatomy

General characteristic is a suppurative inflammation of pia-arachnoid, especially at base of brain. Very acute infections may be fatal before significant meningitis develops.

Blood vessels. Basic lesion is extensive damage to small blood vessels, probably caused by endotoxin. Immune complexes form at sites where meningococci have become attached during septicaemic phase.

Cerebral meninges and brain. Pia-arachnoid injected, and purulent exudate in subarachnoid spaces, especially at base. On cortex often much lymph, especially in larger depressions. Brain substance soft and pink; may be foci of haemorrhages. Ventricles distended with fluid or even with pus. Microscopically, infiltration along vessels and other channels, and may be foci of encephalitis.

Spinal cord. Always affected, especially posterior surface, and in dorsal and lumbar regions. Pus may surround the cord, and even nerve roots.

In more chronic cases *meninges* are thickened and remains of exudate present. Cranial nerves usually involved. *Ventricles* may be greatly distended with clear or turbid fluid, and foramen of Magendie closed.

Meningococcal encephalitis. May occur without meningeal involvement in fulminating cases.

Other organs. In fulminating cases haemorrhages often present in adrenal cortex (Waterhouse–Friderichsen syndrome). Spleen occasionally enlarged. May be terminal pneumonia. Tubular necrosis may develop in kidneys.

Duration of Infectivity
Until nasopharyngeal swabs give negative result.

Quarantine Period
Seven days.

Symptoms
Incubation period. From 1 to 4 or 5 days.
General course. Commences as septicaemia, subsequent progress being: (1) Fulminating septicaemia without localization; (2) Septicaemic stage transient, followed by cerebrospinal localization— is ordinary type; (3) Septicaemic stage chronic without immediate localization—chronic meningococcal septicaemia.
Modes of onset. (1) *Ordinary type*: Sudden onset. Condition becomes progressively worse, suggesting cerebrospinal meningitis in 24 h, signifying progress from septicaemia to meningeal localization; (2) *Fulminating septicaemia*: Abrupt onset. May be mania. Progress very rapid. Comatose within few hours; (3) Chronic meningococcal septicaemia.

Ordinary Form
Onset: Sudden, with cardinal symptoms of *headache, vomiting and pyrexia*, with rigors, and, in children, convulsions. Temporary improvement occasionally follows onset. *Stiffness of neck*, head retraction and general irritability develop. General condition of irritation of the nervous system and increased intracranial pressure. Symptoms usually take 1–5 days to develop, and remain at height for 1–3 weeks in absence of chemotherapy. Rash often develops after 1 week. Spleen may be palpable.

Motor symptoms
  1. *Head Retraction*. May be extreme. In infants, opisthotonos.
  2. *Rigidity*. (i) Kernig's sign, rarely absent; (ii) Brudzinski's 'neck sign'; if the head is flexed by the hand, with the patient lying on his back, flexion of the knees and thighs occurs (a valuable sign of meningitis); (iii) Brudzinski's 'leg sign': if one leg be flexed, flexion also occurs in the other leg.
  3. *Reflexes*. Deep reflexes (knee jerks) usually increased but may be absent. Babinski's sign in about 10%.
  4. *Spasms*. Commence as twitching, increasing to clonic or tonic spasms. Spasms or paralysis of face muscles. Tremor common.
  5. *Ocular Symptoms*. (i) Pupils: Usually dilated, from irritation of sympathetic; may be contracted, in severe forms. Inequality and sluggish reaction common. Hippus not infrequent; (ii) Strabismus: In about 20%; (iii) Optic neuritis:

uncommon; about 10%. Photophobia, conjunctivitis, ptosis, nystagmus occasionally.

Sensory symptoms. Headache often very severe, especially occipital. Pain may extend along spine and limbs; may be severe lumbar pain with hyperaesthesia. General hyperaesthesia may occur.

Physical symptoms. At onset restlessness, mania, or delirium, later stupor and coma.

Vomiting. Of the cerebral type, very frequent at onset, may continue to subside later.

Temperature. Irregular, no typical course, remissions and intermissions common; may rise to 40·5 °C (105 °F) or over; about 39·4 °C (103 °F) usual.

Pulse. Slow in relation to temperature, may be irregular.

Respiration. Towards termination may be Cheyne–Stokes. Only increased with pulmonary complications.

Eruptions

1. *Haemorrhagic rash*. Onset early, first or second day. Either (*a*) petechial, or (*b*) purpuric (fulminating cases only). Rare.

2. *Erythema and papular eruptions*. Pink papules may resemble typhoid or macular eruption like measles.

3. *Herpes labialis*. In 25–50%. Onset not before fourth or fifth day.

Blood. Polynuclear leucocytosis 25 000–50 000/mm^3. Leucocytosis may be absent in fulminating cases.

Emaciation. Often very rapid.

Other Clinical Types

1. Fulminating form. Acute meningococcal septicaemia. Dramatic onset and course. Patient may go from health to death in a few hours. Headache, vomiting, collapse: purpuric rash common. Temperature high or low. *Rapid coma*. CSF may be clear and contain no cocci. Recent work suggests that most cases are not due to haemorrhage in adrenals (Waterhouse–Friderichsen syndrome); meningeal symptoms slight or absent; abdominal symptoms may occur. Meningococcal encephalitis may also be fulminating.

Note: Treatment of this disease forms an urgent medical emergency.

2. Chronic meningococcal septicaemia. Not uncommon; often overlooked.

Onset usually sudden: intermittent headache, rigors, arthritis with muscle and joint pains. Blood cultures positive only intermittently.

Eruption: Usually within few days, rarely absent. Appears in successive crops, often tender. Various types, e.g.: (1) Erythema nodosum, may be indistinguishable but often wider distribution; (2) Papular, may be petechial; (3) Pink macules, resembling enteric.

Temperature: No distinctive course. Often higher periods. May closely simulate malaria.

If untreated may persist for weeks or months without serious malaise. May suggest influenza, typhoid, rheumatism, erythema nodosum, or trench fever.

Terminates dramatically with chemotherapy, but, if untreated, meningitis may develop.

Mild and abortive forms. Symptoms mild or subsiding in a few days.

Chronic forms. Recrudescences may occur over many months. Other chronic forms are associated with closure by meningitis of the foramina of Magendie and Luschka: the ventricles are distended either with pus, turbid fluid, or clear fluid, constituting 'closed ventricular meningitis' or hydrocephalus. Complex nervous manifestations, emaciation, disturbances of pulse and respiration: recovery impossible. Common in posterior basal meningitis.

Posterior basal meningitis. Cerebrospinal meningitis in infants. Onset sudden or insidious. *Note*: (1) Head retraction and opisthotonos marked; (2) Rash rare; (3) Loss of vision without optic neuritis common; (4) Often very chronic; (5) Sequelae usual in non-fatal cases: deafness and hence deaf-mutism, blindness, mental deficiency, general spasticity of extremities (hydrocephalus). Lumbar puncture in chronic cases often gives 'dry tap', from closure of foramen of Magendie. Possibly many cases are sequel of overlooked acute attack with closure of foramen of Magendie.

Prognosis. Poor when chronic symptoms present: in acute stages amenable to sulphonamides.

Complications and Sequelae

Nervous system. Facial paralysis, hemiplegia and paraplegia occur rarely: recovery usual. In the chronic forms and hydrocephalus, attacks occur with headache, vomiting, mental dullness and dilated pupils.

Arthritis or synovitis. Occurs in 5–10%: a previous haemorrhagic rash is almost invariable. Suppuration is rare and prognosis good.

Ear. Deafness not uncommon, and often permanent, from affection of labyrinth. Otitis media also not uncommon.

Disseminated intravascular coagulation. May complicate fulminating meningococcal septicaemia. Causes multiple haemorrhages. Serious and often fatal.

Rare complications. Pericarditis. Pneumonia. Epididymitis.

Recrudescences. Common in untreated or inadequately treated cases. True relapses rare.

Cerebrospinal Fluid

Characters. N.B. Previous antibiotic treatment tends to diminish number of cells and increase proportion of lymphocytes. (1) *Amount increased* and under abnormal pressure; (2) Fluid *turbid* or purulent; (3) *Protein increased*; (4) *Polynuclear leucocytes* present in deposit (lymphocytes in early stages); (5) *Meningococci* present, intra- and extracellular—but may be present even with turbid fluid; (6) *Dextrose absent*: the cause of this is doubtful, possibly fermented by meningococci, or due to action of leucocytes. The fluid may be clear for the first 24 h. In later stages, with closure of foramen of Magendie by meningitis, amount of fluid may be scanty. Mixed infections occasionally occur, usually pneumococci.

Diagnosis

Clinical characteristics. At onset: headache, vomiting, pyrexia, stiffness of neck and delirium: development of head retraction. Eruption.

Special methods. (1) Lumbar puncture: pathognomonic except occasionally in first 24 hours and in acute meningococcal septicaemia in which it is clear or in which cells only slightly increased. (2) Blood count and blood culture: of less value.

Differential Diagnosis

1. Other forms of meningitis. Commonest causes of meningitis:

   1.1 In neonates *Escherichia coli* or sometimes *Streptococcus pyogenes* group B.

1.2 Aged 1–12 months *S. pneumoniae* or *H. influenzae*.
1.3 Aged 6 months – 3 years *H. influenzae*.
1.4 Older children and young adults *N. meningitidis*.
1.5 Elderly persons *S. pneumoniae* (the pneumococcus). Other important causes of meningitis include tuberculosis and *S. typhi*. Extension of infection to meninges from otitis media should be kept in mind.
2. Acute poliomyelitis.
3. Typhus and rarely other conditions with purpuric eruptions.
4. Subarachnoid haemorrhage (may recur).

Course and Prognosis

Mortality approaches 50% in fulminating meningococcal septicaemia. Usually in meningococcal meningitis mortality is under 10%. *Serious features*: (1) Infancy; (2) Fulminating forms with early coma; (3) Purpuric eruptions. Temperature has little prognostic value. Condition of cerebrospinal fluid of little value: pus and cocci may disappear rapidly. *Mortality without sulphonamides*: not under 30%; many complications and sequelae.

Prophylaxis

1. General hygiene. At least 6 feet between beds in barracks and institutions.
2. Isolation of patient. For 2 weeks from onset of chemotherapy. Attendants should wear masks and gloves.
3. Contacts. Immediate contacts only (as decided by responsible medical practitioner) should be kept under observation for 6 days: little practical value in swabbing throats.
4. Carriers and close contacts. Sulphonamide, 2 g/day for 3 days or 6 g for one day for adults in epidemics or rifampicin 10 mg/kg daily for 3–4 days in areas where penicillin resistance occurs. Penicillin ineffective for prophylaxis. Vaccination with group A and C meningococcal polysaccharides effective in older persons but of limited value in children. Group B is poorly immunogenic but vaccines against it are in preparation.

Treatment

N.B. Approximately 30% of strains in America and many strains in Africa, particularly in the Western part of the meningitis belt, are now resistant to sulphonamides.
Sulphonamides. Commence immediately on clinical diagnosis. High dosage at onset to obtain high concentration in blood and CSF (10–15 mg and 5 mg/dl respectively).
Dosage (adults) (1) Intravenous: initial loading dose 2 g sulphadiazine or sulphadimidine. (2) Continue 1 or 1½ g 6-hourly till improvement justifies giving the doses orally.
Dosage (children) I.m. or i.v. initial dose 75 mg/kg followed by 50 mg/kg every 6 h until oral therapy possible.
Penicillin. Effective, but inferior to sulphonamides in areas where sulphonamide resistance is not present. Usually combined with sulphonamide. Give to adults 1·2 g i.v. or i.m. every 6 h until clinical recovery then tail dosage off and half this amount to children.
Shock, hypotension and disseminated intravascular coagulation. Most important

measure is to restore blood pressure and obviate peripheral circulatory collapse. Infusions of plasma or dextran may be used to keep systolic blood pressure above 100 mmHg. Dopamine infusion (rate 2–5 µg/kg/min) or dobutamine (rate 2·5–10 µg/kg/min) can be given to increase myocardial contractility and improve renal perfusion.

Heparin is no longer recommended by most authorities for disseminated intravascular coagulation in meningococcal infections but some recommend 100 units/kg 6-hourly i.v.

Corticosteroids. Not recommended for meningitis, but in fulminating meningococcal septicaemia with shock and low blood pressure may be given as hydrocortisone 100–500 mg i.v. or i.m. up to 4 times in 24 h or prednisolone 25–100 mg i.v. or i.m. Methylprednisone has also been given in very large doses but its value is not proved. *General sedation*. For adults diazepam orally 5–10 mg 1–3 times daily or 10 mg i.m. For children 1–2 mg 1–3 times daily orally or i.m. or paediatric chloral elixir or chloral mixture (*see* p. 172). Photophobia if present requires reduction of light in room.

Chapter 40   # GONOCOCCAL INFECTIONS

Infection by gonococcus (*Neisseria gonorrhoeae*), with primary lesion usually in urethra, various lesions in genital tract due to direct extension, and a liability to systemic infection. Lesions in genital tract are not described here. The infection is particularly common in the tropics where poor socio-economic conditions associated with urban migration favour it but it has increased world wide in recent years due to greater permissiveness.

Aetiology
In newborn; occurs as ophthalmia neonatorum, due to vaginal infection of conjunctiva. Amenable to early treatment, but neglected cases are a common cause of blindness. In infants and children: as vulvovaginitis from accidental infections by sponges, etc. In adults: spreads by sexual intercourse with infected individuals.

Bacteriology
Gonococcus was isolated by Neisser in 1879.
Principal characteristics: (1) Diplococcus, bean-shaped with flat sides almost in apposition; (2) Gram-negative, but stains with ordinary stains; (3) In pus and body fluids mainly intracellular; (4) Characteristically present only in a few cells amongst many, such cells each containing a large number of cocci; (5) Grows best on blood-agar and media containing serum or blood. Growth is delicate: does not grow on many ordinary media; (6) Monoclonal antibodies and iso-enzymes enable strains to be identified by specialist laboratories and study of epidemiology facilitated. Life outside body tissues and media is very short.

Clinical Conditions in Adults
(1) *Primary lesion* in man is a urethritis, in women a cervicitis and urethritis. May be simulated by *Trichomonas vaginalis* infections; (2) *Direct spread* may occur to prostate, epididymis, Fallopian tubes, ovaries, and even by this route to

peritoneum. In males gonorrhoeal peritonitis is extremely rare. Proctitis is not uncommon in females and in homosexual men. *Conjunctivitis* is not very common; (3) *Systemic infections* occur in small proportion of cases. Although gonococcus is not commonly isolated, local lesions are due probably to presence of organisms, and not to toxins absorbed from distant focus. Systemic infections may be:

1. Septicaemia. Rare: more frequent in women than men: organism sometimes isolated from blood. Clinical types: (1) General septicaemia, condition may resemble typhoid; (2) Pyaemic or haemorrhagic abscesses or necrotic skin lesions; (3) Gonorrhoeal puerperal septicaemia; (4) Infective endocarditis and pericarditis: very rare. Fatal termination is rare, except in infective endocarditis.

2. Gonorrhoeal arthritis

Time of Onset. Usually within few weeks or months of initial urethritis, but may be later when there is chronic urethritis. In rare cases follows the vulvovaginitis of infants and ophthalmia neonatorum. Onset usually sudden.

Morbid Anatomy. Changes mainly in *peri-articular tissues*, oedematous swelling and infiltration. Synovial membrane hyperaemic and joint may contain increased and turbid fluid: polynuclear cells often numerous but suppuration rare. In chronic stages, peri-articular tissues thickened, but bony changes rare. Gonococci may be present in fluid: usually absent. Mixed infections very rare.

Joints Affected. Knee especially frequent. *Usually more than one joint. Large joints most common. Temporomandibular* and, rarely, sternoclavicular and sacro-iliac joints may be affected. (These escape in acute rheumatism).

Physical Signs. Variable. May be stiffness and vague pain, without swelling, or with synovial effusion. More typically, red, hot and tender, with *peri-articular swelling*, with or without much effusion. *Suppuration rare.* Mixed infections very rare.

Clinical Course. Untreated duration of joint affection several weeks: as one clears, another often becomes affected. Often very obstinate. Rapid shifting, as in acute rheumatism, does not occur.

Complications, Sequelae and Variations in Lesions. The peri-articular tissues are especially affected, and spread may occur along the tendons. Gonorrhoea tends also to attack fibrous tissue. The following are important:

1. *Fibrous adhesions*: Commonly form around affected joint, in absence of suitable treatment. Cause contractions and limitation of movement. Bony ankylosis rare.

2. *Flat-foot*: Common sequel when foot and ankle affected. Caused by yielding of ligaments and plantar fasciae.

3. *Tenosynovitis*: Joint may be unaffected. Tendo Achillis most frequent site.

4. *Bursitis*

5. *Painful heels*: Pain in calcaneus on walking: probably periostitis of calcaneus, or certain plantar fasciae affected.

Conditions sometimes Gonorrhoeal

Spondylitis deformans

Acute myositis: Painful muscles: usually, but not always, near an affected joint.

Diagnosis. Initial lesion usually makes diagnosis easy in males. Important symptoms are involvement of unusual joints, peri-articular thickening, obstinate nature, slight fever, and uselessness of salicylates. Diagnosis especially from acute rheumatic fever, arthritis deformans, and gout.

Prognosis. Condition obstinate; prognosis good. Recurrences frequent.

3. Other gonococcal conditions. These include myositis, iritis, meningitis, endocarditis, pleuritis, rarely keratodermia blennorrhagica and in women with gonococcal pelvic infection perihepatitis (Fitz-Hugh–Curtis syndrome). Anorectal infection may occur due to extension from vagina, or in men from homosexual practices. Gonococcal pharyngitis may also occur as the result of aberrant sexual practices.

Treatment of Disseminated Gonococcal Infections

Penicillin-resistant strains now common especially in Africa and Asia. Usually safe to give an initial dose of ampicillin 3·5 g or amoxycillin 3·0 g and probenecid 1 g orally and continue with ampicillin or amoxycillin 500 mg orally 6-hourly for 7 days or with erythromycin 500 mg orally 6-hourly for 5 days. An alternative when the organism is known to be penicillin resistant is spectinomycin 2 g i.m. b.d. for 2 days but expense limits its use. For arthritis, meningitis or endocarditis up to 24 g benzylpenicillin may be infused daily. For gonococcal meningitis in patients allergic to penicillin chloramphenicol 2–4 g daily or tetracycline 500 mg i.v. 6-hourly for 10 days may be given.

Chapter 41　　### BRUCELLOSIS *(Undulant Fever; Malta Fever)*

Specific infectious fevers caused by strains of the *Brucella* group of organisms, and characterized by a series of pyrexial attacks with sweats, muscular pains, arthritis and enlarged spleen.

Described under (1) *Brucella melitensis* infection; (2) *Brucella abortus* and *Br. suis* infections.

Brucella Group of Organisms

Bruce, 1887, discovered causal organism of Malta fever, considered to be a coccus, and named *Micrococcus melitensis*. Bang, 1896, isolated organism of contagious abortion of cattle considered to be a bacillus, and named *Bacillus abortus*. All group markedly pleomorphic and may be described as coccobacilli. Evans, 1918, discovered these two organisms to be almost identical serologically and genus named Brucella. Subsequently human infections recognized to be widespread in temperate climates, often with ill-defined clinical features. Localization of lesions in placenta and testes of animals now known to result from presence in these tissues in them, but not in man, of erythritol, or growth stimulant.

Main Varieties

1. *Brucella melitensis.* Primarily infects goats but also infects other animals: conveyed by goat's milk: organism of Malta fever.

2. *Brucella abortus.* Infection of cow, causing abortion: conveyed by milk. *Brucella suis*: allied strain in pigs.

Antiserum of each organism agglutinates others of group, but titre in general is not identical.

3. *Brucella canis*. Isolated 1969. Causes abortion in beagles.

4. *Br. ovis* causes epididymitis in rams. May be a biotype of *Br. abortus*. Now known to arise from *Br. abortus* when cultured with progesterone.

5. *Brucella neotomae* isolated from desert wood rats in Utah in 1957. Not known to infect man.

Francisella tularensis (*B. tularense*) closely related. Antisera to *F. tularensis* agglutinate *Brucella* in low titre. *Brucella*, however, do not adsorb agglutinins from tularense serum.

Brucella Melitensis Infection

Geographical Distribution
Widespread throughout world. Farmers, veterinarians and abattoir workers particularly exposed. The main cause of brucellosis around the Mediterranean, Central and S. America and the Far East.

Bacteriology (applies to *Brucella* group)
Morphology. Minute coccobacillus; markedly pleomorphic; occurs singly, in pairs, or (in cultures) in short chains. Non-motile. Stains with ordinary stains. *Gram-negative*.

Cultural characteristics. Grows on ordinary media but colonies not visible before third day, often much later: anaerobic culture may be necessary. No fermentation of carbohydrates. Growth usually improved under increased CO_2 concentration but CO_2 requirement less than that of *Br. abortus*.

Occurrence in human body. Numerous in spleen: can be isolated at autopsy. Present in blood during attack. Excreted in urine after fifteenth day in 10% of cases, usually for many weeks or months in untreated patients.

Immunology. Agglutinins appear in second week; persist through course, often in high titres. Result from development of IgM and IgG. The IgM can be destroyed by 2-mercapto-ethanol and this forms the basis of the 2-ME diagnostic test. The IgG is monovalent and nonagglutinating but it and some IgA which is formed can be detected by the Coombs' test. Agglutinins remain for long periods: titres about 1:50 suggest past infection, and titres over 1:100, in presence of pyrexia, suggest present infection, but diagnosis on basis of agglutination reaction very unreliable.

Mode of Infection
From infected animals, especially goats, and their products, milk, unmatured cheese, butter. Veterinarians and abbatoir workers may be infected through skin abrasions. Laboratory infections common. One attack apparently confers immunity.

Morbid Anatomy
Organisms localized in reticulo-endothelial system which hypertrophies and may exhibit non-caseating granulomas. Liver, spleen and lymph nodes may therefore be enlarged.

Symptoms
The condition is a septicaemia, characterized by irregular undulations of temperature but many infections are asymptomatic.

Incubation period. Usually about 15 days, but limits uncertain, at least 6–20 days.

Early symptoms. Insidious and vague. Malaise, often pain in eyes and jaws, muscular pains and gastric disturbances. May be ambulatory for several weeks.

Characteristic attack. Period of fever with symptoms lasting 1–3 weeks. *Period of defervescence* follows: may be slight pyrexia or normal temperature and convalescence from 10 to 12 days. *Relapse* occurs for shorter period. *Longer apyrexial period*, which may be again followed by yet milder relapse. Number of undulations variable, often three in mild case: in untreated cases may be numerous. *Duration*: very variable and course erratic; often 3–6 months in untreated cases, but may be more prolonged, 2 years.

Moderate attack or first undulation. (1) *Pyrexia*, 38·9 °C (102 °F) to 40 °C (104 °F) or 40·6 °C (105 °F), typically step-like rise and fall, but may be markedly irregular or even intermittent; (2) *Gastric disturbance*. Nausea and vomiting not infrequent. (3) *Profuse sweats*; (4) *Muscular pains*; (5) *Headache, restlessness*; (6) *Spleen* may be enlarged and tender; (7) *Pulse* relatively slow. Patient does not appear so ill as temperature suggests.

Severer symptoms. Occur more frequently during relapses. (1) *Headache* severe. (2) *Arthritis*: may be large effusion. Tends to be transient, but reappears in other joints. No redness. Pain may be agonizing. (3) Neuralgia pains and sciatica. (4) *Fibrositis*. Especially around ankle-joint. (5) *Anaemia*: progressive.

Complications and other symptoms.

1. *Bones and joints*. The transient arthritis of the acute stage may become purulent and involve bones. Large joints, particularly hip, affected. Spondylitis of the spine particularly important in longstanding untreated cases as found in tropics. Bone destruction and new bone formation lead to 'parrot beak' deformity of vertebrae and intervertebral disk damage to root pain.

2. *Nervous system*. Brachial and sacral neuritis have been reported, as have meningitis and encephalitis.

3. *Brucellar endocarditis*. Tends to affect aortic valve.

4. *Bronchitis and lung affections* occur in late stage.

5. *Orchitis and epididymitis*: rare but painful.

6. *Uveitis* occasionally reported.

7. Rashes rare and not specific: erythema, rarely purpura.

Progress
When relapses are numerous, great debility and mental depression develop, with anaemia and tachycardia.

Varieties
(1) *Ambulatory Form*: Evening pyrexia and slight malaise: recognized in Malta; (2) *Intermittent Form*: Daily variations of temperature, with chills followed by sweats. May suggest malaria; (3) *Malignant Form*: Fatal in 1–2 weeks. Typhoidal state develops. Very rare.

Diagnosis
Consider in prolonged pyrexia without obvious cause. Often difficult clinically, specially from sarcoidosis (when lymphadenopathy present), enteric (never rose-spots) also rheumatic fever, Pel–Ebstein syndrome, amoebiasis, malaria. Many cases of collagen disease and of the more obscure forms of pyrexia erroneously diagnosed as undulant fever on basis of agglutination test in absence of positive blood culture.

Cultures. Certainty in diagnosis depends on isolation of organism. Success more likely in early than in late stages of illness and when pyrexia marked. Should be repeated up to 5 and 6 times if negative in suggestive cases. Urine culture may remain positive when isolation of organisms from blood no longer possible. Isolation from faeces difficult.

Agglutination reaction. Unreliable, *see above.*

Blood count. Leucopenia with relative lymphocytosis.

Complement-fixation test. Usually positive after 6 months of infection.

Fluorescent antibody test. Useful for examining organisms in impression smears from biopsy tissue.

2-ME test. see p. 183.

Prognosis
Tends to spontaneous cure even without specific treatment. Mortality low.

Prophylaxis
Control of milk-supply. Pasteurization sufficient. In developed countries many agricultural areas and herds are made brucella free.

Treatment
Most antibiotics other than penicillin effective. Tetracycline in adult dosage of 2–3 g daily for 21 days much used. Trimethoprim 10 mg with sulphamethoxazole 50 mg (Septrin) per kg body weight daily for 21 days also effective. Most cases diagnosed as undulant fever and which fail to respond to such treatment ultimately found to have another disease. In many such patients reliance on agglutination reaction for diagnosis has been source of error.

For patients with bone or joint complications, streptomycin 1 g i.m. daily for 10 days in addition to tetracycline has been found effective.

Brucella Abortus and Brucella Suis Infections

General Features
A. Brucella abortus

1. Human *Brucella abortus* infections are widely spread. Is the cause of brucellosis in Britain.

2. In Britain most milch herds now tested and certified brucella free but formerly many affected. In developing countries infection of herds still common.

3. Pasteurization of milk, properly carried out, kills *Br. abortus* and renders milk safe for consumption, but does not destroy the agglutinins in milk.

4. Human infections are due to: (*a*) Consumption of infected milk; (*b*) Contiguity to infected animals, cattle and pigs, especially applying to slaughtermen, farm labourers and veterinarians. These may also become hypersensitive to the organism and develop a rash after removing uterine contents from an infected cow or local inflammation following exposure to the veterinary brucella vaccine S. 19.

5. Clinical symptoms develop in only a small proportion of those drinking infected milk, but existence of mild or latent infections is revealed by frequency with which healthy sera agglutinate with *Br. abortus* in low dilutions, e.g. 1:40.

6. No proof that *Br. abortus* has caused abortion in human beings.

B. Brucella suis
  1. Agglutination by monospecific serum differentiates *Br. suis* and *Br. abortus*, which are antigenically closely related, from *Br. melitensis*.
  2. *Br. suis* affects swine, hares, wild rats, cattle and dogs.

Clinical Manifestations
Br. abortus infections tend to be milder than *Br. melitensis*, pyrexia irregular or continuous and less often undulant, arthritis less marked. May be long ambulatory period.
  Br. suis infections clinically resemble *Br. melitensis*. Tend to be chronic. Bacteriological confirmation often difficult.

Treatment
As for *Br. melitensis*.

Chapter 42	*CHOLERA*

Acute infective disease due to presence of *Vibrio cholerae* in alimentary tract, and characterized by profuse diarrhoea followed by extreme dehydration and collapse. Infection is usually water-borne. The current 7th pandemic is caused by the El Tor biotype and since 1961 has spread from Suluwasi (the Celebes) through Asia and Africa to Europe.

Aetiology
Climate. Endemic and epidemic in tropics. Prevalence greatest in India. In temperate zones occurs as epidemics, but never endemic.
Season. Favoured by hot weather in temperate zones, especially in early autumn.
Age. Apart from infancy during which maternally transmitted antibodies and breast feeding protect, all ages affected. One attack does not always confer immunity.

Bacteriology
Organism discovered by Koch in 1883 in outbreak in Egypt.
Morphology. Small, motile, curved rods, about 2 μm long. In cultures mostly single, but two may join together like an S. A single terminal flagellum is usually present, but in some varieties may be two. Correctly it is a spirillum, and in liquid media growth tends to spirillar forms. The short forms are called vibrios. In old cultures numerous involution forms are seen; many are circular but are not spores. Gram-negative, but stains with ordinary stains, preferably weak carbol-fuchsin, one part to four of water.
  Strain Types. Three original strains known as Inaba, Ogawa and Hikojima distinguishable by agglutination with anti-sera against the organisms somatic (O) antigens. Antiserum O I agglutinates all cholera organisms including the El Tor vibrio which, is distinguished by: (*a*) being resistant to cholera bacteriophage, (*b*) causing rapid haemagglutination of sheep erythrocytes, and (*c*) forming a pellicle when grown in heart extract broth, (*d*) being resistant to polymyxin B. The El Tor vibrio can cause severe clinical cholera.

Other vibrios (NAG vibrios) not agglutinable with antisera to classical strains, mimic cholera but produce a less severe illness. This group includes *V. parahaemolyticus* (q.v.) whereas *V. cholera* is not invasive and produces its effects by enterotoxin acting on the small intestine, *V. parahaemolyticus* produces illness principally by invading the colon.

Cultural characteristics. Grows on all ordinary media. Classical characteristics are:

1. *Gelatin Stab*. On fifth day air bubble on surface, with funnel of liquefaction below.

2. *Gelatin Plates*. Colonies have granular surface with irregular outline like fragments of broken glass. Later, medium liquefies, with appearance of concentric rings.

3. *Cholera-red Reaction*. Growth in broth forms both indole and nitrite. Addition of pure sulphuric acid gives a pink colour from nitroso-indole. The culture must be 12 h old. Reaction increases up to 2 or 3 days. Not all broth preparations give reaction. Sulphuric acid used must be free from nitrites.

On broth growth forms no pellicle. In milk grows well without apparent change in medium.

Bacteriological diagnosis

1. Prepare a film from the stools and stain with weak carbol-fuchsin. Organisms may be present in large numbers.

2. Inoculate broth with loopful of stools. Incubate for 2 h, and subculture into media as described under cultural characteristics.

3. *Agglutination of cultures* with specific cholera antiserum. Essential for identification—over 100 non-cholera vibrios now known.

Distribution in the body. Localized to intestines, especially small gut. Vibrios do not penetrate deeply in mucosa. Occasionally in gallbladder; very rarely in other organs. Numerous in stools, especially in rice-water type. In preparations from stools, organisms tend to lie with long axes parallel, 'like fish in a stream'. When the intestine has been colonized cholera toxin stimulates secretion of an alkaline, bile-rich solution in which the organism multiplies profusely. Cholera toxin binds the organism to the cells and continues to act for many hours. It is not easily discarded by the cells.

Resistance. Life in ordinary drinking water very variable, and depends partly on the temperature and amount of organic matter present. Varies from a few days to 3 weeks. Can multiply in water. *Drying* kills in a few minutes. Can live several weeks on moist linen. In stools, rapidly overgrown by bacilli. El Tor vibrio more resistant than classical strains and survives longer in the environment.

Reservoir of infection. *V. cholerae* survives long periods in water of salinity 0·25–3·0% and pH about 8·0. Recent hypothesis is that between epidemics the cholera reservoir is in such estuarine environments and that shellfish from such waters transmits to man.

Agglutinins, antisera. *Agglutinins* appear in blood 8–10 days after onset, and reach maximum in 2–4 weeks, agglutinating *V. cholerae* in high dilution. Consequently of no value *for immediate diagnosis*, but agglutination is usually positive in cholera carriers.

Anti-cholera inoculation. Vaccine gives approximately 50% protection for about 3 months. Two injections, 4000 and 8000 million organisms, at interval of 1 week. No longer recommended by World Health Organization but many countries in endemic zones insist on travellers having vaccination.

Mode of Infection

All large epidemics water borne. Infection may be due to: (1) Water. Drinking water commonest vehicle. Ingestion of 10^{11} organisms required for infection in most healthy persons. Most surface water in endemic areas contains less than 10^2 organisms/litre. Organisms readily killed by HCl and achlorhydria is a predisposing factor. Vegetables, etc. washed in infected water; of less importance in view of large number of organisms normally needed for infection. Food as a vehicle thus contrasts with shigellosis where only 10^2 organisms are needed to cause disease. (2) *Cholera 'carriers'*. Virulent vibrios may be present in stools of clinically healthy persons but usually only for few weeks following an attack, which may, however, have been mild or unrecognized. Other 'carriers' include those incubating infection and asymptomatic contact carriers; (3) *Flies* may carry infection to food but *direct contagion negligible*. Doctors and nurses rarely affected. Is not air-borne. (4) Organism readily killed by acid. Thus those with achlorhydria or hypochlorhydria specially susceptible.

Duration of Infectivity

Vibrios are rarely passed for more than 2 or 3 weeks after an attack, and usually not more than 1 week.

Quarantine Period

Seven days.

Pathology

Intestinal mucosa relatively intact even in patients who have died from cholera. Cholera toxin now known to consist of 5 binding B units surrounding a central A_2 linking subunit and an adenylate cyclase stimulating subunit A_2. This becomes attached to intestinal cells especially crypt cells in the small intestine and stimulates profuse secretion as well as disturbing the delicate endocrine function of the intestine. Half or more of patient's bodily sodium content (usually whole content approx. 170 g in adult weighing 70 kg) may be lost in 24 h in stool and vomit. This causes great extracellular dehydration, haemocentration, hypotension, diminished glomerular filtration rate, oliguria or anuria, uraemia and muscular cramps. Diminished blood flow through kidneys may cause tubular necrosis. Much potassium also lost in stools. Metabolic acidosis also is usual—more sodium than acid lost. The symptoms in cholera are almost all explicable as a result of severe dehydration, potassium loss and metabolic acidosis upon relief of which successful treatment depends. When fluid loss accounts for 12% of body weight death usually ensues.

Symptoms

Incubation period. One to 3 or 4 days or up to 7 days. May be so-called 'premonitory diarrhoea', only recognizable during epidemics.

Clinical course usually described in three stages: (1) Stage of evacuation; (2) Stage of collapse (algid stage); (3) Stage of reaction.

Clinical Features

Onset abrupt: (1) *Severe purging*, followed rapidly by (2) *Vomiting*—often becomes incessant. (3) *Muscular cramps*, especially in legs; may be agonizing. (4) *Progressive exhaustion*. (5) *Thirst* becomes extreme. *Stools* at first yellow, rapidly become white, so-called *rice-water stools*, consist of vibrios and mucus. When frequent, usually odourless. *Tenesmus* usually absent. *Temperature* generally subnormal. *Pulse* feeble. Exhaustion and collapse increase. *Consciousness* usually retained but, particularly in children, hypoglycaemia of undetermined origin may cause drowsiness, unconsciousness or convulsions. Alertness for and correction of hypoglycaemia is therefore important. Duration 3–12 h. Recovery may now commence, or more advanced collapse follow — eyes sunken, skin wrinkled, restlessness, cyanosis, clammy perspiration, semi-consciousness or coma. Anuria may be complete. *Temperature* subnormal; may be high in rectum. *Pulse* rapid, may be impalpable. The collapse is due to dehydration and concentration of blood; sp. gr. of blood rises to 1060 and may reach 1072 or 1078 (normal 1058). Blood thick, polycythaemia and leucocytosis. Pressure low. 70 mm or under.

Convalescence. Usually rapid. Complications arising may be: *Recrudescences*, frequent and sometimes fatal. *Erythema* and numerous forms of skin eruptions.

Sequelae. Unusual, recovery generally complete: (1) Kidney damage; (2) *Cramps in muscles*; (3) Inflammations of mucous membranes, intestine, fauces and genitals; (4) Results of weakness; (*a*) Psychical, e.g. insomnia; (*b*) Tendency to boils, pneumonia, etc.

Clinical types. All grades of severity occur. *Ambulatory* cases without symptoms constitute 'carriers'. In mild types or *cholerine*, collapse slight but vibrios present in dejecta. In most severe form, *cholera sicca*, death from shock occurs before diarrhoea has developed, but large amounts of fluid are present in intestines.

Diagnosis
During epidemics diagnosis simple; confirmed by: (1) Vibrios in stools; (2) Agglutinins in blood. In sporadic cases confusion may arise with other conditions of diarrhoea and dehydration: (1) Arsenic poisoning; (2) Food poisoning; note abdominal pain, faecal stools, no suppression of urine; (3) Acute bacillary dysentery; note character of stools. Also fireman's cramp.

Prognosis
Unfavourable with very rapid onset, low temperature, and especially with high sp. gr. of blood, 1065 or over. Mortality formerly about 70%, but greatly diminished by saline infusions.

Prophylaxis
Preventive methods in checking epidemics: (1) Isolation of patients and disinfection of excreta. (2) Search for 'cholera carriers'. For individuals important to drink only boiled water and milk, and protect all food from flies. Inoculation with anti-cholera vaccine advisable. *Quarantine prevention*: Needs careful organization. Doxycycline, a long-acting antibiotic with activity similar to tetracycline reported useful. Use 100 mg orally daily for adults and for children less than 45 kg 2·2 mg/kg body weight.

Treatment
General treatment. Rest in bed and warmth, and replacement of water and salts lost. Give water by mouth frequently but in small amounts.
Intravenous therapy of highest value.

Intravenous fluid for cholera patients (Carpenter)

	Adults	Children
Sodium (mEq/1)	133	94
Chloride	98	64
Potassium	13	15
Bicarbonate	48	–
Acetate	–	45
Glucose (g%)	–	2

(Fluid prepared by dissolving 5 g sodium chloride, 4 g sodium bicarbonate (or for children sodium acetate) and 1 g potassium chloride in water to make 1 litre.)

Amount of i.v. fluid required. Blood pressure and specific gravity plasma useful guide in epidemics. Give 50–100 ml/min till radial pulse strong, then either measure stools and replace volume lost, or keep radial pulse adequate and skin elastic. Avoid crepitations in lung bases and abnormal distension of neck veins. If systolic blood pressure 80–90 mmHg adults usually need 3–5 litres fluid and up to 8 litres if below 80 mmHg.

Specific gravity plasma much used as a guide but its observation directs attention from clinical observation of patient which is best guide. Also correlation not a straight line and sampling errors considerable. If plasma specific gravity 1030 isotonic fluid deficit approximately 50 ml/kg body weight, if specific gravity 1040 deficit approx. 80 ml/kg body weight.

Children: Avoid excessive rate or volume of infusion as cerebral oedema in them may readily cause permanent brain damage and convulsions.

Oral fluid therapy. In mild cases or when i.v. fluid has restored adequate circulation oral fluid therapy possible. Dissolve in 1 litre water, 3·5 g sodium chloride, 2·9 g trisodium citrate dihydrate, 1·5 g potassium chloride, 20 g glucose. Give 750 ml/h for first 4 h in untreated cases. For maintenance give amount equal to volume of stool passed plus 50 ml/h for insensible loss as water, breast milk, tea.

Drugs. When vomiting ceases tetracycline helps to make stools vibrio negative. Dose, 40 mg/kg body weight per day after 2 days. Chloramphenicol and furazolidone less effective.

Other Species of Vibrios
Numerous species of vibrios have been isolated in varying circumstances.
Paracholera. Strains have been isolated from stools in mild or moderately severe cases of cholera-like illness. Distinguished from *Vibrio cholerae* by agglutination with antisera. *Vibrio parahaemolyticus* has caused such outbreaks. Infection may be conveyed by shellfish from salt water lagoons into which sewage drained, *see also* Chapter 33.

Chapter 43   **PLAGUE**

Specific infective disease caused by *Yersinia pestis*, conveyed by rat-fleas, and occurring in three clinical forms, bubonic, pneumonic and septicaemic. It occurs in vast epidemics. The three members of the *Yersinia* genus belong to the

Enterobacteriaceae family. *Y. enterocolitica* and *Y. pseudotuberculosis* are animal pathogens that infect man causing septicaemia and abdominal illnesses.

Aetiology
Present pandemic commenced in 1860s in Yunnan, China, near Burma border. It reached Hong Kong in 1894 and hence by ship to India.

Mode of spread. Principal factors: (1) Disease primarily affects rats, and in these is always septicaemic; (2) Rat-fleas suck blood containing bacilli; (3) Rat-fleas, leaving rats dead of plague, attack man and inoculate when biting; (4) Maintenance in rats is due to rat-fleas; (5) From rat to man, infection is solely by fleas. Infection is very rarely direct from man to man. Spread of epidemic is almost entirely due to spread in rats and thence to each human being individually (*Pulex irritans* possibly transmits direct from man to man). (6) Epidemic is always preceded by epizootic in rats or, less commonly, other ground animals, e.g. ground-squirrel in Californian epidemic, marmots in Siberia and multimammate mouse and four-striped grass mouse in Kenya. Fleas from these and other rodents may transfer to domestic rats. Sudden heavy mortality among rodents is warning of human epidemic and precedes human cases by about 2 weeks.

Rat-fleas in tropics are *Xenopsylla cheopis, astia*, and *brasiliensis: cheopis* bites man readily, *astia* less so and not when temperature of air exceeds 26·7°C (80°F). Prevalence of plague in a district is influenced by frequency of the different species. In temperate regions common rat-flea is *Ceratophyllus fasciatus*: does not bite man readily. *Y. pestis* secretes a coagulase enzyme that causes blood ingested by flea to clot in proventriculus, thus preventing entry into stomach of next blood meal. The 'blocked flea' in biting regurgitates *Y. pestis* into bite wound while attempting to feed. Now known that the coagulase is not active above 28°C and this explains why transmission of plague ceases in very hot weather.

Rats involved are *Rattus rattus*, small black house rat, and *R. norvegicus*, large grey sewer rat.

Pneumonic Plague; forms an exception to some of above statements. Spreads directly from man to man. Bacilli present in sputum in large numbers. Spread very rapid, but life of bacilli outside the body very short, hence no epizootic of rats occurs, and epidemic may be readily extinguished. Haemorrhage into the intestinal canal of infected rats has been postulated to cause pneumonic plague from inhalation of faecal-containing dust. Though pneumonic forms in rat-borne plague are rare they are relatively common in wild rodent-borne plague.

Distribution. Mainly a disease of tropics, but few countries have entirely escaped since present cycle commenced in 1894. *Frequency* greatest in cool weather in the tropics, and in 'hot' weather of temperate regions. Vietnam, Burma, Brazil, Kenya, Peru and Sudan have reported most cases in recent years. Some cases in South-Western U.S.A. transmitted from sylvatic rodents.

Bacteriology
Y. pestis isolated by Kitasato and by Yersin in 1894.

Morphology. Short fat bacillus with rounded ends and marked 'polar staining'. Non-motile and non-sporing. Stains with usual stains but *gram-negative*. Numerous involution forms occur in cultures, and in them bipolar staining less distinct. In tissues, mainly single; in liquid media may form chains.

Cultural characteristics. Optimal growth on agar and ordinary media at 28 °C. Killed readily by heat and antiseptics. At 37 °C but not at 28 °C and below produces a toxin, Fraction 1, which is antiphagocytic and activates complement. This virulence factor is pronounced in human but not in flea's body because of lower temperature of latter. *Y. pestis* cell walls also produce a lipopolysaccharide endotoxin which causes fever and disseminated intravascular coagulation. An endotoxin is also mitogenic for B lymphocytes.

Methods of isolation. (1) Bubonic plague: Puncture bubo with hypodermic needle, make and stain smears, and inoculate media. Attendant to wear gloves and mask and avoid spraying material from syringe into atmosphere. (2) Pneumonic plague: Smears from sputum; inoculate media. (3) Septicaemic type: Culture from blood; sometimes seen in blood films. Post mortem, bacilli present in every organ. Wayson's stain shows bipolar staining of organism best.

Serological diagnosis. Antibodies appear 8–14 days after onset of disease. Haemagglutination and fluorescent antibody tests performed in specialised laboratories.

Susceptibility of animals. Guinea-pigs, mice, rats, rabbits and most animals are susceptible. *Subcutaneous* or *cutaneous inoculation* results in: (1) Oedematous swelling at site of inoculation; (2) Nearest lymph nodes enlarge, haemorrhages present; (3) Septicaemia: bacilli present in blood. Death usually in 2–4 days. Bacilli in most tissues, especially spleen.

Morbid Anatomy

Bubonic type. *Enlargement of lymph nodes*, usually commencing in one group most commonly axillary or inguinal, forming the 'primary bubo'. Other groups subsequently enlarge, forming 'secondary buboes', but to less extent. *Bubo*: Inflammation of nodes, with extensive periglandular oedema; on section, haemorrhages present; in early stages, masses of bacilli; later, advanced necrosis of cells, bacilli often few or absent.

Suppuration not uncommon, but does not occur until second week, and hence never in the rapidly fatal cases.

Haemorrhages and focal necroses common in other organs, and cloudy swelling. *Pneumonic type*. Patchy bronchopneumonia. Lung may cavitate and heal completely if patient recovers.

Septicaemic type. General appearances of septicaemia with haemorrhages.

Spleen. Commonly enlarged.

Skin. Haemorrhages may be either *petechial* or *diffuse and extensive*. Over a bubo, the skin may be discoloured by hyperaemia.

Duration of Infectivity

Isolate for 7 days after start of antibiotic therapy.

Quarantine Period

Ten days—for those having had contact with pneumonic plague. Is internationally quarantinable and suspected patients should be reported to World Health Organization.

Symptoms

Incubation period. Two to five or possibly 10 days. Usually no symptoms. May be malaise. *Y. pestis* has been found in blood.

Clinical types. (1) Bubonic; (2) Pneumonic; (3) Septicaemic. Bubonic is the commonest epidemic type.

1. *Bubonic plague. Sudden onset*: chill, headache, backache, restlessness, rapid pulse and respiration, high fever. Symptoms often fully developed in a few hours. Great prostration occurs rapidly, and sometimes a typhoidal condition with coma and convulsions within 1–2 days. *Bubo*: usually in 1–2 days from onset. Femoral glands most common, next axillary. Cervical not uncommon in children. Swelling 2–10 cm. Very tender. Oedema may be extensive. Fever may fall slightly on appearance of bubo. Secondary buboes form later. Spleen usually palpable.

Symptoms usually *progress*: extreme prostration and cardiac weakness, tongue brown, sordes, vomiting common and delirium. Death in 2–7 days: usually 3 or 4 unless treated. Mortality in untreated cases at least 70%.

In certain epidemics, *petechiae and haemorrhages* common ('plague spots'). Haemorrhages from mucous membranes in severe cases.

Meningitis may complicate bubonic plague usually between the 9th and 17th days of the illness. *Y. pestis* may be found in CSF. Rarely the infection may present with meningitis.

In children, convulsions at onset, often so severe as to mask diagnosis.

Blood: polynuclear leucocytosis. Bacilli often numerous before death.

Temperature: High at onset 39·4–40 °C (103–104 °F). Subsequent variable: not uncommonly falls after 3–4 days, and rises rapidly again in 1–2 days.

During convalescence, a tragic fatal cardiac failure is known. Prolonged tendency to boils.

2. *Primary pneumonic plague. Sudden onset*: Rigors, pain, cough, fever and extreme prostration. Rapid pulse and respiration. Cyanosis. Sputum watery and bloody. Patchy consolidation in both lungs. Spleen palpable. Numerous bacilli in sputum. Fatal if not treated early. May be few physical signs in a patient gravely ill.

3. *Septicaemic type.* All forms of plague become septicaemic, but this type specially includes cases without bubo or local signs. General symptoms severe and mortality high if not treated early. Haemorrhages common. Does not occur as distinctive epidemic.

Pestis minor. Slight cases occur, especially towards end or beginning of epidemic and in inoculated persons. Bubo may form. Death from cardiac failure may occur.

Diagnosis

During epidemic easy. When suspected, bacteriological proof simple. Early cases in epidemic easily overlooked. Suspect *outbreaks of rapidly fatal pneumonia, especially with several cases in one household*: also buboes from tropics and seaports. In tropics, buboes occur from filariasis, lymphogranuloma venereum; also from syphilis and suppuration. *See also* p. 192 for serological diagnosis.

Prophylaxis

Vaccine treatment. Gives considerable immunity. Inactivated vaccine for 3–6 months: live attenuated vaccine for much longer: severe reaction. Recommended only for plague workers specially exposed, not for mass prophylaxis. Contacts should take tetracycline 250 mg 6-hourly for 7 days or sulphadiazine or sulphamerazine in doses of 3 g daily for 6 days, or 6 g daily for 3 days.

In large epidemics, a wide organization is necessary. The destruction of rats and examination of their bodies for bacilli, cleanliness of houses, and protection of uninvolved areas by quarantine are initial measures; dead rats must not be handled or closely approached except by trained personnel. Fleas are killed by dust containing 10% DDT. Contacts no longer ordinarily isolated; kept under surveillance and given prophylactic drug—*vide supra*. Bedding and clothing fumigated or destroyed.

Treatment

Streptomycin, chloramphenicol and tetracycline very effective. In India single intramuscular injection 1 g streptomycin found sufficient for adults in some outbreaks (0·5 g for children). Usual courses: streptomycin 12–20 g intramuscularly over 10 days; tetracycline or chloramphenicol 0·5 g intravenously followed by 0·5 g orally 3-hourly for 3 doses then orally 6-hourly to a total of 20 g. Tetracycline now generally preferred as severe toxic reaction may follow streptomycin therapy because of sudden massive destruction of bacilli.

To bubo, ice or fomentations but incision harmful. During convalescence, *avoid cardiac strain*.

Chapter 44   *TETANUS (Lockjaw)*

Infective disease caused by toxins of *Clostridium tetani*, and characterized by spasms of voluntary muscles, commencing usually in jaw and neck, and extending to rest of body.

Aetiology

Organism's prime habitat is soil to which it is conveyed in faeces of many species of animals, particularly horses. Tetanus occurs as a sequel to wounds and abrasions throughout the world particularly where soil is manured. More common and more severe in the tropics where tetanus neonatorum may result from severance or dressing of the umbilical cord with contaminated instruments or materials. Wounds of operations carried out during dust storms liable to be contaminated. Latterly, drug abuse has been a significant cause. Tetanus spores sometimes present in crude heroin and disease may develop when injected subcutaneously. *Warfare* in cultivated regions is always accompanied by tetanus. In the 1914–18 war, it was prominent among all armies until greatly controlled by prophylactic injections.

Modes of Infection

Contamination of wounds with infected soil containing bacilli or spores: septic and lacerated wounds more liable to infection than clean cuts, destruction of tissue forming anaerobic medium for bacilli. Never by ingestion. Occasionally from catgut (postoperative) freedom from spores difficult. May be no visible wound when causative lesion heals.

Bacteriology

C. tetani discovered by Nicolaier, 1885, and isolated by Kitasato, 1889, in pure culture anaerobically.

Morphology. Slender bacillus. Forms a terminal spore wider than bacillus, thus producing characteristic 'drum-stick' appearance. Stains with ordinary stains. Gram-positive. Weak methylene blue, followed by carbol-fuchsin, stains bacillus blue and spore as a red ring. Slightly motile. Numerous flagella: need special stain. When spores present, bacilli may be recognized in pus. Some of the 'gas gangrene' bacilli are closely similar, but shorter and thicker, and spores rarely quite terminal.

Cultural characteristics. *Strict anaerobe.* Isolation very difficult owing to simultaneous presence of other spore-bearing anaerobes. Methods mainly depend on resistance of spore to heat and subsequent growth anaerobically on numerous subcultures, trusting that one may be in pure culture.

Spores extremely resistant to heat and antiseptics; resist autoclaving at 121 °C for 10–15 min. Virulent for many years in dried cultures.

Occurrence of bacilli. Usually a few centimetres below surface of soil.

Distribution of bacilli in tissues. Present only at site of inoculation or in wound: seldom, if ever, present in organs or blood.

Pathological effects due to toxin produced.

Tetanus toxin. Injection of a filtered culture, i.e. pure tetanus toxin, produces all symptoms of tetanus. The toxin tetanospasmin produces the features of tetanus.

Mode of Action. An *incubation period* is always present between injection and onset of symptoms, even with enormous doses. The period varies with dose, mode and site of injection, but, for similar methods, varies with size of animals, e.g. guinea-pigs few hours, monkeys about 4 days, horses about 5 days.

Site of Action. Much animal and clinical research over the past 80 years indicates that tetanus toxin is absorbed at the local motor nerve endings and carried in nerves to the anterior horn cells where it interferes with synaptic junctions of inhibitory neurones and induces motor hyperactivity. Toxin also reaches the brainstem via the bloodstream, and there causes 'descending' tetanus. The masseters and facial muscles are first affected followed by more general spasms. Central action of the toxin appears to account for most of the features of clinical tetanus.

Autonomic nerves are also interfered with and the result is excessive sweating, fluctuating hypertension, periodic tachycardia and cardiac arrhythmias and increased secretion of catecholamines.

Susceptibility of animals. Nearly all animals are susceptible, degree varying greatly. Birds and cold-blooded animals very resistant.

General Tetanus

Symptomatology

Incubation period. Very variable. *Commonest 8–12 days.* Very rare under 5 days: never under 48 h. Upper limit doubtful; definite cases of 100–200 days. With central and cephalic wounds incubation period tends to be short, with distal wounds longer.

Premonitory symptoms (rarely observed except after prophylactic injections of serum). Stiffness, twitching, irritability, spasms and pains in muscles near wound, especially flexors.

Symptoms. Characterized by the development of tonic spasm of muscles, with frequent paroxysms. *Relaxation of muscles is not complete between spasms*.

Initial symptoms. May be slight sore throat, difficulty in swallowing, and fleeting pains in neck and back developing into stiffness of neck.

Onset of definite spasm. (1) *Masseters* and muscles of mastication. Often noted first on waking; (2) *Muscles of back .of neck*. *Spasm* extends, in order to: (3) Abdominal muscles, especially recti; (4) Back; (5) Limbs.

Condition developed. Tonic spasm and rigidity of muscles produce characteristic phenomena: (1) *Trismus*: severe spasm of muscles of mastication, teeth clenched, difficulty in feeding increased by spasm of pharyngeal muscles. Unable to open mouth or speak; (2) *Risus sardonicus*: lips stretched over closed teeth in ghastly smile; (3) Eyes partly closed: forehead wrinkled; (4) Head retracted to varying degree. Spine may also be extended (opisthotonos); (5) Lower extremities usually extended, very stiff: knees sometimes flexed; (6) Elbows may be flexed. *Hands usually escape*; (7) Abdomen very rigid.

Paroxysmal exacerbations of spasms, usually with agonizing pain, occur as result of stimuli, e.g. movements, sudden noises, or apparently spontaneously.

Pulse usually rapid, 100–120.

Sympathetic nervous system. Usually in severe cases. Profuse sweating, hyperpyrexia, tachycardia, labile hypertension, ventricular irritability and peripheral vasoconstriction.

Progress in favourable cases. Paroxysms diminish in severity and frequency: in severe cases which recover duration of spasms often about 3 weeks. Tonic spasm slowly passes away.

Progress in unfavourable cases. Paroxysms and rigidity increase in severity. Pulse often very rapid. *Temperature* often high but irregular; occasionally low. *Urine* may contain acetone bodies, albumin and casts.

Death may occur from: (1) Exhaustion: in these the spasm may have continued several days without alteration: starvation often a factor; (2) Asphyxia; spasm of respiratory muscles and glottis; (3) Cardiac failure: pulse very rapid; (4) Bronchopneumonia, patient drowns in own secretions.

Mental condition may remain clear: usually (and properly) obscured by sedatives.

Duration: death usually within 7 days: uncommon after 10 days.

Complication and Sequelae
Compression fracture of spine in severe spasms and hernia from increased intra-abdominal pressure. Affected muscles may remain stiff for longer periods, especially jaw muscles. *Recurrences* are on record, following shortly after apparent recovery.

Neonatal Tetanus
Continues to be very important in tropics. May develop 3–24 days after birth. the cause is almost always (i) cutting the cord with a contaminated object, e.g. a blade of elephant grass; (ii) dressing the stump with cow dung or contaminated earth; (iii) tying the cord with stringlike roots contaminated with soil. The first sign is usually failure to suck. Ideally should be treated with neuromuscular blocking agent and positive-pressure respiration (*see* p. 198) but these are often not available in tropics. Treatment with diazepam (p. 198) and tetanus human hyperimmune antitoxin or failing that equine tetanus immune globulin are then

the best alternatives with the other measures discussed in section on treatment (p. 198). The mortality in the tropics is of the order of 80–90% but in countries where muscular blockade can be practiced mortality is much reduced.

Localized Tetanus
Comparative frequency due to result of prophylactic injections of serum, probably preventing generalized tetanus but not completely neutralizing toxin.
Incubation period usually many weeks.
Onset with stiffness near wound: slight spasms follow: finally may be extreme chronic rigidity. In rare cases becomes generalized, and all intermediate forms occur.
Prognosis. Death very rare when spasm remains localized.
Treatment. For first day or two full treatment of tetanus, but rapidly relaxed, especially serum, when condition remains localized.

Cephalic Tetanus
Rare. Occurs only in wounds of head and neck or following middle ear disease. One or more cranial motor nerves involved, usually unilaterally. Commonly 7th nerve. Also spasm of masseters, and usually of pharynx, with *facial paralysis.* Almost invariably fatal if wound severe. May progress to generalized tetanus.

Prognosis
Varies with:
   1. *Length of incubation period.* Improving in general as period lengthens; but specially marked in contrasting durations over and under 11 days. Approximate mortality: 10 days and under, 60–70%; 11 days and over, 40–50%.
   2. *Rapidity of spread* of stiffness and spasms, and also frequency and severity of spasms. Paroxysms may commence at any interval from 12 h to 7 days after onset of trismus, the shorter the interval the more severe and fatal the disease: if interval less than 48 h, death usually within 6 days (Cole).
   3. *Frequency of convulsions.* If 2–3/h—favourable; if every few minutes— poor.
   4. *Severity of wound.* (Site of wound of less influence.)
   5. *Hyperpyrexia and very rapid or irregular pulse* are serious signs.
   6. *Age.* High mortality in very young and in the aged.
   Mortality of all cases 40% but recently considerably reduced as result of endotracheal intubation, positive-pressure respiration, and aspiration of bronchial secretions.

Diagnosis
Onset in jaw and posterior neck muscles: note also sweating, early abdominal rigidity and rise of temperature (rarely absent).
Trismus. Reflex from teeth, Vincent's angina, tonsillitis, etc., or osteoarthritis of jaw. No rigidity of neck muscles, or very slight. Difficulty rare.
Strychnine poisoning. (1) Jaw and neck not specially affected; (2) Complete relaxation between spasms; (3) Temperature normal.
Tetany. (1) Predisposing causes; (2) Extremities mainly affected, with characteristic posture.
Rabies. Physical disturbances prominent. Spasms specially affect larynx. History of being bitten.

Hysteria. Nervous wounded men with knowledge of symptoms occasionally develop trismus: other symptoms absent.

Bacteriological methods. Inoculation of mice alone reliable. Never delay treatment to await result.

Treatment

Immediately on diagnosis. Constitutes a formidable medical emergency. In many cases spasms are agonizing.

Antitetanic serum. Inject intramuscularly immediately on admission 3000–10 000 u of human tetanus hyperimmune antitoxin, infants 1000 u, to counteract any unbound toxin. If human material not availabile 10 000 u equine tetanus immune globulin. (For precautions, *see* Diphtheria, p. 167.) With severe wounds, repeat at weekly intervals before operation. Daily and frequent injections not indicated. *Intrathecal* injections contra-indicated, induce or accentuate muscular spasms: aseptic meningitis with severe cerebral symptoms not infrequent; also little evidence of efficiency. Serum injections have only limited value not comparable with diphtheria: can neutralize circulating toxin, but no appreciable effect on toxin which has already reached nervous tissue.

Wound. Cleanse carefully 1 h after serum injection.

Sedatives and muscle relaxants. Many regimes used. Diazepam currently drug of choice as it reduces spasms and sedates while being rapidly metabolized. Up to 1000 mg/day have been given i.v. in divided doses; initially 200–600 µg/kg (max. 25 mg) over 2–6 min; preferably a maximum of 3 mg/kg should be used over 24 hours. Number of spasms and tension of abdominal wall used as guide to amount required. If diazepam is not available sodium amylobarbital may be given intramuscularly in doses of 5 mg/kg body weight and repeated as required to produce relaxation. Chlorpromazine has sedative and antispasmodic effects. Up to 1000 mg daily has been used but danger of toxicity. If possible limit dose to 50 mg 6-hourly.

Neuromuscular blocking agents. In appropriate centres and with the help of one trained in their use—usually an anaesthetist—pancuronium or other curare-like substance, usually combined with tracheostomy and positive-pressure respiration can give excellent results.

Morphine is contraindicated as dangerously large doses are required to control spasms.

Tracheostomy. Perform if spasm of larynx or difficulty in breathing.

Nursing. Isolate in darkened room. Shoulders raised to aid respiration and relax abdominal muscles. Head supported. All disturbance and examination to be reduced to minimum.

Nutrition and hydration. Of great importance. Difficult owing to spasm of jaw. Nasal tube or tube through teeth if necessary. Fluids, milk and glucose. If this not possible, maintain intravenously.

Chest complications. Many deaths due to bronchopneumonia as patients cannot adequately clear bronchial secretion and infection follows. A major advance in treatment has been use of tracheostomy with positive-pressure ventilation and suction of mucus as required. Such treatment also obviates laryngeal spasm as cause of death and is particularly valuable for tetanus neonatorum. Should only be carried out in properly equipped and staffed centres.

Chemotherapy. May be indicated by condition of wound or respiratory infection. *C. tetani* sensitive to penicillin but injections of doubtful value once symptoms started and precipitate additional spasms. Logical to give a single large dose of depot penicillin to kill organisms and limit further toxin production.

Prophylactic Treatment
Active immunization. Injection of tetanus toxoid: 2 injections of 1 ml at interval of 6 weeks and third injection after 10–12 months. No reaction. High degree of immunity for several years. Give booster every 5 years.

Prevention of Neonatal Tetanus. Active immunization of pregnant woman during last trimester reduces incidence of neonatal tetanus as antibody crosses placenta. Valuable in highly endemic areas.

Prophylaxis after wounding. If the patient has had two or less doses of tetanus toxoid in the past a full course of active immunization (*vide supra*) should be given. If 3 doses have been given no further toxoid is essential unless, in the case of a minor wound the last dose had been 10 or more years previously and in the case of other wounds, 5 years previously.

Prophylaxis after clinical tetanus. A standard course of toxoid is recommended as clinical tetanus may be brought about by amounts of toxin too small to immunize.

Passive immunization. Inject 3000 u tetanus immune globulin i.m. for punctured or severely lacerated wounds, especially if contaminated with soil or clothing. After injury to those who have been previously fully immunized with tetanus toxoid, immune globulin is not required.

Chapter 45   # GLANDERS

Rare infectious disease due to *Pseudomonas mallei*, and primarily affecting horses and asses. Characterized in man by inflammatory and suppurative lesions arising especially in nasal mucous membrane and subcutaneous tissues, and occurring in an acute and a chronic form.

Bacteriology
Pseudomonas mallei discovered by Loeffler and Schutz in 1882. Isolated from man by Weichselbaum in 1885.

Morphology. A non-motile, non-sporing bacillus, in shape resembling turbercle bacillus, but thicker: is often beaded. Stains with ordinary stains: gram-negative. In tissues, mainly extracellular: numerous in acute and scanty in chronic forms.

Cultural characteristics. Grows readily on ordinary media: best on blood serum or potato at 37 °C. Growth visible in 2 days. On potato, a yellowish growth, which by eighth day becomes a characteristic chocolate colour. Easily killed, except by drying. Does not ferment carbohydrates.

Glanders in animals. Eradicated from Britain and USA. Present in much of tropics. Horses, asses and mules especially affected. Cattle immune. Occurs in two forms: (1) Glanders, involving nasal mucous membrane; (2) Farcy, involving the lymphatics.

Mode of infection in man. Direct infection of nasal mucosa or skin abrasion with bacilli discharged from the nostrils or from sores of diseased animals. Laboratory infection occurs with exceptional readiness, and many deaths are on record. Infection from patients also occurs, and extreme care necessary.

Morbid Anatomy
In acute forms lesions show ordinary suppurative changes. In chronic forms, an early glanders nodule resembles a tubercle, with greater acute inflammatory changes and less proliferation. Glanders is considered to be an infective granuloma.

Symptoms
In man, infection being through the nasal mucous membrane, occurs in acute and chronic forms.

1. *Acute glanders. Incubation period*: usually 4–8 days. *Onset*: sudden or insidious with general malaise and pains in muscles and joints. Constitutional symptoms and evidences of general infection in 2 or 3 days:

Nasal mucosa. Nodules form, ulcerate and discharge, with subsequent necrosis and foul discharge; nose becomes extremely swollen and red. Process extends to palate, mouth, larynx, pharynx and bronchi.

Eruption of papules. Especially on face and joints, rapidly becoming pustular, as in smallpox.

Abscesses form: subcutaneous, muscular and in joints.

Bronchitis. Common, and frequently pneumonia.

Extreme collapse and *acute septicaemia* follow. Liver and spleen often enlarged. Typhoid state may occur.

Death in from 1 to 3 weeks. Mortality 95% in untreated cases. Albuminuria usually present. Secondary infections common, but lymph glands and testes not specially affected in man.

2. *Chronic glanders. Incubation period* 10 days or upwards. At *onset* may be rash, papular, pustular, or erysipelatous.

Formation of abscesses is characteristic symptom, subcutaneous and intramuscular, especially near joints. Abscess ruptures: irregular ulcer results: discharge often very offensive. Abscesses often heal, and with great frequency break down again, or fresh abscesses form. Condition *often extremely chronic*: may be latent for months or years and then relapse and fresh abscesses form. *Recovery* in 50% of untreated cases, but at any stage, even after apparent cure, may develop symptoms of acute form and be fatal. In chronic condition nose and lungs usually escape, but there may be purulent nasal discharge.

Farcy. Also occurs rarely in man, from infection through skin. A spreading lymphangitis, with subcutaneous nodules—'farcy buds'—which form abscesses. May be acute or chronic.

Diagnosis
Occupation. Often suggestive.

Clinical diagnosis. Extremely difficult. At onset, usually mistaken for acute rheumatism or influenza.

Bacilli. These may be present in discharges, and recognized in films and cultures. Occasionally isolated from blood cultures.

Inoculation into animals. Intraperitoneal injection in guinea-pigs results in *suppuration of testes* in 2–3 days. Inoculation may be made from cultures or direct from discharge, but in later case secondary pyogenic organisms may cause acute peritonitis rapidly.

Injection of mallein. Of great value *diagnostically* for animals and man. Mode of preparation and technique resembles tuberculin.

Complement-fixation and haemagglutination tests. Of value in man and animals.

Treatment
Prophylaxis. Detect with mallein and destroy glandered animals. Disinfect premises. Warn attendants. Use protective clothing. Destroy or autoclave soiled linen, etc.

Acute and chronic cases. Good results may follow standard courses of absorbable sulphonamides, chloramphenicol, tetracycline or streptomycin.

Melioidosis
Rare disease resembling glanders, caused by *Pseudomonas pseudomallei* also known as Whitmore's bacillus. It is akin to *Ps. mallei.*

Epidemiology
Mainly in S.E. Asia. There were more than 300 cases with 36 deaths among American forces in the Vietnam war. The organism occurs saprophytically in still surface water and in rice fields in S.E. Asia and although it affects many animals, infection is now thought mainly to occur from soil contamination of skin abrasions. Inhalation of organisms is a possible infective route.

Morbid Anatomy
Scattered abscesses, particularly in lungs, liver and spleen.

Symptoms
Variable, septicaemic and pyaemic types known. Former characterized by fever, delirium, pulmonary involvement and hepatosplenomegaly. Later by abscesses in lungs and other organs, occasionally in skin. The infection may remain inapparent and latent for many years.

Diagnosis
Clinically may resemble typhoid, tuberculosis or mycoses. Organism cultured from blood, urine, pus, or CSF. Guinea-pig inoculation valuable. Haemagglutination, agglutination and complement-fixation tests are available.

Treatment
Chloramphenicol, tetracyclines and co-trimoxazole may be valuable but prolonged courses necessary. Ideally the organism's sensitivities should be assessed to ascertain the most effective agent. Abscesses, if superficial, should be incised.

Chapter 46   *ANTHRAX (Malignant pustule; Wool-sorter's disease. (In animals) Splenic fever)*

Acute infectious disease, caused by *Bacillus anthracis*, occurring in man in a cutaneous form as malignant pustule; in a pulmonary form; and very rarely in an intestinal form.

Aetiology and Epidemiology

Primarily a disease of animals, especially sheep and cattle, causing a septicaemia, with enlarged spleen, pulmonary congestion and bloody mucus discharge from nose and mouth. Occurrence is worldwide. Organism was discovered by Pollender in 1849, and investigated chiefly by Davaine, Koch and Pasteur. It is the organism in connection with which Koch first enunciated his postulates.

Diseased animals contaminate the soil which is the main reservoir of infection. Spores form, may remain viable for many years and infect grazing animals.

Human infection. Almost entirely from contact with animals or their products, very rarely from man to man. Wool and shaving brushes used to be sources of infection but legislation in developed countries ensures that these and other similar commodities are sterilized. Occurs among tanners, workers handling hides, raw wool, bone meal and cheap furs. In tropics, among cattle-rearing tribes, e.g. Maasai and Dinka of Africa, consumption of lightly cooked meat from infected animals is a source of intestinal and even tonsillar anthrax. Cultures with spore formation form a significant hazard to laboratory workers.

Bacteriology

Morphology. Large rod-shaped bacillus with clear-cut ends, length 6 µm and upwards. Non-motile. Forms spores readily. Bacilli in cultures often joined end to end in a chain. Stains with ordinary stains, and is gram-positive. Capsulated strains are always virulent, colonies rough: independent of spore formation.

Spores and spore formation. Never present in living tissues. Probably due to absence of free oxygen. Form readily in media and are always present in cultures. Especially frequent when organism is under slight adverse conditions, e.g. lying on soil or in dead animals. Spores are seen in body of bacillus or lying free. Stain with weak carbol-fuchsin, while body of bacillus may be stained by methylene blue.

Extremely resistant. When dry, alive after a year. Withstand boiling for 5 min. Very resistant to dry heat: also to gastric juice.

Cultural characteristics. Grows readily on all ordinary media. Most characteristic are: on agar plates at 37°, in 12 h, colonies visible with wavy outline like locks of hair. Medusa's head colonies. In broth forms long spiral threads. In deep gelatin stab, radiating spikelets and slow liquefaction, commencing at surface. Bacillus not very resistant apart from spores.

Filtered cultures non-toxic.

Clinical Features

The symptoms vary according to mode of inoculation, external or internal.

Usual varieties are: (1) *Cutaneous anthrax*: forms 90% of all cases. An erysipelatous anthrax, or anthrax oedema, also occurs rarely; (2) Pulmonary anthrax or wool-sorter's disease; (3) Gastrointestinal anthrax, rare.

1. Cutaneous anthrax or malignant pustule. Site of inoculation most commonly face, back of neck, and arms, being rubbed by hides carried on back. Incubation period from less than 1 to 7 days. Onset with *itching* at site of inoculation. *Papule* forms in 1–3 days: rapidly becomes a vesicle containing clear or bloody fluid and surrounded by area of congestion: *central necrosis* occurs. Typical *malignant pustule* present in 1½–3 days—viz. central black eschar surrounded by a ring of vesicles, and outside this an area of congestion. The pustule never contains pus. Subcutaneous oedema spreads from the pustule. Local lymph nodes enlarged.

General symptoms. Often mild but may rapidly become severe, with malaise, faintness, weak pulse and collapse. *Temperature* is high. Severity of general symptoms out of proportion to size of local lesion. Pain usually slight. Septicaemia develops as in internal forms, but modified. Death, when it occurs, usually does so in 3–5 days in absence of treatment. The mind is usually clear to the end. Cases vary in severity. Eschar may slough out, and recovery occur without treatment.

Mortality. Very low with treatment.

Anthrax oedema. No pustule occurs. Infection possibly from hair follicle. Oedema commonly commences on eyelid and spreads rapidly. Rarely diagnosed. Rare.

2. *Pulmonary anthrax*. Results from inhalation of organism. Incubation period 1–5 days then often cough without sputum and malaise, fever and aching limbs for a few days. This is followed by rigors, cyanosis, profuse sweating, stridor, rapid respiration, pain in chest, rapid and feeble pulse. Cough and bronchitis worse.

Temperature high. Oedema of chest wall develops, of gelatinous consistency. Much frothy mucus. Extreme collapse and death in 1–3 days unless treated. Mind usually remains clear.

Prognosis. Improves with longer duration. In some cases marked cerebral symptoms—convulsions, delirium, etc., due to bacilli in capillaries of brain. Diarrhoea occasionally severe.

Morbid anatomy. Main lesion in trachea and large bronchi, with oedema and haemorrhages. Lungs oedematous. Pleural and pericardial effusions. Great enlargement of thoracic glands. Apart from thorax, changes in the organs slight. Bacilli are numerous in the affected sites, in pleural fluid, blood and cerebrospinal fluid.

3. *Intestinal form*. Known in tropics from eating diseased meat. Tonsils may be affected. Resembles acute food poisoning. Chills, vomiting, bloody diarrhoea, convulsions, enlarged spleen.

4. *Anthrax meningitis*. A complication of the bacteraemia accompanying any form of anthrax. Collapse and toxic signs are marked and death virtually invariable. The cerebrospinal fluid is bloodstained.

Diagnosis

Cutaneous anthrax. Diagnostic features are: (1) Occupation; (2) Appearance of pustule. Rapid onset, eschar, oedema, no pus, no pain; (3) Sometimes severe symptoms with small local lesion and vice versa. (4) *Bacteriology*. Bacilli are present in edge of eschar, and in cultures. Inoculation of cultures or material from pustule into guinea-pig causes malignant gelatinous oedema at site of inoculation, with haemorrhages into organs, and bacilli present in large numbers especially in capillaries.

Immunofluorescence enables rapid and precise identification of bacteria in smears etc.

Indirect microhaemagglutination test is sensitive in detecting anthrax antibodies.

Differential diagnosis from *chancre* by rapid onset: from *cellulitis* and *erysipelas* by absence of pain; from *boils* by absence of pus; from *gas gangrene*, no gaseous crepitations; from *glanders* (no nasal discharge and no red vesicles).

Pulmonary anthrax. Enquire for occupational exposure. In early stages difficult. Examine sputum.

Intestinal anthrax. Consider in very ill patients with bloody diarrhoea and a history of possible exposure. Culture stool but treat immediately.

Anthrax meningitis. Distinguish from subarachnoid haemorrhage and from meningitis due to naegleria, pseudomonas, listeria, herpes simplex, and in America Rocky Mountain spotted fever. Careful CSF examination required, but give appropriate treatment immediately.

Prophylaxis (Man)
Protective vaccination of specially exposed persons possible.

Prophylaxis (Animals)
Infected animals burned or buried: in Britain post-mortem of animals suspected of anthrax illegal. An ear may be cut off using protective clothing and sent in a secure container to specialist laboratory.

Treatment
Local lesions to be kept clean, but no surgical treatment, as septicaemia may follow.
Antibiotic therapy. Penicillin continues to be the drug of choice, resistance is rare. For small lesions 0·6 g i.m. 6-hourly till lesion begins to improve—usually in 2 days. Then phenoxymethylpenicillin (Penicillin V) orally in similar initial doses then tailed off. For more severe cutaneous lesions and for pulmonary, intestinal and meningeal infections up to 24 g benzylpenicillin (penicillin G) may be required i.v. daily. In these severe forms a danger is that such treatment may be delayed because the diagnosis is overlooked. It is imperative to treat immediately any suspicious case; even so the prognosis is very poor. For these severe internal forms streptomycin 1–2 g i.m. daily should be given concomitantly with the penicillin. Erythromycin, tetracycline and chloramphenicol are also effective against anthrax but less so than penicillin.
Steroids. Where there is oedema of chest wall, neck or elsewhere associated with shock and/or respiratory difficulty, hydrocortisone 100–300 mg i.m. or i.v. daily or dexamethasone 10–20 mg i.m. or i.v. daily may be helpful.

Chapter 47   # LEPROSY

Infective disease of marked chronicity caused by *Mycobacterium leprae*, and characterized particularly by lesions in the skin, mucous membranes, nerves, and eyes. The nature of the lesions varies with the host's degree of cell-mediated immunity.

Epidemiology
Referred to in most ancient literature of the East. The clinical picture is so distinctive that most early descriptions probably refer to the disease itself. Most prevalent in the tropics, but distribution is not limited geographically. Has occurred in temperate countries and still occurs in Japan and Korea. Most frequent in India, Africa, and China. Formerly spread over the entire Old World, but commenced to decline in the fifteenth century. In Great Britain now only imported cases. Infection mainly occurs from nasal secretions of untreated or relapsed lepromatous leprosy patients though bacilli are also found in breast milk

of lepromatous women. Close contact, especially in childhood is important in transmission, the most probable portals of entry being the nasal mucosa, the skin and the gastrointestinal tract but the exact mode of transmission is not known.

Aetiology
The *Mycobacterium leprae* was discovered by Hansen in 1871. Slender, non-motile bacillus, resembling tubercle bacillus in appearance and staining reactions. Gram-positive and acid-fast (in 12% acid). Stains with ordinary stains more readily than tubercle bacillus. Bacillus has never been cultivated in vitro but in vivo growth is obtained in foot pads of mice, hamsters and rats; this may in part be explained by the organism preferring slightly lower temperatures than 37 °C (98·4 °C) for growth. Hence cooler peripheral sites both in man and experimental animals are those that best support the organism's growth. Systemic infections develop in thymectomized or irradiated mice, in nude mice and about half of normal nine-banded armadillos. From the latter most leprosy bacilli are now obtained for research.

Pathology
Histological appearances vary according to resistance of patients.
Indeterminate leprosy. An initial reaction to infection in many persons especially children. May disappear in a few months without further development or may progress to a defined type. Histologically there is lymphocytic cuffing of neurovascular bundles in the skin and very scanty *M. leprae*
Tuberculoid leprosy. Develops in those with high resistance.
   The lesions commence in nerve twigs where the Schwann cells engulf them and coalesce to form giant cells, later surrounded by lymphocytes, eptheliod cells and histiocytes. In the dermis similar lesions follow neurovascular bundles and are surrounded by fibrous tissue. The clear zone normally present beneath the epidermis is encroached upon by inflammatory cells and the rete cones are flattened and irregular. The lepromin test is strongly positive.
Lepromatous leprosy. Develops in those with low resistance. In this, bacilli break out from the nerve fibrils in which they have developed in the early stages of the disease—usually the nasal mucosa and adjacent skin—they multiply profusely and are engulfed by enormous numbers of histiocytes which infiltrate the dermis fairly uniformly, their long axes may be parallel and the occurrence has been referred to as 'fish in a stream'. Bacilli multiply within the cytoplasm of these cells and produce lipoid material giving the cell cytoplasm a foamy appearance. Such cells may coalesce to form 'globi'. The epidermis becomes thin and rete cones are flattened. A zone clear of cellular infiltration occurs just below the epidermis. There is little invasion of nerves by inflammatory cells and lymphocytes are scanty. A bacteraemia is usual and bacteria are carried to the spleen, the Kupffer cells in the liver, the lymph nodes and the reticulo-endothelial system generally. They become numerous in the testes but not in kidneys, heart, lungs and central nervous system.
Borderline types. In those with an intermediate degree of resistance borderline types may occur in which the histological features range through a 'spectrum' of which tuberculoid leprosy (TT) is the polar type at one end of the range and lepromatous (LL) at the other. Between them are borderline-tuberculoid (BT), borderline (BB), and borderline-lepromatous (BL).
   Immunology. In untreated lepromatous and borderline lepromatous leprosy

there is great depression of cell-mediated immunity both specifically against specific leprosy and non-specific stimuli. The latter slowly improves with treatment in lepromatous patients but the former does not. Some borderline lepromatous patients develop partial specific cell-mediated immunity after a year or two's treatment. In lepromatous patients circulating T lymphocytes are diminished. Albumin-globulin ratio in the blood is reversed, IgG is increased and IgM and IgA may be increased. There may also be false positive tests for syphilis, thyroglobulin antibodies, LE cells, antinuclear factor and cryoglobulins.

Lepromin test. Helps differentiate lepromatous from tuberculoid and related forms. The antigen contains leprosy bacilli and is injected intradermally. The late (Mitsuda) reaction is read at 3–5 weeks and is positive in tuberculoid states when an erythematous papule 3–10 mm or more develops. It is not a diagnostic test—many uninfected persons give a positive result.

Clinical Features

Clinical like pathological features vary according to the resistance of the patient and the type of leprosy which accordingly evolves.

Age. Commonest between 10 and 30 years.

Incubation period. Usually 3–10 years. Longer for lepromatous than tuberculoid.

Nerves particularly involved. Nerves of predilection are the ulnar, the radial and median at the wrist, great auricular, lateral popliteal and posterior tibial.

Initial symptoms (indeterminate leprosy). Sometimes a period of recurrence of indefinite symptoms: fever, malaise, sweating, vague pains, and appearance of fleeting macular lesions. May progress to tuberculoid, lepromatous or borderline forms or may heal without recurrence.

Tuberculoid leprosy

   Onset: Insidious. Progress very slow.

   Prodromal symptoms: Indefinite. Malaise and occasional pyrexia. Vague pains in limbs. Areas of hyperaesthesia.

   Tuberculoid eruption: Erythema appears in localized areas; lesions affect the body asymmetrically; size varies from 1 cm to several centimetres. Edge of lesion is clear cut and elevated. Lesions are few in number. Usually situated on outer aspect of limbs or on face or buttocks. Lesions do not involve hairy scalp. On subsiding, area may be pigmented or white; local paraesthesia. As erythema extends central portion heals leaving a ring of inflamed skin. Nerves supplying affected skin thickened and may be nodular. Ulnar and peroneal nerves often affected. Loss of sensation over lesion but may be difficult to demonstrate on face. Corneal anaesthesia may follow injury due to local anaesthesia (Vth cranial nerve) or lagophthalmos (VIIth cranial nerve). Anaesthetic digits liable to repeated injury. Seldom demonstrable bacilli in lesions. May heal spontaneously, seldom if ever regresses to lepromatous or dimorphous type.

Lepromatous leprosy. A leproma is formed by infiltration of deeper layers of skin; size varies; commence as small papules or thickened skin in multiple patches—some of them hypopigmented—remaining from erythemata. Areas grow and multiply. Ill-defined macular erythematous areas develop on cooler parts of body and have shiny surface; they are not anaesthetic. Nose becomes blocked early. Anaesthesia develops late and is of 'glove and stocking' type.

   Fully developed. Marked changes are:

Face: Natural lines obliterated and replaced by creases between masses of growth—leonine facies. Hair on face and eyebrows drops out, but scalp not affected. General expression sombre. Ears, especially lobes, much thickened.

Mucous membranes: Nasal discharge. Nose flattened. Pharynx and larynx affected. Vocal cords infiltrated—voice hoarse, or only whisper. Tongue infiltrated or ulcerated.

Limbs: Covered with nodules and masses to varying degrees. Nerves thickened, muscular wasting and anaesthesia of 'glove and stocking' type due to nerve fibrosis and damage.

Eyes: Affected commonly. Conjunctivitis, keratitis, iritis common. Caused by fine lepromatous deposits.

Subsequent Progress. Variable: (1) Quiescent for many years, or marked remissions; (2) Exacerbations; more common. Pyrexial attacks occur, with spread of growth. Ulceration of masses common, with discharge: cicatrix on healing: often chronic; (3) 'Mixed' form frequently develops, with symptoms of 'neural' leprosy.

Late lepromatous leprosy

Contractions. Ulnar nerve especially affected, whence 'claw hand'.

Trophic Changes. (1) Perforating ulcers arising from bullae or injuries resulting from anaesthesia; (2) Loss of fingers, toes from injury due to anaesthesia. Also absorption of phalangeal bones from leprotic endarteritis. Both processes cause fingers to become shortened.

Eyes. Affections result from lesions of Vth and VIIth nerves and fine lepromatous deposits.

Borderline forms. *Borderline tuberculoid*: lesions are similar to those of tuberculoid but are more numerous and smaller. Nerve involvement and consequent deformity is common.

Borderline: the typical lesion is annular with a broad irregular rim and an inner raised edge within which is a hypopigmented, anaesthetic and 'punched out' centre. There is considerable damage to and enlargement of nerves.

Borderline lepromatous: the lesions at first are similar to those of the borderline type but are more numerous and later many erythematous nodules or plaques develop with other features similar to those of the lepromatous form.

Reactional states

1. *Related to increase in cell-mediated immunity*. Swelling, erythema and sometimes ulceration of lesions, particularly in the three borderline types. Often associated with painful reaction in local nerves and nerves of predilection. Associated with increase in delayed-type hypersensitivity and usually an increase in specific cell-mediated immunity. Most commonly occur in patients being treated.

2. *Erythema nodosum leprosum*. Usually occurs after some months of treatment in lepromatous or borderline lepromatous patients. Fever and painful pink nodules develop in subcutaneous tissue, often associated with painful neuritis, due to immune complex formation with antigen derived from dead leprosy bacilli. Local vasculitis results but circulating immune complexes are the cause of glomerulonephritis and probably of the fever.

Diagnosis

Suspect in patients with skin lesions as described above plus nerve lesions, thickening and/or anaesthesia: Diagnosis in advanced cases is usually obvious—even to lay persons.

Early lepromatous leprosy. Bacilli present: (1) in nasal secretion; (2) in skin smears or in excised piece of skin. Stain with Ziehl–Neelsen technique. Clinical diagnosis from syphilis, tuberculides, erysipelatoid attacks from septic foci. Wassermann reaction is often positive in leprosy.

Early tuberculoid leprosy. Diagnosis depends on erythematous lesions with clear-cut outer margins, thickened nerves, and anaesthesia. Often no bacilli in nose or skin. Tubercles present in biopsied affected skin.

Differential Diagnosis

Thickened nerves have to be distinguished from those of amyloidosis and familial progressive hypertrophic interstitial neuritis of Déjérine and Sottas. The depigmented skin in leucoderma (vitiligo) often causes fear of leprosy and very occasionally so does that of onchocerciasis and yaws. The lesions in leprosy are, however, hypopigmented, not depigmented, and usually are anaesthetic which the others are not. Sarcoidosis and diffuse cutaneous leishmaniasis may occasionally be confused clinically but not histologically.

Prognosis

Tuberculoid and indeterminate forms are usually self-limiting. Other forms have an excellent prognosis with treatment but usually are steadily progressive without it.

Treatment

General treatment. Diet, hygiene, follow up, attention to deformities and provision of well fitting shoes of importance.

Chemotherapy. Treatment best carried out by institutions with special facilities. Combined initial therapy now recommended to reduce resistance of *M. leprae* to drugs.

WHO now recommend two main regimes depending on whether bacilli are scanty or numerous. The drugs are taken orally.

For paucibacillary leprosy: rifampicin 600 mg monthly for 6 months plus dapsone 100 mg daily for the same period.

For multibacillary leprosy: Dapsone, 100 mg daily; rifampicin, 600 mg once monthly; clofazimine, 50 mg daily or a 300 mg dose monthly.

This treatment should continue for a minimum of 2 years and preferably till smears are negative.

Clofazimine: Has anti-inflammatory and anti-leprotic activity. Stains skin red but stain disappears on ceasing drug administration.

Ethionamide and prothionamide: Either of these may be given in monthly doses of 500 mg in addition to the standard regimes. One of them may be used in doses of 250–375 mg daily in place of clofazimine if the latter is unacceptable to the patient because of its skin-staining effect.

Reactional states. May be controlled with prednisolone 30–40 mg daily but once on steroids it may be years before leprosy patients can be weaned off them. Attempt therefore to control reactional symptoms with simple analgesics or failing them stibophen which has a steroid like effect (2 ml daily i.m. or i.v. for 5-day courses). Thalidomide 200 mg daily initially then reduced, is very effective and may be given to males and postmenopausal females. Clofazimide because of its anti-inflammatory effect is very valuable and may be used up to 300 mg daily for 3 months, then reduced.

Prophylaxis
Tuberculoid type is generally accepted as non-infective and segregation is unnecessary. Segregation indicated in lepromatous type in active stages only. Local prejudices and administrative difficulties often great. Compulsory notification often causes concealment. Children of leprous subjects should be seperated from infected parent or parents until their disease is under control and bacilli granular.
Note: In Great Britain leprosy is a notifiable disease. Notification and consultation with one of the experts listed in the Department of Health and Social Security '*Memorandum on Leprosy*' should precede treatment.

Chapter 48   **TULARAEMIA**

Specific infectious disease caused by *Francisella tularensis*, and characterized by fever, glandular enlargement and septicaemic symptoms.

Aetiology
Primarily a disease of rodents, squirrels, rabbits, hares and also sheep. It is transmitted to man and by handling (and possibly consuming) infected animals, by bites of ticks and other blood-sucking insects, especially in America, the deer fly. Laboratory infections occur with exceptional ease, causes infection when inhaled.
   Francisella tularense: minute gram-negative coccobacillus: difficult to culture: serological affinities with *Brucella* group. All isolates are serologically homogeneous but may be divided into two categories. Type A is isolated from rodents and is highly virulent in rabbits; type B from water and aquatic animals and is less virulent in rabbits.

Geographical Distribution
Reported in America, Japan, Russia, Norway, Sweden and Austria but not from Great Britain. Probably widespread but unrecognized.

Symptoms
Incubation period: 1–10 days.
1. Ulcero-glandular type. From infected bites. Papule forms at site and necroses, leaving ulcer. Lymph nodes in area enlarge and may suppurate. Onset of symptoms sudden: fever, scattered pains: duration 2–3 weeks. *Oculo-glandular type*: Conjunctivitis, oedema of lids, from rubbing eye with infected fingers, enlarged glands in neck. Mortality low.
2. Typhoidal type. From infection intradermally, or via respiratory or gastrointestinal tracts. Constitutional symptoms without local lesions: pyrexia, pains, lassitude. Pulmonary complications common: many fatal cases. Otherwise recovery in weeks or months: relapses common.

Diagnosis
From enteric, rat-bite fever, plague. *Agglutination reaction*: positive in second or third week. Organism obtained by injecting blood ulcer or lymph-node juice into

guinea-pigs. Only done under special circumstances because of risk of causing laboratory infections. *F. tularense* may also be identified by fluorescent antibody tests. Blood cultures negative.

Treatment
Streptomycin is drug of choice given i.m. in doses of 0·5 g every 12 h for 72 h or until temperature becomes normal and then daily for 5 days. Chloramphenicol and the tetracyclines also very effective in standard dosage regimes. Homatropine drops used for ocular tularaemia. Sulphonamides and penicillin: no effect.

Chapter 49   # BARTONELLOSIS *(Oroya Fever; Verruga Peruana; Carrion's Disease)*

An acute specific fever characterized by rod-shaped *Bartonella bacilliformis* in the red cells and by two distinct phases in man, the first, Oroya fever, and the second, verruga peruana, which follows after 4–6 weeks and is characterized by eruption of granulomas.

Distribution
Confined to certain narrow hot valleys on western slopes of the Andes.

Aetiology
The rod-shaped *Bartonella bacilliformis* present in erythrocytes and reticulo-endothelial cells cause the disease. The infective nature of the disease was established by Carrion, a medical student, who experimentally gave himself a fatal infection. *B. bacilliformis* can be cultivated on blood-agar, on Noguchi's medium, and in tissue culture. Transmitted by female *Lutzomyia* (*Phlebotomus*) *verrucarum*. All ages and both sexes susceptible.

Pathology
Basic concept is that Oroya fever is initial form of infection and verruga peruana results from a change in host-parasite relationship.
Oroya fever. Erythrocytes heavily invaded by bartonellae have a short lifespan and are engulfed by reticulo-endothelial cells in liver, spleen and lymph nodes which consequently enlarge. In liver, sinusoids choked with parasitized cells and centrilobular necrosis occurs. *Bartonellae* invade the endothelial cells lining blood and lymph vessels.
Verruga peruana. Granulomatous eruption in skin with many new blood vessels of small diameter relative to the thickness of their lining endothelium. Results from proliferation of invaded reticulo-endothelial cells and increased immunity to the infection which prevents its more general manifestations.

Clinical Features
Oroya fever
   Incubation period. Three weeks
   Onset insidious, but progress rapid in severe cases.
   Temperature rises: irregular. Falls in fourth week.

Pains, diffuse and severe. Bones often tender.

Anaemia develops very rapidly: red cells may fall to 500 000/mm^3 in days. Anaemia usually normocytic but haemolysis increases the demand for folic acid and secondary megaloblastosis may result. There is also leucocytosis (20 000); many abnormal cells. Bartonellae numerous in severe cases during pyrexia. Skin waxy pale due to anaemia.

Lymph nodes enlarge. Liver and spleen palpable, and tender.

No eruption.

Prognosis. Good with antibiotic treatment. Mortality in pre-antibiotic epidemics 30–40%. Now known that most deaths were due to secondary infection with salmonella, especially *S. typhimurium*, to which these patients particularly susceptible.

Verruga peruana. A later phase of Oroya fever in those surviving initial stage.

Incubation period. 30–40 days after a previous attack of Oroya fever.

Onset. Pyrexia. Rheumatic pains.

Eruption. Miliary papules or larger nodular excrescences; are granulomas. On skin and mucous membranes. Haemorrhages often extensive, e.g. from alimentary tract. Smaller lesions dry up and fall off. Larger ones may lead to permanent fibrotic nodules.

Mortality. Low.

Diagnosis

Bartonella in stained blood films. Also complement-fixation and agglutination reactions.

Complications

Patients prone to salmonella infections.

Treatment

Acute manifestations cease dramatically with penicillin therapy but infection not eradicated. Chloramphenicol preferred to penicillin lest salmonella infection also present. Dose 500 mg 6-hourly for 5–7 days.

Relief from anaemia by blood transfusions. Folic acid 5–10 mg orally per day may be helpful if there is megaloblastosis.

Chapter 50 **ACTINOMYCOSIS, NOCARDIOSIS AND MADURA DISEASE**

Organisms causing actinomycosis and madura disease have latterly been reclassified. *Actinomyces* formerly regarded as fungi are now classed as prokaryotic bacteria as their cell walls lack the chitin found in fungal cell walls and they reproduce by fission, never by spore formation as do true fungi. Also, important to the clinician, they are sensitive to antibiotics but not to amphotericin B which is a specific antifungal agent. *Actinomyces* are microaerophilic and anaerobic. The closely related *Nocardia* are aerobic and have been placed in a separate family Nocardiaceae. They are classed as actinomycetes.

Madura disease can be caused either by true fungi, e.g. *Madurella mycetomatis* or by *Actinomycetes* including *Nocardia*.

Actinomycosis and Nocardiosis

For many years the syndromes produced by *Actinomycosis* and *Nocardiosis* have been considered together and indeed have often been confused. A case can be made for giving each a separate chapter but the diseases they cause and the methods of diagnosing and managing them are so similar that to consider them together provides a clearer picture of the spectrum of disease produced and of its management.

Chronic granulomatous lesions, tending to suppurate, produced by *Actinomyces or Nocardia* species.

A. bovis occurs in cattle and is similar to *A. israelii* the commonest actinomycete infecting man. It was long thought to be transmitted from cattle to man but this is not now considered to be so and the two organisms are distinct and separate.

The Organisms
Related both to bacteria and to higher filamentous fungi or moulds. Characterized by true branching; *vide supra.*
Actinomyces israeli. The commonest actinomycete in man. Occurs in normal mouth in pleomorphic rod-shaped bacterial form and in tissues as a mycelium. In pus mycelial clumps form white or yellow 'sulphur granules'.
Nocardia asteroides. Closely related to *Actinomyces* but do not form clubs though

213

they may occur in granules when they cause mycetoma lesions but not in visceral nocardial disease. They usually develop into interlacing branching threads. It is aerobic and grows readily on 1% dextrose agar at 37 °C. On this produces long branched and fragmented forms and pale yellow colonies. In tissues hyphae 0·5–1·0 μm in diameter and may fragment into rod-shaped or coccoid particles.

Character of Pus
From an abscess pus is thin, greenish-yellow, *containing small clumps, size of a pin's head*, visible to the naked eye, usually yellow, and formed of Actinomyces so-called 'sulphur granules'. (Old pus may be thicker.)
Examination of pus. Pick out granule and place on microscope slide: tease or squeeze clumps flat under cover-slip, stain with Gram or carbol thionin. Centre composed of branching filaments with outer layer of club-shaped bodies.

Culture
Actinomyces israelii grows on blood-agar or brain-heart medium containing 2% agar. Grows best anaerobically with 5% carbon dioxide for 4–6 days at 37 °C. It produces opaque white lobulated colonies.

Mode of Infection
Actinomyces israelii, probably from human contact and organism gains entrance to body via damaged tissue, especially carious teeth. Various *Actinomyces* formed on grain or in soil no longer considered pathogenic.

   Nocardia asteroides is widely distributed in nature and in the soil and usually enters the body via the lungs or by wound infection leading to mycetoma. Latterly many opportunistic infections have been suspected in those with lymphoreticular neoplasms, debilitating diseases and persons with impaired cell-mediated immunity.

Changes produced in Tissues
Chronic inflammatory reaction, little granulation tissue: spreading suppuration: mainly filamentous forms. In dense tissues more granulation; in soft tissue, e.g. liver, more pus formation.

Clinical Characteristics
Usually in males. Three chief sites, possibly corresponding to paths of infection:
1. *Jaw and neck. Chronic* unilateral swelling of jaw and neck; later superficial *abscesses* on skin, which discharge pus. Mode of infection: probably through carious tooth or tonsil. Forms approximately 50% of cases.
2. *Intestinal.* Especially appendix and following acute appendicitis, also caecum and large intestine. Great tendency to spread in various directions ignoring anatomical boundaries: to peritoneum, forming abscesses between coils; to abdominal wall, causing superficial oedema and abscesses; to retroperitoneal, retrocaecal and perirectal tissues. Occasionally in oesophagus. Infection: probably with food.
   Symptoms. Depend on site: septic phenomena, chronic appendicitis, often indefinite nature. Comprises approximately 25% of cases.
3. *Pulmonary. Nocardia* spp. show special tendency to affect lungs. Form about 25% of cases. Various types of chronic pulmonary disease may be confused with tuberculosis: (*a*) Chronic bronchitis; (*b*) Resembling miliary tuberculosis; (*c*) Bronchiectasis, fibrosis, foetid bronchitis; (*d*) Formation of small but rarely of

large cavities. Great tendency to involve pleura, ribs with bone destruction, sternum, and thoracic wall, forming empyema or abscesses. Infection: usually via respiratory tract. Acute forms with confluent bronchopneumonia are particularly likely to occur in nocardia infection and in the immunologically compromised host.

Symptoms. Irregular pyrexia, cough, wasting, sputum which not always contains the organisms. Physical signs often unilateral.

Metastases and formation of secondary abscesses occur in many directions, possibly by leucocytes engulfing filaments. Of importance are:

Liver. Not uncommon: characteristic 'honeycomb' appearance, containing pus.

Cerebral abscesses, especially in pulmonary cases.

Skin infections have been recorded. Also kidneys, etc.

Diagnosis
Depends on identification in pus, tissues, or sputum of the causal organism. Involvement of ribs and bony structures suggests these infections rather than tuberculosis as does sinus formation.

Prognosis
Greatly improved by modern therapy. Depends on extent of spread and on site: (1) Jaw and neck: recovery usual. (2) Intestinal: prognosis fair. (3) Pulmonary: more severe. Tendency to recurrence after apparent cure: but rare after 2 years' freedom.

Treatment
Combined surgical and medical:

Medical. For *A. israelii* penicillin preferred in high dosage—5–12 g daily i.m. or i.v. for 6 weeks or until good response obtained then phenoxymethylpenicillin 2–6 g orally daily or 2 g tetracycline orally daily for 6–12 months. Erythromycin is an alternative to penicillin or tetracycline. *N. asteroides* usually responds well to high doses of sulphonamides given for at least 6 weeks and preferably 6–12 months to prevent recrudescences. Long-acting sulphonamides and sulphones also used.

Surgical. Usually impossible to remove focus entirely. Aspirate small and drain large abscesses.

Mycetoma (Madura Foot, Madura Disease)

A chronic granuloma, almost confined to the foot, and characterized by great enlargement, formation of cavities, and discharge of granules. Due to infection with *Madurella* or *Nocardia* spp. Prevalent in India, Sudan and other parts of the tropics. Occasionally hand or other parts affected.

The Organisms
Caused by *Actinomyces* and *Nocardia* species, *see* pp. 213–5, and by true fungi. The actinomycetes include *Actinomadura madurae*, *Streptomyces somaliensis* and the nocardia, *N. braziliensis* and *N. asteroides*, and the disease they cause is termed an actinomycetoma. The true fungi include *Madurella mycetomatis* and *M. grisea* and the disease they produce, an eumycetoma.

Aetiology
Organisms found in soil and may enter foot through injury, e.g. treading on thorn. From some cases thorns have been recovered but mode of entry of organism often obscure. Recent evidence suggests patients often have impaired cell-mediated immunity.

Clinical Description
Extremely chronic: progress very slow.
Incubation period. Experimentally 10–16 days.
Onset. Swelling of foot: irregular nodular character: slowly softens in centre: discharges *granules* or granule-free oily pus or serosanguineous fluid in infections with *Nocardia* spp.
Progress. Great enlargement of foot: numerous sinuses and cavities: caries of bone. Gradually destroys all tissues but tendons long survive. No tendency to heal or to become cured. Death from exhaustion after many years. Internal lesions never occur (unless terminally). Lesions in actinomycetoma are less defined than in *Nocardia* infections, they progress more rapidly and involve bone earlier.

Diagnosis
Granules are present in cavities: larger than in actinomycosis: collections form definite nodules. Organisms may be identified in sections of biopsy material or in culture from discharges.

Precipitin reactions are also carried out in specialised laboratories.

Treatment
If causal organism an actinomycete, it may respond to penicillin and if a *Nocardia* to a sulphonamide, *vide* Actinomycosis. If caused by a *Madurella*, antibiotic therapy is of no or limited value, complete surgical removal of the lesion is imperative.

6

Chapter 51   **MALARIA**

Conditions due to infection with certain specific protozoa of genus *Plasmodium* conveyed by bite of mosquitoes, and characterized by fever, often periodic, splenomegaly and anaemia.

Geographical Distribution
Most of tropics with extensions into subtropics. Malaria in travellers arriving by air from endemic regions is now an important cause of death and morbidity in non-malarious regions. Physicians world-wide must suspect malaria in febrile patients and routinely ask all patients if they have travelled recently.

Susceptibility of Animals
Plasmodium malariae occurs naturally in chimpanzees which are also partially susceptible to *P. vivax* and *P. ovale*. Aotus monkeys and young howler monkeys (*Alonatta palliata*) can be infected with *P. falciparum*. Otherwise malarial parasites occurring in man are not found in and are generally not transmissible to animals. Numerous other plasmodia occur in animals, especially birds and monkeys, but are not found in man. *P. knowlesi*, parasite of monkeys, is transferable by inoculation to man and can be used therapeutically. *P. cynomolgi* also transmissible from certain monkeys to man.

The Mosquito

Genus *Anopheles* is sole host of malarial parasite: but not every species of anopheles can transmit it. Numerous vector species exist, especially *A. maculipennis*. Of this species there are many varieties differing in breeding grounds, sexual behaviour, feeding habits and in geographical distribution. Habits of strains of the same species may differ in different localities. A given species does not always transmit all types of malaria. The mosquito vector must be carefully studied in every malarial country and special local methods devised for extermination. Certain species prefer brackish water.

Anopheles. Feeds only at night or in twilight. Rests with body sloping forward as though standing on head.

A. maculipennis: bites man fairly freely.

A. gambiae: breeds freely in tanks, etc., near dwellings: bites man freely. Causes large epidemics when transported to new localities.

Culex (Culices). Common mosquito in houses: breeds in tanks, etc. near dwellings: bites man freely. *Never conveys malaria*. Rests with body parallel with surface and *one pair of legs elevated above body*.

217

Note: Female mosquitoes only are blood-suckers: males feed solely on vegetable juices. Antennae in females are very sparsely haired: in males are bushy and plume-like. Flight is very limited, not exceeding 1–2 miles; wind and mechanical transport increase range.

Mode of Infection of Man
(1) Bite of infected mosquito: injects sporozoites. Is natural mode of infection.
(2) Inoculation of infected blood: introduces trophozoites into circulation, whence merozoites develop.

The Protozoon

Four species infect man:
1. *Plasmodium vivax*. Benign tertian. Most extensive distribution: predominant infection in temperate zone, also widespread in tropics and subtropics. Acute attack easily controlled but infection difficult to eradicate.
2. *P. ovale*. Ovale tertian. Restricted distribution: East, Central and West Africa only. Attacks often mild.
3. *P. malariae*. Quartan. Wide distribution but less common. Difficult infection to eradicate, may relapse for many years.
4. *P. falciparum*. Malignant tertian or subtertian. Wide distribution in tropics and subtropics. Commonest African malaria. Associated with hyperendemic malaria and with great regional epidemics. Early and moderately early infections easily controlled and eradicated by modern therapeutics but in those with low immunity may be rapid transition to severe case with hopeless prognosis.

Life Cycle
Two phases: (1) *In man*: Intermediate host. Characterized by recurrent asexual cycles and production of sexual forms. Stage is mainly intracorpuscular (in red cells); (2) *In mosquito*: Definitive host. Single sexual cycle developing from human gametocytes.

Cycle in Human Body
Infection by sporozoites from mosquito.
General course
1. Pre-erythrocytic and exo-erythrocytic stages in *P. vivax* and *P. ovale* infections but no exo-erythrocytic stage in *P. falciparum*, or it is now considered *P. malariae*.
2. Intracorpuscular cycle, in red cells. (2.1) Recurrent asexual cycles, sporulation corresponding with clinical paroxysms. (2.2) Production of sexual cells (gametocytes) which only develop in the mosquito: they enable them to infect man, and preserve the life of the parasite.
Pre- and exo-erythrocytic stage. Sporozoites from bite of mosquito reach the liver through the circulation and enter parenchymatous cells (are present in no other tissue): there develop into schizonts with many thousand merozoites. Liver cell then ruptures, discharging merozoites—so-called cryptomerozoites.
Fate of cryptomerozoites. May: (1) Be engulfed by phagocytes and destroyed; (2) Re-enter liver cells and repeat cycle or lie dormant for a latent period (except *P. falciparum* and *P. malariae*). Reactivation of dormant forms responsible for long-term relapses of *P. vivax* and *P. ovale* infections. Relapses of *P. falciparum*

and *P. malariae* due to persistence of parasites in circulation. Recent evidence suggests that dormant forms are smaller than others and the term hypnozoites has been suggested for them. They may represent a subpopulation of the parasite; (3) Enter circulating red corpuscles and produce blood infection, and symptoms of malaria.

Incubation period. Following infection by mosquito sporozoites are present in blood for 30 min and then disappear, having entered liver cells. Periods follow: (1) Blood non-infective during development in liver, in *P. falciparum* 6 days, *P. vivax* 8 days. (2) Blood then becomes infective but no protozoa discoverable ('submicroscopic' infection) for further 3 days. Incubation period is sum of these two phases. (3) Protozoa become recognizable in red cells: *primary attack* follows.

Recurrent cycles and malarial paroxysms. With above phases, merozoites are repeatedly produced in liver, reach circulation, enter red cell and cause clinical malaria. But if subject is under prophylactic treatment drug destroys merozoites entering circulation and thus prevents a malarial paroxysm. While drug is being given, no attack occurs but if exo-erythrocytic cycle in liver persists, further attack develops on omission of drug. This applies to *P. vivax* and *P. ovale*. In *P. falciparum* and *P. malariae* there is only one cycle in liver, no merozoites re-enter liver cells: hence if the primary infection is completely destroyed by drugs, no relapse or recrudescence occurs.

Intracorpuscular cycle

1. *Merozoite.* Enters the red cells either from: (1) production in blood cycle; or (2) exo-erythrocytic development in liver.

2. *Development of trophozoite.* Merozoite grows within red cells forming a trophozoite. Young forms have their cytoplasm arranged crescentically around a central vacuole within the red cell, thus producing 'ring' forms. Protozoon grows in size, exhibits amoeboid movement, pigment appears as granules and increases in amount, forming from haemoglobin. *'Fully-grown parasite'* thus develops: no amoeboid movement: roughly circular. Protoplasm stains blue: intense red chromatin in nucleus: dark pigment (haemozoin).

3. *Schizonts. Stage of sporulation.* Protoplasm of 'full grown parasite' divides into segments, into which the red chromatin scatters: pigment collects in centre. Red cell ruptures, dispersing the spores named 'merozoites': pigment enters leucocytes. *Malarial paroxysm* coincides with sporulation.

4. *Merozoites* (spores). Round: about 2 μm: protoplasm stains blue: red chromatin in nucleus. Merozoite attaches to and enters red cell, and a fresh cycle commences.

Gametocytes. Sexual cells. Certain trophozoites become sexual cells, developing no further unless ingested by a mosquito. Appear in blood in irregular waves and survive about one week. Never produce asexual forms. Resistant to most schizonticidal anti-malarial drugs. Two forms: (*a*) Macrogametocytes: female cells. (*b*) Microgametocytes: male cells; smaller.

Pigment. Trophozoites digest haemoglobin and form malarial pigment: is a compound of haematin. May or may not contain iron. Does not occur normally in body: is not an intermediate product between haemoglobin and bile. When liberated from parasites, is taken up by circulating polymorphs and monocytes and deposited in reticuloendothelial cells of viscera, producing a slaty-grey discoloration and contributing to enlargement and fibrosis of liver and spleen.

Varieties of Protozoon
Main differences in human stage:
1. *Plasmodium vivax. Benign tertian.*
    Intracorpuscular cycle: 48 h.
    Young trophozoite: 'ring' forms of various sizes in early stage.
    Partly grown forms: in varying stages' of development. Active amoeboid movements. Outline indistinct.
    Fully grown forms: red cell filled; no amoeboid movement; enlarged, pale, may be basophilic degeneration.
    Schüffner's dots: often present in red cell containing protozoon in middle stages: stain pinkish.
    Pigment: fine, light brown granules.
    Schizont: 'rosettes', containing 15–20 regularly arranged merozoites.
    Gametocyte: resembles large round or ovoid fully grown parasite. Females larger than males, stain deeper, pigment coarser central nucleus. Larger than red cells.
2. *Plasmodium ovale. Ovale tertian.*
    Cycle: 48 h. Resembles *P. vivax*, but gametocytes oval.
3. *Plasmodium malariae. Quartan.*
    Cycle: 72 h.
    Trophozoite: often grows across red cell producing 'band' forms in early stage, otherwise resembles benign tertian, but movement slight, outline distinct, and pigment coarse, dark brown granules.
    Red cells: unaltered in size and appearance. No Schüffner's dots.
    Schizont: 'daisy-heads', contain 6–12 regularly arranged merozoites.
    Gametocyte: as benign tertian, but smaller than red cell.
4. *Plasmodium falciparum. Malignant tertian, Subtertian, or Aestivo-autumnal.*
    In peripheral blood, parasites scanty and are mainly sexual 'crescents' and asexual 'ring forms'.
    Cycle: 48 h.
    Trophozoite: chiefly as small 'rings'. Full-grown forms smaller than red cell. Actively amoeboid. Pigment: scanty dark granules.
    Red cells: shrivelled and dark. No Schüffner's dots. Maurer's dots: larger, less regular, stain violet.
    Schizont (in spleen): contain 6–20 small irregularly arranged spores.
    Gametocytes: only appear in blood after 7–10 days' fever.
    'Crescents': distinct outline, pigment and chromatin in centre, remains of red cells often visible. Male form is fatter, stains lighter, and has pigment more scattered than female.

Cycle in Mosquito
Extracorpuscular and sexual. Single cycle. Cycle commences from *gametocytes* taken from man into stomach of feeding mosquito: asexual forms from human blood take no part in mosquito cycle and disintegrate. Parasites must have been present in blood 15 days before gametocytes develop.

1. Development of gametocytes
    Male cell (microgametocyte): vibratile movements of pigment granules become visible, then flagella are extruded forming 'flagellated body'. 'Flagella' are long, thin, often with a bulbous end, and have a deep red chromatin core covered with protoplasm; they are spermatozoa, 'microgametes', and are not true flagella.

Female cell (macrogametocyte): maturation occurs by separation of portion of nucleus, resulting in a 'macrogamete'.

In *P. falciparum*, first stage is conversion of crescent into a sphere.

2. *Impregnation of female macromagamete*. Formation of zygote: 'Flagella' become free, enter and impregnate female gametes. Resulting cell has power of movement, the 'travelling vermicule' or *zygote*.

3. *Formation of oocyst*. Zygote penetrates mucous membrane of stomach, settles beneath it, acquires a definite wall and is then named an 'oocyst'.

4. *Formation of sporozoites*. 'Oocyst' grows by division into numerous cells, and these further divide, until finally the oocyst, now 60 µm in diameter, is full of fine spindle-shaped 'sporozoites' staining blue, with central chromatin nucleus. Oocyst ruptures, and sporozoites are freed into insect's body cavity or haemocele and reach salivary glands of mosquito through which they pass and on biting are injected with saliva into skin, thus causing infection and commencing human asexual cycle.

Infectivity of mosquito. Not infectious until cycle complete: for *vivax*, 11 days; *malariae*, 18–22 days; *falciparum*, 10–12 days. Sporozoites remain viable, and infectious, in mosquito for many weeks.

Epidemiology

Depends on number and efficiency of mosquito population, climate, rainfall, virulence of parasites, mortality from the disease, immunity of population and their living habits. Defined levels of endemicity are:

Hypoendemic—spleen palpable or parasites in blood of less than 10% of children between 2 and 10 years.

Mesoendemic—spleen palpable or parasites in blood of less than 11%–50% of children between 2 and 10 years.

Hyperendemic—spleen palpable or parasites in blood of more than 50% of children between 2 and 10 years.

Holoendemic—spleen palpable or parasites in blood of more than 75% of children between 2 and 10 years.

Malaria said to be *stable* when it is transmitted in a region throughout the year and *unstable* when not transmitted continuously.

Pathology

Basic pathological processes. Tissue anoxaemia and shock are important factors. With the exception of nephrosis most changes more severe in *P. falciparum* than in other infections.

Destruction of erythrocytes. This results from growth within them of parasites and also from haemolysis which continues when parasites eradicated. This haemolysis results from a complement-mediated immune process. Depression of erythropoiesis also contributes to resultant anaemia.

Shock. Follows fever caused by haemolysis and by release of parasites from erythrocytes and possibly also toxins similar to bacterial endotoxin. The latter are thought to cause cytotoxic anoxia and release from endotoxin sensitive macrophages of mediators of various pathological processes. Disseminated intravascular coagulation develops in very severe infections. It is probably brought on by products of disintegration of erythrocytes.

Circulating blood volume is reduced; there is generalized vasodilatation and hypotension. Aldosterone secretion is consequently increased causing conservation of sodium and water.

Vascular stasis. May lead to thrombosis and haemorrhage from small vessels. Blood within them sludged. Results partly from shock and hypotension and partly from obstruction to blood flow caused by masses of parasitized erythrocytes adhering to internal walls of vessels. Leakage of fluid and protein through damaged capillaries causes oedema of tissues and aggravates anoxia.

Protuberances on parasitized erythrocytes now thought to contain malarial antigens which react with malarial antibodies and cause the erythrocytes to agglutinate and adhere to vessel walls. Hence in *P. falciparum* infections sporulation occurs in internal organs, rarely in peripheral blood.

Immunity
Inherited immunity
Due to absence of Duffy blood group. Most Negroes immune to *P. vivax.* Receptors for invasion of erythrocyte by *P. vivax* associated with Duffy blood group determinant and most Negroes are Duffy negative. They thus lack the mechanism whereby this parasite invades erythrocytes. Rarity of *P. vivax* in Africa due to this.

Due to sickle-cell disease. Moderate resistance to malaria conferred by possession of sickling gene. This resistance becomes overshadowed by acquired immunity in later life resulting then in no difference in malaria incidence between sicklers and non-sicklers. In childhood, however, before immunity is acquired, the inherited immunity resulting from sicklaemia reduces morbidity and mortality from malaria. Sicklaemic children therefore are more able than non-sicklers to survive the period of heavy childhood mortality from malaria. The incidence of the sickling gene thus increases in highly malarial regions.

Haemoglobin C and Thalassaemia. Possession of the haemoglobin C and/or the thalassaemic gene act in a similar way to possession of that for sicklaemia. *Glucose-6-phosphate dehydrogenase.* Hereditary deficiency of this enzyme is thought but not proved to confer some resistance against malaria.

Acquired immunity
Humoral—Merozoites contain soluble antigens and, particularly when liberated into plasma, stimulate production of antibodies effective against them. IgG probably contains most important antibodies. It damages the dividing nucleus of parasite. IgM and IgA probably assist phagocytosis of parasites. Antibody-coated merozoites usually fail to enter erythrocytes.

Cellular immunity—Also operates. Antigens involved in activation of T and B lymphocytes. Plasma cells develop from B lymphocytes and have greater immunoglobulin-producing ability than B lymphocytes.

Morbid Anatomy
Spleen. Enlarged, capsule tense, reticuloendothelial cells hypertrophied, many macrophages containing pigment in sinusoids. Haemorrhages and infarcts common. In chronic cases, fibrosis.

Liver. Enlarged, congested, parenchymal cells swollen, sometimes centrilobular necrosis. Lymphocytic infiltration in sinusoids of those with 'big spleen disease' associated with malaria.

Brain. Hyperaemic and oedematous small vessels blocked with parasitized erythrocytes and haemorrhages around capillaries.

Kidneys. Punctate haemorrhages, congestion and mononuclear and lymphocytic infiltrations. IgM, IgG and complement deposits in glomeruli. In chronic cases and particularly in *P. malariae* infections these may be the basis of nephrotic syndrome. In severe malaria with oliguria and anuria tubular necrosis prominent.

Gastrointestinal tract. Occasionally oedematous and this may rarely lead to diarrhoea in severe infections.

Lungs and heart may be congested.

Placenta. Infected erythrocytes lining sinusoids may precipitate abortion.

Clinical Course and Manifestations

Severity of Attack

Paroxysm coincides with sporulation. Severity of attack and prognosis are closely but not entirely related to density of parasitaemia, which is influenced by immunity and by following factors:

1. *P. vivax* (benign tertian): Invades reticulocytes almost exclusively, mature cells rarely; this limits parasitaemia. Hence attack though severe is rarely dangerous.

2. *P. malariae* (quartan): Invades ageing red cells. Hence attack mild.

3. *P. falciparum* (subtertain): Invades all red cells and produces more merozoites than other forms, hence attack often severe and infection always dangerous.

Clinical Course

In untreated subjects. Includes in sequence:

1. *Incubation period.* Pre-erythrocytic stage.

2. *Stage of primary fever.* Paroxysms synchronous with schizogony of parasites in red blood cells and release of merozoites.

3. *Latent period.* Protozoon dormant or undergoing recurrent cycles in liver cells; latter do not occur in *P. falciparum* or *P. malariae* infections.

4. *Short-term relapses.* Usually occur after primary fever. Are recrudescences of fever caused by parasites persisting in the blood from stage of primary fever. Rarely result from maturation of exo-erythrocytic parasites.

5. *Long-term relapses and chronic malaria.* 'Recurrence' of malarial paroxysms at irregular intervals.

Important variations in the different species of protozoon. In *P. vivax* and *P. ovale* infections usually result from maturation of exo-erythrocytic forms of the parasites. In *P. falciparum* and *P. malariae* from persistence of erythrocytic cycle as a result of inadequate treatment of immunity as no exo-erythrocytic forms of this parasite occurs.

Incubation Period

During pre-erythrocytic stage. Average period is 10 days for benign tertian, 12 days for malignant tertian, and longer for quartan. With blood inoculations limits are 8–23 days.

Premonitory symptoms. May be malaise and vague pains in final 2 or 3 days when blood is infective but parasites too few to demonstrate except by inoculating patient's blood into a human volunteer.

Primary Fever

Related to schizogony (segmentation) of parasites in blood. Manifestations are not pathognomonic of malaria; may be overlooked; course varies greatly depending on degree of immunity. Does not invariably occur. Followed in those with relatively low immunity by typical intermittent attacks of fever.

Fever usually remittent for 3–4 days; rises to 39·4°C (103°F). May be continuous or even intermittent, often irregular. *Liver* often palpable and tender. Herpes on lip common. Parasites in blood: usually scanty.

In P. vivax (*Benign Tertian*) *and* P. ovale *infections*. Primary fever usually occurs and may be prolonged: may sometimes be daily pyrexia for weeks before latent period and recrudescences develop with tertian periodicity.

In P. malariae (*Quartan*) *Infections*. Periodicity develops early: often double or triple infections which may give quotidian fever.

In P. falciparum (*Malignant Tertian*) *Infections*. Primary fever often indefinite but never a lengthy latent period. *Note*: Pernicious forms may occur in primary fever.

Action of suppressive drugs: In persons taking suppressive drugs in sufficient dosage at time of infection with benign tertian, there is no primary fever and a long latent period follows, recrudescence depending on cessation of prophylactic therapy. In malignant tertian if primary fever does not develop, the infection is permanently eradicated.

If suppressive drugs are taken in irregular or insufficient doses, an irregular primary fever may occur.

Latent Period

The phase of latency—either with or without a primary fever—may last for many weeks or even months, especially in benign tertian and quartan, before fever reappears and assumes the periodic form typical of malaria.

Parasites cannot usually be found in the blood in latent period by routine microscopy but inoculations and blood transfusions may be infective, especially in *P. falciparum* and *P. malariae* infections.

Attack of Malaria

Typical attack in non-immune persons or in those with low immunity consists of regularly recurrent paroxysms of fever. A paroxysm has three distinct stages: (1) Cold Stage; (2) Hot Stage; (3) Sweating Stage.

1. Plasmodium Vivax (Benign Tertian) Paroxysm

Premonitory stage. Sensations of discomfort for a few hours.

Cold stage. Onset: lassitude, headache, often nausea and yawning. *Rigor*: commences with chill and rapidly becomes extreme. *Temperature*: rapidly rises to 38·9–41°C (102–106°F). *Skin*: cold and blue. *Pulse*: rapid and weak. *Headache*: often severe. *Vomiting*: common. *Blood*: numerous parasites present. *Duration*: ¼–2 h.

Hot stage. Patient feels very hot, beginning with flushes of heat. Face, hands and skin congested. Complains of intense headache and thirst. Nausea ceases. Temperature begins to fall. Pulse full. Respiration rapid. *Duration*: from ½–6 h.

Sweating stage. Perspiration extreme. Temperature falls to normal. Pulse slows. Feeling of comfort, often sleeps.

Spleen commonly tender and palpable during paroxysm.

Herpes labialis and bronchitis common.

Variation. Rigor and cold stage often slight: hot stage being most prominent. Severity of paroxysms varies greatly.

Total duration. Usually 10–12 h.

Interval. Usually no symptoms. *Length of interval*: Single *P. vivax* infection has cycle of 48 h: paroxysm often commences regularly *at same hour*: most commonly, between midday and midnight. 'Quotidian' (daily) paroxysm may result from (1) double benign tertian, (2) triple quartan infection, (3) often in malignant tertian infections, or (4) single infections, plasmodia sporulating at different times.

2. Plasmodium Ovale Fever
Milder. Relapses unusual. Tends to be self-limited after a few paroxysms.

3. Plasmodium Malariae (Quartan) Fever
Clinically resembles benign tertian fever, but cycle is 72 h. Paroxysms shorter but sharp and temperature high, may be 41 °C (106 °F). Tendency to relapses prolonged. Cachexia not marked. *Nephrosis*: Special tendency in children, with or without oedema and ascites.

4. Plasmodium Falciparum (Malignant Tertian, Subtertian or Aestivo-autumnal) Fever
Character of fever, symptoms and course tend to be irregular and vary greatly.
Pyrexia. May be: (1) Recurrent rises, tertian or quotidian, with paroxysms; (2) Continued, irregular or remittent pyrexia, either with or without paroxysms. May be several strains of parasites.
Paroxysms. Temperature rises abruptly. Cold stage slight without rigor. Hot stage prolonged. Sweating slight. Duration of attack varies; may be 16–36 h. Temperature falls slowly; may be few hours' interval before next paroxysm, or may remain high. Headache, nausea, vomiting, more severe than in benign types.
Clinical features. Very variable. Illustrative types are (1) Weakness. Tongue furred. Temperature 38·3–39·4 °C (101–103 °F): often not higher. Pulse full. Spleen enlarged. Closely resembles enteric fever; but diarrhoea rare; (2) Paroxysms; (3) Haemolytic anaemia develops. Headache often severe. May be vomiting, delirium, jaundice.
Course and progress. If untreated: (1) May subside in one or two weeks, only in mild cases; (2) May simulate enteric fever (so-called 'typhoid remittent type'); (3) Anaemia and weakness increase, condition becomes serious. High mortality. Various pernicious forms may develop.
Bilious remittent fever. Result of severe blood destruction. Fatal if untreated. Two types:
   1. *Haemolytic jaundice.* Bilious vomiting, spleen enlarged. Anaemia. Haemorrhages and haematemesis may occur. Hyperbilirubinaemia. Direct van den Bergh negative.
   2. *Hepatitis.* Jaundice early. Liver enlarged and tender. Van den Bergh biphasic. Other symptoms as above.
Complications in severe, pernicious or malignant malaria. May develop with great rapidity, often with no previous warning, or may be slight malarial manifestations. Occurs in hyperinfections, viz. more than 5% red cell infected. Nearly always fatal in absence of efficient treatment or partial immunity.
   Pathogenesis. Parasites in enormous numbers localized in internal organs, therefore parasites in peripheral blood sometimes scanty: small vessels blocked with parasites, red cells, fibrin and pigment. Any site in body may be attacked,

and thus *can simulate nearly every acute condition*, cerebral, spinal, abdominal, cardiac, respiratory, etc.

Cerebral malaria. Onset with cerebral disturbances, or with hyperpyrexia or acute mania or quiet delirium, occurring separately or passing through all such stages and progressing to (or commencing directly with) coma. May be convulsions and paralyses of various types. Temperature variable: hyperpyrexia, 38·3–39·4 °C (101–103 °F), or normal. May regain consciousness and lapse again into coma. Parasites always present in blood. Fatal ending common. The form with hyperpyrexia and rapid coma is often mistaken for 'heat stroke' or cerebrospinal fever.

Algid type. Parasites concentrated in gastro-intestinal mucosa. *Intense sudden collapse.* Vomiting, diarrhoea, anuria. Feels cold. Pulse feeble. Temperature usually subnormal. Blood pressure very low. Peripheral circulatory failure. May be conscious until death. Due to lesions in adrenal glands.

Cardiac. May be congestive failure or sudden death.

Alimentary tract. Rare. *Bacillary dysentery* may be simulated, stools may contain blood but no cellular exudate: no ulceration on sigmoidoscopy. *Choleraic*: when small intestine attacked, but stools brownish. 'Gastric malaria': severe bilious vomiting. Intussusception and acute abdominal diseases imitated.

Renal. Impaired blood flow to renal cortex and vascular stasis in medulla lead to diminished glomerular filtration rate and to tubular necrosis respectively. Former causes oliguria or anuria with uraemia. Often fatal, is special indication for treatment by haemodialysis.

Sequelae. Cerebral malaria may be followed by lack of concentration, amnesia, or psychosis; or blindness. *Cerebral or spinal forms* may leave paralyses, neuritis, or conditions resembling disseminated sclerosis, or ataxia. Orchitis may occur.

Chronic Infections
Due to partial immunity and no, or inadequate, treatment. Patient anaemic, skin pale, wasted, cachectic, hepatosplenomegaly, occasional irregular fever.

Other Complications and Sequelae

Mainly from malignant and malarial cachexia. Sequelae of anaemia and debility, e.g. tuberculosis, pneumonia.

Ocular Complications
Corneal ulceration, iritis, retinal haemorrhages.

Spleen
Rupture: when soft in acute or hard in chronic malaria. Subcapsular haematoma. Perisplenitis.

Hepatitis and gallstones in malignant tertian.

Blackwater fever (q.v.) is most serious complication.

Relapses

In *P. falciparum* infections, in absence of adequate treatment or immunity, parasites persist only in blood (no exo-erythrocytic stage in liver) and hence relapses usually occur within a few weeks of primary attack. Occasionally have occurred up to 18 months after primary attack.

In *P. vivax* and *P. ovale* infections exo-erythrocytic forms in liver may mature up to 3 and 1½ years respectively after primary attack and cause recurrence of symptoms.

In *P. malariae* relapses develop up to 20 years after primary attack. Now considered to result from persistence of erythrocytic forms of parasites. Exo-erythrocytic forms now believed not to occur.

Prognosis

Plasmodium Falciparum Infections
Formerly high mortality from blackwater fever and pernicious forms. Suppressive and prophylactic treatment available. Adequate treatment of acute attack eliminates this infection entirely. Progress is excellent in uncomplicated cases.

Plasmodium Vivax and P. Ovale Infections
Attacks easily controlled therapeutically and convalescence short. Long-term relapse may occur from persistence of exo-erythrocytic parasites in liver but these may be eradicated by 8-aminoquinolone drugs.

Plasmodium Malariae
If initial attack thoroughly treated there are no relapses. Otherwise may relapse for many years. Nephrosis may be a complication, especially in children.

Mortality

Greatest in pregnancy, infancy, old age.

Immunity
Following repeated infections, partial immunity acquired but only to the specific infecting strain. Associated with high γ-globulin (IgG and IgM) values in serum.

Diagnosis

Malaria may simulate many diseases: also is often a complicating factor as any illness may stimulate a recurrence. Various infections may complicate malaria.

General Diagnosis
Note: (1) Opportunities for infection; (2) Character of fever and symptoms; (3) Presence of parasites in blood; (4) Fluorescent antibody test for past malaria.

Differential Diagnosis
Primary fever. Enteric, influenza, dengue, typhus, sandfly fever. With splenic enlargement: brucellosis, relapsing fever.
With icterus. Infective hepatitis, yellow fever.
Malarial coma. Heat hyperpyrexia, cerebral haemorrhage, diabetes, alcohol, drugs.
Pernicious forms. See p. 226.
Examination of blood for parasites. (*Note*: examination most valuable shortly *before* a paroxysm is due, and not during height of attack, when sporulation has lately occurred, except for malignant forms.)

1. Film of blood stained by Romanowsky method. Stain buffered to pH 7·2.

2. Thick film method. Six drops on a slide evenly spread: dried: red cells carefully haemolysed with distilled or tap water: dried and stained by Giemsa diluted 1 : 20 or by Field's method. (Rapid and effective if parasites scanty.)

Species of Plasmodium. Malignant tertian is proved by presence of 'crescents', and strongly suggested if 'ring forms' are numerous. (*See also* Varieties of Protozoon, p. 220.)

Prophylaxis

Malaria can be controlled and in some areas completely eradicated. Prophylactic measures vary with locality and habits of mosquito (*see* p. 217).

Anti-mosquito Measures
Object: to destroy mosquitoes and prevent breeding:

1. Breeding sites eradicated by drainage, filling in shallow pools, etc.

2. Pools, shallow streams and banks treated with oil and larvicides to destroy mosquitoes in aquatic larval stage. *Gambusia* (minnows) useful in wells and limited areas.

3. Dwelling houses sprayed with residual insecticides to kill adult mosquitoes.

Individual Prophylaxis
Object: to prevent transmission of infection.

Prevention of mosquito bites: screened house, mosquito nets over beds. Wear garments covering body, especially ankles and arms after dusk. Apply insect repellent to exposed skin.

Drug Prophylaxis
See section on treatment.

Endemic Index: Estimation of Prevalence
Prevalence of infection in a district can be estimated by: (1) 'Parasite rate': percentage with parasites in blood; time-consuming, but accurate, especially in adults in whom splenomegaly may be absent. (2) 'Spleen rate' *see* Epidemiology, p. 221. (3) Number of bites from infected mosquitoes sustained in given period.

Treatment

No one drug acts on all stages of malaria, and no drug acts on sporozoites. Different species of parasites show different responses; this is also true for certain strains within a given species.

General Treatment
Rest in bed. Much fluid. Watch urinary output.
Cold stage. Apply warmth.
Hyperpyrexia. Tepid sponging. Cool with a fan.

Specific Treatment
Objects

1. *Suppressive treatment.* To prevent acute malaria—viz. clinical attacks resulting from bites of infected mosquitoes.

2. *Treatment of acute malaria.* To eradicate asexual blood-borne cycle of parasites. *Note*: Treatment of cerebral and severe forms of *P. falciparum* infection are described separately (*see* p. 231).

3. *Prevention of relapses.* To free patient from long-term relapses by eradication of exo-erythrocytic parasites.

Specific antimalarial drugs. Nine groups at present in use:

1. *4-Aminoquinoline compounds.* Chloroquine (aralen, resorchin, Avlochlor and Nivaquine) Amodiaquine.

2. *Cinchona alkaloids.* Quinine.

3. *Biguanide compounds.* Proguanil.

4. *Diaminopyrimidines.* Pyrimethamine (Daraprim).

5. *8-Aminoquinoline compounds.* Primaquine.

6. *Sulphonamides and sulphones.* Action limited but useful for chloroquine-resistant strains. Sulphormethoxine the most useful in combination with other drugs for acute cases and sulphone for prophylaxis.

7. *Mefloquine.* Newly developed 4-quinoline-carbinolamine.

8. *Tetracycline.* Has slow schizonticidal action.

9. *Quing Hao Su.* Isolated in China; a sesquiterpene lactone and trials indicate considerable value. Not yet generally available.

Action of specific drugs. At various stages of parasitic cycle.

1. *Sporozoites*: No drug effective.

2. *Pre-erythrocytic stage in liver*: Primary tissue phase in *P. falciparum* infections only. Not effective with other species. Proguanil, pyrimethamine.

3. *Asexual parasites in erythrocytic stage* ('schizonticidal action'). All groups except that 8-aminoquinolines have limited action.

4. *Sexual parasites in erythrocytic stage*: Only 8-aminoquinolines, e.g. pamaquin. Proguanil has partial action, also preventing development in mosquito. Of limited public health value only.

5. *Late exo-erythrocytic stage* (prevention of relapses): Primaquine.

Prevention and Treatment of Acute Attacks

Drugs and their Uses
(*see also* Cerebral and Severe Infections, p. 231)

Chloroquine
Most rapidly acting schizonticide known. Drug of choice for treatment of acute attack. Does not precipitate blackwater fever in *P. falciparum* infections. Toxic effects slight. For rheumatism and some collagen diseases has been used in doses greatly in excess of those used in malaria therapy and has then sometimes damaged retina and caused temporary opacity of cornea due to deposition of minute crystals in it. May have similar action if used in maximal prophylactic dosage for several years.

Valuable suppressive, does not stain skin. Some strains in S. America, the Far East and recently in tropical Africa have become resistant to it.

Chloroquine hydrochloride, sulphate and diphosphate available; 250 mg diphosphate and 200 mg sulphate and hydrochloride contain 150 mg chloroquine base. Dosage usually measured in amount of base.

Acute malaria. Initially 600 mg (base) and 300 mg (base) 3–6 h later followed by 300 mg on each of 2 successive days.

Suppressive treatment. 300 mg (base) weekly or 150 mg (base) twice weekly. Duration of administration as for proguanil (*below*). In hyperendemic areas or where there are chloroquine-resistant parasites is sometimes used in double this dosage. If so change to alternative drug after 2–3 years.

Amodiaquine

Another 4-aminoquinoline with action similar to chloroquine. Dosage 600 mg (base) initially and 400 mg (base) on each of 2 successive days.
Suppression. 400 mg (base) weekly.

Quinine

Suppressive action. Doses less than 1200 mg daily ineffective. This dosage suppresses and eradicates *P. falciparum*, but only suppresses growth of *P. vivax*, overt attacks occur on omission. Dose is toxic if prolonged. Action not completely reliable and other drugs better. Carries risk of causing blackwater fever in those infected with *P. falciparum*.
Acute malaria. Satisfactory by mouth except in patients vomiting and in those with severe and cerebral types. Dosage: 600 mg thrice daily for 3 days or until fever subsides; then 600 mg daily for 6–8 weeks. Replaced mainly by other drugs.
Mode of action. Destroys asexual forms. No action on gametocytes or sporozoites.
Severe and cerebral malaria. Quinine if used must be injected. Usual i.v. dose 500 or 650 mg. Inject slowly over 10–20 min or preferably administer in drip infusion.
Toxic effects. In therapeutic doses causes vomiting and tinnitus. May also be deafness (rarely permanent), palpitations, cutaneous eruptions. In persons with idiosyncrasy or glucose-6-phosphate dehydrogenase deficiency: haemoglobinuria, amblyopia.
Preparations. (1) Bisulphate: by mouth only, poorly soluble. Tablets must be crushed; (2) Bihydrochloride: soluble. Can be injected i.v. if indicated or i.m., but latter involves risk of abscesses.

Proguanil

Least toxic of all antimalarial drugs. Has partial action on gametocytes, preventing development in mosquito. Schizonticidal action too slow for use in treatment of acute malaria. Parasite resistance occurs.
Suppressive treatment. Dose: 0·1–0·2 g daily. Commence on day of entry into malarial area and continue until been away from the area 6 weeks.

Pyrimethamine

Used only for prophylaxis. Dose 25 mg weekly. Is a folic acid antagonist and in large doses causes megaloblastic anaemia. It is tasteless and fatalities have been caused by children eating the tablets as sweets; appropriate storage precautions therefore needed. Parasite resistance occurs and cross-resistance with proguanil.

Primaquine

Acts in gametocytes and the exo-erythrocytic stages of *P. vivax* and *P. ovale*. The gametocidal action is of no benefit to the human host but helps to prevent mosquitoes becoming infected. The action on exo-erythrocytic forms prevents long-term relapses of the relevant infection. Primaquine readily produces haemolysis in glucose-6-phosphate dehydrogenase-deficient persons.

Sulphonamides and Sulphones
Sulphormethoxine (sulphadoxine) in doses of 1·0 g with 25 mg pyrimethamine used for treatment of chloroquine-resistant strains of *P. falciparum*. Diamino-diphenylsulphone (dapsone) is used in dosage of 100 mg weekly in combination with 12·5 mg pyrimethamine weekly in the preparation Maloprim. Useful for prophylaxis in areas where resistance of *P. falciparum* to chloroquine occurs.

Mefloquine
Still under trial in treatment of multi-drug resistant *P. falciparum* in South-East Asia. In acute attacks single dose of 1·5 g orally. For prophylaxis 180–250 mg weekly, preferably in combination with 500 mg sulphadoxine and 25 mg pyrimethamine to reduce rush of resistant strains emerging.

Tetracycline
Used against resistant *P. falciparum* infections in doses of 500 mg four times daily for 7–10 days but its slow action necessitates simultaneous administration of rapidly acting schizonticide.

Cerebral and Severe Infections
Parenteral treatment indicated instantly: take blood film then commence treatment without waiting for findings of film. Either: (1) Chloroquine i.v. in doses of 200 mg (base) repeated in 2–3 h, if necessary. The *British Pharmacopoeia* lists chloroquine sulphate and phosphate for parenteral injection each dispensed in concentration of 40 mg drug per ml saline or water; the 200-mg dose should be diluted to 20 ml and injected slowly or given in a drip to obviate marked reduction in blood pressure. Children given 5 mg (base) per kg body weight. Or: (2) Quinine bihydrochloride: 600 mg in 20 ml distilled water, inject slowly in 10 min; i.v. infusion given over 20–30 min preferable. Blood pressure may fall suddenly: add to above injection, ephedrine, 0·6 ml of 1:1000 solution. One injection usually sufficient: repeat in 8 h if indicated. Continue with drugs by mouth.
Fluid replacement. Usually advisable in serious malaria to combat dehydration. Avoid excess sodium.
Blood transfusion. If severe anaemia. Washed packed cells in normal saline solution give good results.
Corticosteroids. Intravenous injection 10 mg dexamethasone or 100 mg hydrocortisone i.m. often followed by immediate and dramatic improvement. Some studies in Far East have questioned the value of such treatment.
Children. Dosage: One-fifteenth of standard dose for each year: full dose at 15 years. Quinine well tolerated.
Pregnancy. Chloroquine and amodiaquine well tolerated. Quinine may cause abortion.

Suppressive Treatment
Proguanil, pyrimethamine and 4-aminoquinolines are complete suppressants of sensitive *P. falciparum* strains, no attacks occurring under treatment and no relapses subsequently: pernicious malaria and blackwater fever are eliminated

and malarial mortality reduced almost to zero. For benign tertian these three drugs are also suppressants of about equal value: no attacks under treatment but subsequent relapses.

Method. Commence on day entering malarial area and continue at least 14 days after leaving endemic area.

Relapses

Should receive efficient antimalarial treatment. Relapses can be prevented in almost all cases by course of primaquine 15 mg base daily for 14 days. (Usually dispensed as phosphate of which 26·5 mg equivalent to 15 mg base.) Has largely replaced pamaquin which is more toxic and less effective. (Pamaquin dosage 10 mg (base) t.d.s. for 10 days). Both are 8-aminoquinolines and this group of drugs may cause haemolysis and methaemoglobinaemia in G-6-PD deficient persons. Patients so treated should be kept in hospital or under very close medical supervision. The drugs destroy exo-erythrocytic forms of *P. vivax, P. ovale* and *P. malariae*.

Chloroquine-resistant Malaria

Usually also resistant to proguanil and pyrimethamine but resistance seldom absolute.

Acute attacks. Quinine in dosage of 1·3 g daily for 10 days effective or quinine i.v. (*see* p. 231) if attack severe. Sulphormethoxine 1·0 g and pyrimethamine 25 mg an alternative with 50 mg pyrimethamine on following day.

Tetracycline or *Meflaquine* could be used (*see* p. 231) *Artemetherin* an extract of the plant Quin (or Quing) Han Su grown in China has recently been used in the Far East and appears to be effective against chloroquine-resistant strains. It is prepared in oily suspension and 200 mg are injected i.m. followed by 100 mg i.m. 12-hourly for 4 injections. A watery extract Artemesinin is under development.

Suppression. Diaminodiphenylsulphone with pyrimethamine (Maloprim) *see* p. 231.

Chapter 52   ## BLACKWATER FEVER (Malarial Haemo-globinuria; Haemoglobinuric Fever)

Acute condition produced by *Plasmodium falciparum* infection, characterized by pyrexia, haemoglobinuria, vomiting, jaundice, rigors and frequently diminution or suppression of urine. Immediate cause is great haemolysis of red cells.

Relation to Malaria

Occurs only in persons resident in *P. falciparum* endemic areas for at least 2–3 months and usually 2 or more years. Result of repeated attacks of or continuous infection with insufficiently treated *P. falciparum*. (*P. vivax* infection may also be present but is not a factor.)

Presence of malarial parasites during attack. If examined before attack, parasites are nearly always present: rapid disappearance during attack observed on many occasions. Rarely present, or very scanty, after first 24 h: due to dissolution of red cells which have contained and been damaged by plasmodia.

Relation to Quinine
Attacks are almost invariably preceded by irregular administration of quinine insufficient to cure infection. Occasionally occurs during treatment of overt attack with quinine. Have become rare since quinine has been largely replaced by synthetic drugs for prophylaxis.

Note: Quinine without malaria can, though rarely, cause haemoglobinuria in G-6-PD deficient persons but not to extent or with symptoms of blackwater fever.

Theory of Pathogenesis
Enormous numbers of red cells haemolysed thus producing haemoglobinaemia.

Disintegrated products of red cells, altered by plasmodia and quinine thought to form antigen which adheres to erythrocyte membrane on which complement is then deposited.

Anuria. Tubular necrosis as in severe *P. falciparum* infections (*see* p. 226).

Onset in Temperate Climates
Attacks not infrequently occur on return to cooler climates: often within few days, rarely more than 6 months. Often follows quinine taken after an interval for recurrence of malaria or a chill or even in tonic water.

Morbid Anatomy
Spleen. Enlarged and soft. Active phagocytosis present.
Liver. Enlarged and soft. Often degenerate foci.
Kidneys. Tubules degenerated: contain debris and casts.

Symptoms
Consumption of quinine may immediately precede an attack.
Prodromal symptoms. Often a slight attack of malaria treated with quinine. In others: more vague—general malaise, digestive disturbances, spleen painful, urobilin increased. May be none, until rigor and red urine passed.
Onset. Characteristic symptoms usually commence suddenly. Onset with rigors in 50%: often recurrent for several hours.

Haemoglobinuria. Urgent desire to micturate after a rigor; dark urine passed. Duration of dark urine few hours to 1 day; rarely exceeds 2 days.

Temperature. 39·4–40·5 °C (103–105 °F): irregular. May be 37·8 °C (100 °F) or lower. Falls as urine clears.

Vomiting. Much retching and epigastric pain.

Icterus. Within 24 h of onset: becomes intense in severe cases.

General symptoms. Restlessness. Pain in loins. Great thirst. Exhaustion. Liver and spleen enlarged and tender.

Progress. (1) *Recovery*. Urine clears, and temperature falls: patient sweats and symptoms pass. (2) Symptoms increase. Restlessness, rigors, high temperature. *Thirst extreme*. Hiccup serious. Urine diminished: final anuria common: fatal termination. Blood urea raised.

Death from: (1) *Cardiac failure*—secondary to peripheral circulatory failure caused by extracellular dehydration and haemoconcentration; (2) *Anuria*; (3) *Hyperpyrexia*. Coma or delirium common. *Mortality*. Varies: at least 25%.

Urine
In early stages, micturition often frequent, later oliguria or anuria as renal

failure develops. Urine, on standing, separates into two layers: (1) Clear and dark. Gives spectrum of oxy- and methaemoglobin; (2) Large, dark sediment, consisting of much debris and casts. Albumin present: almost solid on boiling. Bile rarely present.

Blood
Red cells reduced to, in severe cases, 1 000 000. Haemoglobin 20%. Red cells little changed, but 'ghost' cells present. During attack: polynuclears form 90% of leucocytes. During recovery: mononuclear increase, leucopenia, nucleated red cells, punctate basophilia.

Plasma urea increases when oliguria present.

Sequelae
Post-haemoglobinuric fever. Occasional pyrexia frequent for several weeks: may end in hyperpyrexia.
Relapses. Shortly after attack, quinine will often cause relapse.
Recurrences. May occur: do not increase in severity.

Differential Diagnosis
From: (1) Yellow fever; (2) 'Bilious remittent fever' of malaria. In blackwater fever, rigor, pyrexia, and haemoglobinuria occur together at onset; (3) Haemolytic anaemia and haemoglobinuria caused by drug administration to persons deficient of glucose-6-phosphate dehydrogenase. Up to 30% of some African tribes so defective as are some from Middle East and elsewhere. Drugs responsible include 8-aminoquinolines, quinine, sulphonamides, sulphones, nitrofurazone, *p*-aminosalicylic acid, vitamin-K analogues, and in addition, certain constituents of the Fava bean, favism being so caused. Only old erythrocytes haemolysed so initial administration of drug causes illness, then further administration for a period is without additional effect. Glucose-6-phosphate dehydrogenase deficiency can be recognized by Motulsky's and other tests.

Suppressive Treatment (*see* p. 229 et seq.)
Completely prevents blackwater fever if synthetic antimalarial employed.

Treatment
General measures. Rest in bed. Measure urine and vomit. Acute renal insufficiency present when urine volume 300 ml or less/24 h. Give sufficient i.v. saline to replace fluid lost and, in addition, give 0·5–1·0 L.
Corticosteroids. On diagnosis give 200 mg cortisone or its equivalent or other steroid preparation i.m. daily until patient convalescent, then tail off dose.
Blood transfusion. Advisable in all but mild cases. Washed packed cells in normal saline solution preferable.
Suppression of urine or oliguria with uraemia. Use artificial kidney or peritoneal dialysis when plasma urea 32 mmol/L (200 mg/dl) and rising. If necessary fly or otherwise transport the patient to nearest centre where such treatment available. Longstanding practice of avoiding movement of patient to be put aside in view of this consideration. Peritoneal dialysis apparatus easily taken to patient.

Specific malarial drugs. Avoid quinine. Only limited therapy may be needed as so many parasites destroyed by haemolysis, but prophylactic suppression should be continued after attack.

Chapter 53   *TRYPANOSOMIASIS (Sleeping Sickness)*

Infection by trypanosomes conveyed by tsetse flies, producing long-continued pyrexia and glandular enlargement and, if untreated, finally a prolonged fatal lethargic condition.

History
Progress in discovery of trypanosomes has been:
1. Non-pathological and in animals: Gruby, 1843, in frogs; later others found in birds and fishes; Lewis, 1878, in rats (*T. lewisi*).
2. Pathological and in animals: 1880, Evans, in Surra, disease of horses (*T. evansi*); 1895, Bruce, in Nagana, tsetse-fly disease in South Africa (*T. brucei*).
3. Pathological and in man: 1901, Dutton—pathological nature not recognized; 1903, Castellani, followed by Bruce and Nabarro, in blood and cerebrospinal fluid of 'sleeping sickness' (*T. gambiense*). Other human pathological strains described: *T. cruzi* (Cruz and Chagas, 1909); *T. rhodesiense* (Stephens and Fantham, 1910).
   Note: This chapter refers to human trypanosomiasis or 'sleeping sickness'.

Distribution
Patchy, throughout tropical Africa.

Mode of Infection
Infection is conveyed only by tsetse fly of genus *Glossina*:
1. *Glossina palpalis (T. gambiense).* Breeds solely on lake and river banks in bush or forest. In Western Nigeria and Ghana also by *G. tachinoides*.
2. *Glossina morsitans (T. rhodesiense).* Prevalent in Zambia, Zimbabwe. Also *G. swynnertoni*. Breed in any locality. Bites mainly by day.
3. Transplacental infection of newborn known.
   In addition to man, big game form a reservoir.

Trypanosoma Gambiense
Morphology. Protozoa, subclass Flagellata. Stained by Leishman's or similar methods, possess following characteristics:
1. Unicellular. Roughly fusiform shape. Length about 30 μm. Breadth 1·5–3 μm (variable). Protoplasm stains blue and contains two nuclei.
2. *Macro-* or *trophonucleus*: Near middle. Stains purple-red.
3. *Kinetoplast*. Near posterior end. Small. Stains intense deep purple-red.
4. *Undulating membrane*: Commences near kinetoplast. Margin stains purple. Runs entire length, and is continuous with—
5. *Flagellum*. At opposite end to kinetoplast. Since progression is usually in direction of flagellum, this is regarded as *anterior* end.

In fresh blood: actively motile, by movements of undulating membrane and flagellum.

Cultivation. Readily infects laboratory rodents.

Life cycle. Two phases: (1) In blood of vertebrate host (man or big game); (2) In gut of blood-sucking invertebrate host (*Glossina*).

In *Glossina palpalis*: Trypanosomes enter with sucked blood, reach midgut and multiply. None on proboscis after 48 h. They pass between the peritrophic membrane and the gut wall to the proventriculus where they re-enter the gut lumen. They pass forward along the food channel and then are thought to ascend the salivary duct and develop in the salivary glands. Becomes infective after 3–7 weeks; remains so for life.

[*T. lewisi* in rat-flea and also in cultures, passes through spherical stages resembling *Leishmaniae*. Multiplication of trypanosomes can occur by mitotic division, longitudinally, commencing with kinetoplast, flagellum dividing last; thus forming a rosette with numerous daughter trypanosomes united by flagellum before final separation. Before division breadth greatly increases. In all trypanosomiases, forms vary greatly in breadth.]

Trypanosoma Rhodesiense

Morphologically indistinguishable from *T. gambiense*. In rat, produces stumpy forms with nuclei placed posteriorly in non-flagellar end. Resemble *T. brucei*. May be distinct species or a human strain of *T. brucei*, or *T. gambiense* transmitted through *G. morsitans*. Epidemiologically, clinically and chemotherapeutically different from *T. gambiense*.

Morbid Anatomy

Brain. Fluid increased; convolutions flattened. Often a terminal purulent meningitis.

Histology of CNS. A characteristic meningo-encephalomyelitis, most marked at base of brain and medulla; great infiltration of mononuclear leucocytes in perivascular spaces, sufficient to interfere by pressure with circulation and hence with nutrition of nerve cells. Cells and protein in CSF increased.

Lymph nodes. Enlarged in early stages (pea to bean).

Blood. Anaemia with marked haemolytic component recently demonstrated and is associated with splenomegaly. Great increase in plasma globulins, especially IgG.

Symptoms

T. gambiense. Incubation period: 2 or 3 weeks or less; in animals 5 days. At site of bite may be local irritation and formation of a nodule, followed by brawny induration and bruise-like discoloration, 'trypanosomal chancre'; fever develops a few days later. Two stages; transition gradual.

Stage 1: Trypanosomal fever. Onset gradual. Duration: several months, slow progress. Trypanosomes in blood and gland fluid, but not in CSF. Often scanty in blood.

> *Fever*: Irregular. Continuous, intermittent, or remittent, or with apyrexial intervals.
> *Eruption*: Transient pink circinate erythema on trunk.
> *Pulse*: Rapid, 100–120. *Respiration* rapid.

> *Lymph nodes*. General enlargement, especially in posterior cervical triangle (Winterbottom's sign). At first painless, later hard and painful. No suppuration.
> *Oedema*: Local areas: face, ankles, etc.
> *Spleen* enlarged: may be enormous. Also *Liver*.
> *Deep hyperaesthesia* to blows (Kérandel's sign).
> *General symptoms*: Anaemia, tachycardia, debility progressing to muscular weakness and apathy. Intellect clear.

Stage 2: Cerebral Stage (*'Sleeping Sickness'*). Usually develops after about 6 months, but may not appear for years. Trypanosomes in CSF. Progress usually insidious and chronic; occasionally rapid. At onset may be acute symptoms and mania.

> *Expression* becomes vacant and sad. Headaches. *Tremors* of tongue, and later of limbs. Glandular enlargement increases. Cerebration becomes slower; apathy and disinclination to work. Gait shuffling.
> *Further Progress*. Drowsiness marked. Weakness increases until patient is bed-ridden. Emaciation rapid.
> *Final Stage*. Patient is comatose. Lies on side of bed with limbs flexed. Anaemia marked. Temperature subnormal.

Total Duration. Often about a year, but may be much longer.

T. rhodesiense. Incubation period: short, 1–2 weeks. Tends to be acute and more rapid than *T. gambiense* infection. Temperature higher. Glandular enlargement not so marked. Trypanosomes usually more numerous in blood. More resistant to treatment. Cerebral symptoms may develop without glandular enlargement.

Prognosis

T. gambiense: without treatment, spontaneous recovery occasionally occurs in first stage, never in second. May recover even in second stage following treatment.

T. rhodesiense: fatal in 1 year if untreated.

Diagnosis

Suggested by general glandular enlargement. Confirmed by presence of trypanosomes. Earliest: by puncture of lymph nodes in gambian infections and by blood examination in rhodesian. In blood when scanty centrifugalize 10 ml citrated blood. In later stages in CSF also lymphocytosis and increase in protein. *Blood*: increased percentage of lymphocytes and large mononuclears. Trypanosomal fluorescent antibody test reliable and becomes positive few weeks after infection.

Kits now available commercially: (1) for testing ability of patient's serum to agglutinate trypanosome serotypes (Testryp CATT, Smith-Kline); (2) for indirect haemagglutination (Testryp IHA, Smith-Kline and Cellognost Trypanosomiasis, Behring); (3) for rapid screening of plasma for increased IgM (Rapid TexIgM, Behring).

Prophylaxis

Factors to be considered to prevent spread:
Drug prophylaxis. Injection of pentamidine isethionate, 5 mg/kg body weight

every 6 months gives protection in gambian form but dangerous in rhodesian and also less effective. May mask early stages and thus delay effective treatment until brain invaded. If this happens in gambian form treatment still usually ensures good prognosis but *T. rhodesiense* relatively resistant to arsenicals which penetrate blood–brain barrier.

Human host. Prevention of movement of population from infected to uninfected districts. For long periods some persons may carry trypanosomes in blood and occasionally have pyrexial attacks without developing sleeping sickness. Therefore investigate and treat all persons with adenitis or other suspicious signs or symptoms. Houses and persons should be protected against flies.

Tsetse fly. *G. palpalis* breeds on waterway banks: these can be cleared. Breeds within 20 m and rarely feeds more than 60 m from water. *G. morsitans*, however, breeds too widely for this mode of control.

Big game. Big game acts as a reservoir, but the extent of its influence is uncertain.

Spraying of insecticide. From aircraft. Good results indicated.

Treatment
Principal drugs used are: (1) For gambian infections: Antrypol (Suramin), pentamidine, and melarsoprol. Course of first or second plus third recommended; (2) For rhodesian infections: Antrypol (Suramin), melarsoprol B. Course of each recommended.

Suramin (Antrypol, Germanin, Bayer 205). Most effective drug in early stage, in *T. rhodesiense* infections. Little use in second stage. May cause albuminuria.

Dosage. Intravenous injections, 1 g in 10 ml water. Repeat weekly, usually for 4–5 injections followed by melarsoprol.

Pentamidine isethionate. Valuable for early infections with *T. gambiense*. Antrypol preferable for *T. rhodesiense*. Course consists of 7–10 injections of 2–4 mg drug per kg patient's body weight given daily or on alternate days.

Melarsoprol (Mel B, Arsobal). A combination of melarsen and dimercaprol (British Anti-Lewisite or BAL), effective in all stages of *T. gambiense* and *T. rhodesiense* infections.

Dosage. 3·6 mg/kg patient's body weight daily for 3–4 days. Drug dispensed in propylene glycol to make a 3·6% solution and injected intravenously. Courses of 3–4 daily injections are separated by rest periods of 7 days. The drug causes cellulitis or abscess if it leaks from the vein. Therapeutic dose near that at which arsenical toxicity occurs and in some arsenical encephalopathy and convulsions develop. This may be treated with 5 mg diazepam (Valium) i.v.

Nitrofurans. Nitrofurazole (Furacin) and furaltadone (Altafur) may be used if all other drugs fail. Are very toxic. Given orally in doses of 10–13 mg/kg body weight t.d.s. for 7 days. Three such courses may be given, each separated by a 7-day interval. Furaltadone may be given i.v. as 3·5% solution in 5% glucose. Cause haemolytic anaemia in G-6-PD deficient persons.

Dosage regimes. Early *T. gambiense* infections—one course of 3–4 melarsoprol injections commonly used. Similar course can be used for *T. rhodesiense* but 5 injections suramin preferred. Late cases of either infection treated with 8–9 injections either in 3 groups of 3 or 2 groups of 4 injections with 7 days rest between courses.

Prognosis
Almost invariably fatal if untreated. Full cure cannot be presumed till symptom free, blood and CSF free from trypanosomes and CSF protein and cell count normal.

South American Trypanosomiasis (Chagas' Disease)

Infection by *Trypanosoma cruzi*, producing acute pyrexia with glandular enlargement, and in survivors, either no symptoms or a chronic stage with myocardial fibrosis and heart failure and occasionally dilatation of alimentary organs.

Trypanosoma Cruzi
Intermediate host is a flying bug, *'Triatoma'*. In man, trypanosomes in blood for about 2 weeks: then pass into internal organs and assume leishmanial form, occasionally producing trypanosomes which enter peripheral blood. Animals are also hosts (armadillo). Infection is by faeces of bugs containing the organisms.

Symptoms
Infants of 1 year chiefly affected. Acute and chronic stage.
Incubation period: 8–10 days.
Acute stage. Principal symptoms: (1) Pyrexia; (2) Superficial lymph nodes enlarged; (3) Oedema at site of bite which is often orbit or cheek—bitten by bug during sleep; (4) Spleen and liver enlarged and tender. Acute stage may be fatal in 1 month, terminating with meningeal symptoms: may pass into chronic stage.
Chronic stage. Many groups of manifestations, including: (1) Intermittent pyrexia with parasitaemia; (2) Damage to myocardium caused by organism destroying cardiac ganglia and causing dilatation, hypertrophy and ultimate failure. Right bundle-branch block common; (3) Other hollow viscera may similarly be damaged by destruction of their nerve ganglia. Thus mega-oesophagus, dilatation of stomach and colon all encountered.
Diagnosis. Fluorescent antibody test. In early and acute cases trypanosomes may be demonstrated in blood films. Later xenodiagnosis and complement-fixation test.

Treatment
African trypanocidal drugs have no effect.
Nifurtimox (Lampit) used in acute cases. No evidence of benefit in chronic longstanding infections. Dosage 8–10 mg/kg. body weight orally daily for 60–120 days. Toxic effects include haemolysis in G-6-PD deficient persons and nausea common, but serious toxicity unusual.

Chapter 54   ## LEISHMANIASIS (Kala-azar; Cutaneous and Mucocutaneous Leishmaniasis)

Group of chronic diseases with irregular pyrexia caused by flagellate protozoa of the genus *Leishmania*. Two divisions: (1) Visceral leishmaniasis; (2) Cutaneous and mucocutaneous leishmaniasis.

Visceral Leishmaniasis

Kala-azar
Characterized by irregular pyrexia, splenomegaly and cachexia.

Parasite (Leishmania donovani): Leishman–Donovan Bodies
Morphology. In smears from spleen with Romanowsky stain: small 'cockle-shaped' bodies, about 2·5–3·5 μm; protoplasm pink or blue, and contains: (1) small nucleus near periphery, staining intense red; (2) larger nucleus nearer centre, staining less deeply; also usually vacuoles. In smears lie free, but in sections are mainly intracellular in large endothelial cells, known as Leishman–Donovan bodies.

Cultivation. Cultivated in rabbit-blood agar (NNN medium), develops into promastigotes, with a flagellum. Resembles to some extent trypanosomes, but no undulating membrane.

Enzymatic differentiation. Species of leishmania now differentiated by their isoenzyme profile and nuclear and kinetoplast buoyant densities.

Epidemiology
Visceral leishmaniasis is transmitted in 3 main ways:

1. *From canines (including dogs, foxes and jackals) to man.* Especially around Mediterranean, Middle East, China. Also in scattered foci in Mexico, Guatemala, Colombia, Venezuela, Brazil, Northern Argentina and Paraguay.

2. *Predominantly from rodents to man.* In Sudan, Ethiopia, Kenya and Somalia.

3. *From a human reservoir.* In India, Assam and Burma. *P. argentipes* is the vector and causes large epidemics at intervals of a decade or two.

Parasite and host factors determine the clinical and epidemiological pattern.

Pathology
Sandfly inoculates promastigote forms of parasite. If cell-mediated immunity absent parasites spread diffusely and multiply in visceral reticuloendothelial cells especially in spleen, liver, lymphatic tissue, bone marrow and small intestine. Erythrocytes haemolyse due to complement and presumably antigen coating on them. Spleen greatly enlarges partly due to erythrophagocytosis, partly due to multiplication of parasitised cells.

If cell-mediated immunity present, infection limited to skin and cutaneous forms of the disease develop.

Clinical Features
Incubation period. Probably usually 1–4 months: up to 10 years.

Onset insidious or sudden with high fever. Principal symptoms:

1. Pyrexia. Irregular: may be day and night rise twice in 24 h: sweats after each paroxysm. Later in bouts of few weeks, with apyrexial intervals.

2. Spleen enlarges. May reach right iliac fossa in chronic cases. Liver edge palpable. Abdomen becomes prominent.

3. Anaemia of which the aetiology was long problematic. Now a marked haemolytic factor is recognized.

4. Loss of weight, sweats and debility. Loss of hair. Low blood pressure. Oedema. No adenitis.

5. Skin: dusky pigmentation; whence name 'black fever'.

6. Diarrhoea. (Ulcers in intestine.) Rare.

7. Absence of toxaemia striking. Appetite good.

Later, if untreated. Ascites. Oedema. Diarrhoea. Haemorrhages from mucous membranes. Finally: death from exhaustion and secondary infections. Duration: about 1–2 years.

Under treatment with antimony. Symptoms improve and weight increases. Cure is permanent.

Post-Kala-azar dermal leishmanoid. Depigmented patches on skin: nodules later develop, may resemble leprosy. *Leishmania* present in skin, but not in spleen. Occasionally xanthoma. Condition usually develops about 1–2 years after antimony treatment.

Laboratory Features

Leucopenia common with neutropenia and lymphocytopenia. Rarely agranulocytosis. Thrombocytopenia common.

Plasma globulins. Greatly increased and mostly consist of IgG. Little of the immunoglobulin is protective. Albumin fraction diminished.

Liver enzymes in serum increased. Prothrombin and thromboplastin diminished.

Complications

Intercurrent diseases, especially pulmonary tuberculosis, dysentery and cancrum oris. Hepatocellular damage may cause jaundice. Later post-kala-azar dermal leishmaniasis (*vide infra*).

Diagnosis

By symptoms, confirmed by discovery, preferably in culture, of Leishman–Donovan bodies in liver, bone marrow, or splenic aspirate. Only do latter if prothrombin time normal, platelets above $40\,000/mm^3$ and surgical facilities available.

Leishmanial antibodies. Demonstrable in serum by immunofluorescence and precipitation.

Leishmanin skin test. Negative in kala-azar but becomes positive after recovery in 75% cases. It is positive in subclinical self limiting kala-azar. Is of epidemiological value.

Aldehyde test. Add 1 drop formalin to 1 ml serum; shake and stand in room; serum turns viscid and sets solid in few minutes. Useful where laboratory facilities limited but is not specific.

Differential Diagnosis

From various febrile tropical splenomegalies, e.g. brucellosis, malaria, schistosomiasis; also from leukaemia.

Mortality

Formerly 80%. Low with modern treatment.

General Treatment of Leishmaniasis

Antimony Preparations

Specific for all forms, but *L. braziliensis* may be resistant and strains in Sudan and Mediterranean may be relatively resistant. Sodium stibogluconate, marketed as Pentostam, Solustibosan, and Stilbatin administered i.v. or i.m., former preferred as latter may cause necrosis of tissue and is painful. Initial dose 5 mg/kg patient's body weight followed by daily doses of 10–20 mg/kg. Usually marketed as 10% solution and course consists of 10–14 injections followed by a rest of 7 days and then another 10–14 injections. In India urea-stibamine much used, dosage 3 mg/kg body weight i.v. on 10–15 occasions. Courses may be repeated after 2–3 weeks if patient fails to respond. Meglumine antimonate (Glucantine), a pentavalent antimonial also used and contains 85 mg Sb/ml. 0·12 ml/kg body weight equivalent to 10 mg antimony/kg.

Toxic effects of pentavalent antimonials rare but include nausea, vomiting, exfoliative dermatitis and electrocardiographic changes.

In resistant cases more toxic drugs may have to be tried: (1) Pentamidine isethionate (Pentamidine) and pentamidine dimethane-sulphonate (Lomidine). Both marketed in solution containing 40 mg/ml given i.m. in doses of 0·1 ml/kg body weight every 3–4 days. May cause collapse if any given i.v. and later may cause diabetes. (2) Amphotericin B given by slow i.v. infusion in doses of 1 mg/kg body weight in 5% dextrose on alternate days to maximal total of 40 mg/kg body weight. Side effects include vomiting, rigors and thrombophlebitis.

Splenectomy

Sometimes done in resistant cases but is hazardous and best avoided. Such patients commonly later die of intercurrent infection.

Results

Spleen diminishes: blood and general condition improve: parasites disappear. Mortality: less than 5%.

Infantile Kala-azar

Distribution

Shores of the Mediterranean. Widespread.

Characteristics

Occurs in children, ages 2–5 years. Symptoms as in adult form. Parasite named *L. infantum*, but indistinguishable from *L. donovani*. Caused by a canine strain of parasite.

Treatment

Vide supra.

Post-kala-azar Dermal Leishmaniasis

Commonest in India, Sudan and East Africa. Develops 1–2 years after apparent cure of kala-azar. Erythematous or hypopigmented macules develop and contain many leishmania. Later become nodular. Associated with lack of cell-mediated immunity to leishmania. This usually develops after recovery from kala-azar but in post-kala-azar dermal leishmaniasis it fails to do so.

Cutaneous Leishmaniasis

Oriental Sore *(Baghdad Boil; Delhi Sore; Tropical Sore; Aleppo Button)*
Infective granuloma of skin and subcutaneous tissues, originally ascribed to *L. tropica*, but indistinguishable morphologically from *L. donovani*. Recognized in same way as *L. infantum*. *L. tropica* now divided into *L. tropica tropica* (= *L. tropica (minor)*) and *L. (tropica) major*.

Parasite
Present in juice aspirated from spreading edge of sore.

Mode of Infection
Infection conveyed by sandflies (*Phlebotomus papatasii* and others).
Incubation period. Very variable: weeks to many months.

Pathology
Leishmaniae invade local macrophage cells. Lymphocytes cuff small blood vessels. Cell-mediated immunity present from outset of infection and continues after cure.

Symptoms
Commences as small itching papule, forms sore with scab. Surface ulcerates, but margins raised, hard and clear-cut. Satellite papules often present. Multiple lesions may coalesce forming large area. Non-ulcerating warty growths may also form. No general dissemination: glands not enlarged unless cellulitis. Common on, but not limited to, face and hands.
   If untreated, heals in about one year, by granulation, much scarring.

Diagnosis
Organism in tissue juice aspirated from edge of ulcer.

Treatment
Remove crusts by soaking or poultice, dress with tulle gras and give antimony systemically as for kala-azar. Obtains best results. CO_2 snow may be used but painful and usually causes more severe scarring. Local application for 4–5 hours daily of electrically heated pad to raise skin temperature to 40–43 °C. Very effective.

Mucocutaneous Leishmaniasis *(Espundia)*
An infective granuloma with tendency to secondary lesions of buccal and nasal mucosa. Occurs in S. America, especially in Amazonian forests.

Parasite
L. braziliensis, indistinguishable morphologically from *L. donovani*, but distinguished clinically, epidemiologically, by isoenzyme recognition and by poor growth in culture or when inoculated into nose of hamsters.

Mode of Infection
Conveyed by *Psychodopygus wellcomei* and *Lutzomyia* species. Several forest rodents form the reservoir.

Symptoms
Commences as small papule, on arms or often on margins of ears; extends and may suppurate. Heals spontaneously but metastases may remain dormant for months or years and then break down especially in nose or mouth or at their mucocutaneous border, extend, and cause destruction of tissue; bone not affected. No general dissemination. External genitalia may also be affected.

Treatment
Often resistant. Curettage of active areas of lesions often helpful. Full treatment with pentavalent antimonial should be given for at least 21 days (p. 242) and if not successful follow with Amphotericin B in dosage as for diffuse cutaneous leishmaniasis.

Lupoid Leishmaniasis and Leishmaniasis Recivida
Occur when complete immunity does not develop after oriental sore.

Lupoid leishmaniasis occurs in Middle East; affects large areas of skin. Lesions develop slowly and usually heal in their centres forming irregular circinate sores of great chronicity. Responds to systemic pentavalent antimonials.

Leishmaniasis recivida is a chronic relapsing infection associated with delayed hypersensitivity during and after its onset. Responds to systemic pentavalent antimonials.

Diffuse Cutaneous Leishmaniasis (*Leishmaniasis Tegumentiria Diffusa; Disseminated Anergic American Cutaneous Leishmaniasis; Lepromatoid Leishmaniasis*)
A form of the infection recognized only in the last 30 years and occurring in South Central America and East Africa.

Aetiology
Thought to result principally from the lack of patient's cellular immunity and hypersensitivity response to the infection. No cellular immunity or humoral antibodies develop. In Africa *L. aethiopica* and in New World *L. mexicana* spp. now recognized as the infective agents.

Pathology
Epidermis thin and flat but intact with loss of the rete. Clear zone usually present immediately under epidermis and beneath this zone the dermis is much infiltrated with macrophages and thickened. Cytoplasma of macrophages filled with leishmanial amastigotes. Numerous monocytes migrate through walls of small blood vessels in the lesions, appear to develop into tissue histiocytes and deeper in the lesion transform into parasitized macrophages. There is no round cell or plasma cell infiltration. Though leishmania have been recovered from blood and bone marrow there is no general invasion of internal organs.

Clinical Features
Nodule forms on face, arm or leg, enlarges, becomes shiny and inflamed and has

distinct edges separating it from normal skin. Lesion enlarges and numerous others develop. Mucous membranes of nose and mouth not involved. Extensor surface of limbs most commonly affected and skin may become oedematous. Lesions chronic, general health unaffected. Leishmanin test negative.

Differential Diagnosis
Leprosy may be simulated but nodules softer, shinier and more sharply defined than those of leprosy. Nerves not thickened but enlarged lymphatics may be confused with them.

Differentiation from keloids, Kaposi's sarcoma, mycoses and onchocerciasis by demonstration of leishmania in smears from lesions.

Treatment
L. aethiopica is resistant to antimony, therefore for it, use Amphotericin B by slow i.v. infusion in daily doses of 250 μg to 1 mg/kg body weight for 20–60 days. Also pentamidine isethionate i.v. or i.m. in doses of 3 mg/kg body weight daily for 7–15 days is of value but several courses separated by intervals of 2 or 3 weeks at least may be required. For *L. mexicana* infections pentavalent antimony should first be tried (*see* p. 242).

Chiclero's Ulcer *(Bay sore)*

Geographical Distribution
Belize and parts of Mexico.

Aetiology
Reservoir of infection in various forest rodents from which the causative organism *Leishmania mexicana mexicana* is transmitted to man by the bites of sandflies (*Lutzomyia olmeca olmeca*). Particularly affects chicleros who are so named because they collect chicle or latex from forest trees. They spend long periods in the forest usually living under rough conditions.

Pathology
Similar to that of oriental sore. Delayed hypersensitivity present during and after infection.

Clinical Features
Chronic ulcer usually affecting ear and causing considerable destruction of the pinna. Very chronic and alternately heals and breaks down.

Diagnosis
Clinical and epidemiological features characteristic. Organisms may be found in tissue juice aspirated from the edge of the ulcer.

Treatment
Pentavalent antimony as for kala-azar or pyrimethamine orally in adult doses of 25 mg b.d. for 2 weeks or single injection of cycloguanilpamoate (Camolar) in doses of 5 mg/kg body weight. This injection may be repeated if necessary after 1–2 months.

Peruvian Cutaneous Leishmaniasis
Caused by *Leishmania peruviana* and transmitted to man from dogs by *Lutzomyia verrucarum*. Gives rise to simple ulcers which do not invade mucocutaneous junctions. Management as for oriental sores.

Diseases
due to
Metazoan
Parasites

Chapter 55 **TREMATODE OR FLUKE INFECTIONS**
(Distomiasis)

Four principal groups of fluke infections occur in man. All flukes require a specific snail as intermediate host in their life cycle: needs special conditions of climate and irrigation. Transmitted only in tropical and subtropical regions, but disease, if untreated, persists in persons returning to cooler climates. (1) Pulmonary flukes—*Paragonimus westermani*. (2) Hepatic flukes—*Clonorchis sinensis; Fasciola hepatica*. (3) Intestinal flukes—*Fasciolopsis buski; Heterophyes heterophyes*. (4) Blood flukes—*Schistosoma haematobium; S. mansoni; S. japonicum*.

Pulmonary Fluke

Paragonimiasis

Life Cycle
Paragonimus westermani measuring $7–12 \times 6$ mm in lungs of man, canidae and felidae. Ova in sputum release miracidia in fresh water; infect *Melania* snails from which cercariae emerge to infect freshwater crabs and crayfish, consumption of which raw, causes infection in man. Larvae migrate from human intestine to lung and there mature.

Geographical Distribution
China, Far East, West Africa.

Clinical Features
Chronic cough, bloodstained sputum. Occasionally diarrhoea and/or hepatomegaly. Worms may rarely reach brain or spinal cord and cause focal symptoms.

Diagnosis
Ova $100 \times 50\,\mu m$ in sputum. Radiological appearance of lung lesions: groups of small cavities like clusters of grapes. Worms located in cavities. Exclude tuberculosis.

Treatment
Praziquantel orally in doses of 25 mg/kg body weight daily for 2 days. If not available bithionol, 20 mg/kg body weight orally daily for 14 days or chloroquine 600 mg (base) orally daily for 6 weeks.

Hepatic Flukes

Clonorchiasis

Life Cycle
Clonorchis sinensis measuring 11–20 × 3–4 mm in bile ducts and liver of man and fish-eating mammals. Ova 30 × 16 μm passed in bile and faeces. Hatch in fresh water and infect *Bythrynia* snails from which cercariae emerge and enter fish which infect man when eaten raw or undercooked. Parasites released from fish in duodenum enter biliary tract.

Geographical Distribution
China and Far East.

Clinical Features
Often none but in heavy chronic infections, cyst-like cavities in biliary tracts and liver develop; liver enlarges and fibroses, cachexia, cholangitis, jaundice and malignant changes may supervene. Leucocytosis with eosinophilia.

Diagnosis
Demonstration of ova in faeces.

Treatment
As for paragonimiasis; antibiotics, rehydration and blood transfusion may be needed for cholangitis.

Fascioliasis

Life Cycle
Fasciola hepatica measures 3·5 × 1·2 cm, lives in bile ducts of sheep, man and cattle. Ova 140 × 180 μm passed in faeces and in fresh water release miracidia which enter *Limnaea* snails. Cercariae leave snails and encyst on aquatic vegetation as metacercariae. Man infected by eating these on water cress, etc. Larvae liberated from metacercariae in intestine and invade and mature in bile ducts.

Geographical Distribution
Worldwide.

Clinical Features
During invasive phase, fever, hepatic pain, eosinophilia. A long latent period may be followed by biliary obstruction resulting from epithelial proliferation in bile ducts with biliary cirrhosis.

Diagnosis
Demonstration of ova in faeces. Complement-fixation test.

Treatment
As for paragonimiasis.

Intestinal Flukes

Fasciolopsiasis

Life Cycle
Fasciolopsis buski measures 2–7 × 1·4 cm and lives in small intestine of man or pigs. Ova 140 × 80 μm passed in faeces and in fresh water release miracidia which enter *Planorbis* snails from which cercariae emerge and encyst on water caltrop and water chestnut. Man infected by eating these.

Geographical Distribution
Far East, especially China.

Clinical Features
In heavy infections diarrhoea and haemorrhage from abscesses of intestinal wall.

Diagnosis
Ova in faeces.

Treatment
As for hookworm infections.

Heterophyiasis

Life Cycle
Heterophyes heterophyes measures 2 mm and lives in small intestine of man, canidae, and felidae. Ova in faeces measure 30 × 16 μm and in fresh water release miracidia which enter the snail, *Pironella conica* from which cercariae emerge and infect mullet and other fish. Man infected by eating these lightly cooked.

Geographical Distribution
Egypt, Middle and Far East.

Clinical Features
Usually asymptomatic but diarrhoea in heavy infections.

Treatment
As for hookworm infections.

Blood Flukes

Schistosomiasis (*Bilharziasis; Endemic Haematuria*)
Chronic endemic disease due to infection by blood flukes of family Schistosomidae inhabiting the portal vein and producing pathological changes mainly by passage of ova.

Geographical Distribution
S. haematobium. Africa: Mediterranean coast, Nile valley, entire east coast to Natal and Cape, areas on the Congo and Niger. Iraq and Yemen. Not in America.

S. mansoni. Africa: Nile delta, large area across Africa from Zanzibar to Sierra Leone. Northern areas of South America. Not in India or U.S.A.

S. japonicum. Valley of Yangtze Kiang, Japan, Philippines, and areas in South-East Asia.

S. intercalatum. Limited to Zaïre, Cameroon and Gabon.

S. matthei and *S. bovis* occasionally infect man.

Distribution is limited by that of intermediate host. Non-human varieties of schistosomes producing cercariae exist in the USA and elsewhere. Parasites do not mature in man but cercariae may cause dermatitis (swimmer's itch).

The Parasite in Man

Sexes distinct: (1) *Male*, length varies with species 6–20 mm by 1 mm broad, sides curved to form an unclosed cyclinder (the characteristic *gynaecophoric canal*), body covered by spinous prominences; (2) *Female*, much longer but filiform. Both sexes have an anterior and a more posterior ventral sucker by which they maintain their position in bloodstream. When young, sexes are separate, but at maturity female enters gynaecophoric canal of male, projecting at each end owing to greater length. Ovum oval: size 160 by 60 μm.

Life cycle. Has two phases: (1) In man—definitive host; (2) In snail—intermediate host.

Cycle in Man

1. Cercaria discharged from snail reaches skin or mucous membrane of man during washing or drinking, and penetrates, shedding its tail. Thence reaches portal vein.

2. Parasites in portal vein grow to maturity in about 6 weeks; female enters gynaecophoric canal of male, together migrate to smaller veins of bladder or rectum; after copulation thinner female continues alone into smallest veins, deposits ova, and then withdraws.

3. Ova escape through wall of veins, traverse tissues and reach bladder or rectum; an embryo is now present in ovum. On ovum reaching water an active embryo, covered with cilia, escapes (miracidium).

Cycle in Snails: Miracidium penetrates a freshwater snail, reaches liver, forms sporocysts in enormous numbers, whence bifid-tailed cercariae escape into the water. Cycle in snail, 14 days. Cercaria dies in 48 h unless it finds a host.

Life of Parasite: Can remain active and produce viable eggs for 30 years.

Types. Four types occur, with following differences:

    1. *Schistosoma haematobium*.

        1.1. Habitat of worms especially in vesical and prostatic plexuses and less commonly in veins of portal system and rectum;

        1.2. Ovum has a terminal spine;

        1.3. Ova pursue path through vein and tissues to bladder, producing pathological changes in urinary tract and neighbouring tissues;

        1.4. Miracidium set free from ovum enters a snail, genus *Bulinus*. Male worm covered with tubercles.

    2. *Schistosoma mansoni*.

        2.1. Habitat of worms especially in inferior and superior mesenteric veins, haemorrhoidal plexus, and also in portal system;

2.2. Ovum has a lateral spine;

2.3. Ova penetrate tissues to rectum and colon;

2.4. Miracidium from ovum enters a snail, genus *Biomphalaria*. Male worm more coarsely tuberculated. Spleen and liver may be affected (Egyptian splenomegaly).

Note: Habitats described are not absolute. *S. haematobium* ova are common in rectum, and *S. mansoni* ova may occur in bladder lesions.

3. *Schistosoma japonicum*.

3.1. Ovum has no spine, but a lateral knob;

3.2. Ova deposited in large and small intestine;

3.3. Miracidium enters a snail, genus *Oncomelania*;

3.4. Male worm has no tubercles. Spleen and liver may be affected (Katayama disease).

4. *Schistosoma intercalatum* similar to but now recognized as distinct from *S. haematobium*. Eggs longer and broader with long terminal spine but adults live in mesenteric and portal veins and eggs pass through bowel to faeces.

Snails: Intermediate Host

For *S. haematobium*: genus *Bulinus*, spiral snail with sinistral opening; many species, in Egypt *contortus*. For *S. mansoni*: genus *Biomphalaria*, flat whorled snail; many species, in Egypt *B. alexandrina* and in East and West Africa, mainly *B. pfeifferi*. The above snails all die if dried; but have recently been shown to survive relatively dry conditions beneath surface of mud of dried-out ponds. For *S. japonicum*: genus *Oncomelania*: multiple whorls; can live in dried mud. For *S. intercalatum*, *Bulinus globosus* and *B. forskali*.

Pathology

General pathology. Pathological changes are produced by ovum in its passage from the venule to a site of escape from the body. Such changes largely mediated by immune reactions, both cell-mediated and systemic, forming around ovum a pseudo-tubercle with giant cells: cells necrose permitting passage of ovum, and scar formation follows. Many such tubercles fuse, forming visible tubercles; aided by repeated waves of ova and death and calcification of many ova. Local lesions result from agglomeration of tubercles—ulceration, scarring and calcification; formation of polypi, adenomas and neoplastic transformation; and by resulting blockage of ducts and passages.

Urinary tract and genital organs. *S. haematobium* is usual infection: *mansoni* rarely. Tubercles appear on mucosal surface of bladder as papules: granular phosphate deposits forming 'sandy patches'. Trigone earliest affected. Ulceration and scarring of tubercles. Mucosa covered with blood-stained mucus with many ova. Later polypoid excrescences, adenopapillomas which may become neoplastic; gravel and calculi.

Urinary tract: Lower end of ureter first affected: causing renal calculi, hydronephrosis and ureteric reflex. All urinary tract may be involved, e.g. prostatic enlargement; secondary infections common; urinary fistulas.

Deposits of immune complexes demonstrated in renal glomerulus in longstanding infections. Largely responsible for nephrotic syndrome sometimes encountered in such patients.

Genital tract: similarly attacked.

Intestinal schistosomiasis. S. mansoni is usual infection; *S. haematobium* occasionally; may be both. General changes correspond to above description: tubercles, sandy patches. papillomas; polypi may cause obstruction, intussusception, or extrude through anus. *Large pericolic tumours* may form. Mesenteric glands enlarge. Appendicitis not uncommon. Ileum rarely infected.

S. Haematobium Infection

Symptoms
Invasion. Dermatitis and irritation at site of entry of cercariae.
Initial stage: development and ovulation. Four to ten weeks after infection. Constitutional disturbances, fever, abdominal pain, cough, diarrhoea, urticaria; when severe, may resemble typhoid. May be absent. Leucocytosis, with high eosinophilia, 30–50%. Interval of months or years before bladder affected.
Genito-urinary symptoms. Occur in attacks: (1) Haematuria, especially at end of micturition; (2) Aching in perineum and penis; (3) Frequency and urgency of micturition; (4) Ova urine; (5) Symptoms of secondary bacterial infection; (6) Bladder carcinoma may develop.
Progress. Course depends on severity and repetition of infection. May be mild and health maintained under treatment. For complications, *see* Pathology (p. 251).

S. Mansoni Infection

Symptoms
Similar to above initial stage.
Intestinal symptoms. Attacks of blood and mucus in stool and symptoms as in chronic dysentery. In mild cases may be asymptomatic.
Progress. Cirrhosis of liver and splenomegaly in longstanding cases of moderate or severe infection. *See* Pathology (p. 251).

Egyptian Splenomegaly
Occurs in longstanding heavily infected patients, especially those with *S. mansoni* infection. Due to: (1) ova reaching liver and causing multiple granulomas with fibrosis and portal hypertension; (2) haemolysis of erythrocytes with erythrophagocytosis in spleen and consequent hypertrophy of reticulo-endothelial cells. In such haemolysis immune complexes deposited on red blood cells.

Symptoms
Spleen and liver enlarge progressively: abdomen becomes enormous. In later stages liver may shrink but not spleen. Visceral symptoms often slight. Progressive anaemia. Wasting. Final stages of cirrhosis of liver; ascites. May be haemorrhages. Duration: many years in adults; in children rapid.

Cardiopulmonary Schistosomiasis
Ova present in lungs in 33% of autopsies. Lesions usually unimportant. Serious developments in few cases (*vide infra*).

Route traversed to Lungs
Neither worms nor ova can traverse liver. From intestinal lesions (mainly *S. mansoni*) heart only reached through anastomoses due to cirrhosis of liver. From genito-urinary infections (mainly *S. haematobium*) heart can be reached even in early cases through iliac veins.

Changes in Pulmonary Arterioles and Arteries.
Ova reach lung as emboli in pulmonary arterioles. Changes in walls proceed as described under General Pathology. As ova escape from arterioles, necrotizing arteriolitis is produced and proceeds to obliterative arteriolitis. Pulmonary artery becomes dilated from increased pressure: in rare cases aneurysmal.

Cardiac Complications: Cor Pulmonale
Hypertrophy of right ventricle and dilatation of right atrium develop as result of the rise of pulmonary pressure. Congestive heart failure follows.
(Known in Egypt as Ayerza's disease.)

Lesions of Lung
Lungs have scattered foci of fibrosis around affected arterioles. Parenchyma of lung not primarily affected: hence *no cyanosis* until heart fails.
Effects of anti-schistosomal treatment. Antimonials may increase pulmonary hypertension and precipitate right heart failure. Therefore proceed cautiously.
    Note: X-ray foci may temporarily enlarge.
Radiographs. Scattered foci of thickened arterioles throughout lungs (resemble silicosis but not in lung tissue). Shadow in right hilum due to enlarged pulmonary artery.

S. japonicum Infection

Symptoms
Initial stage. Pyrexia, urticaria, cough, eosinophilia, muscle and joint pains. Symptoms more severe than in other schistosomal infections. Long latent period follows.
Second stage. Intestinal and dysenteric symptoms.
Third stage. Spleen and liver enlarged. Wasting. Anaemia and ascites. Latter only with severe infections. Duration: many years.

Diagnosis of Schistosomiasis
Concomitant infections and malnutrition common and complicate manifestations, e.g. amoeba, ankylostoma, ascaris. Differential diagnosis is from other causes of haematuria and dysentery: in splenomegalic type from kala-azar and other splenomegalies.
Diagnostic methods. (1) Search for eggs in urine and stool. In *S. haematobium* search often most productive in terminal portion of urine expressed, and collection of such specimens over 24 h valuable. Urine allowed to sediment and deposit examined. If ova scarce centrifuge deposit. (2) Biopsy and direct examination rectal mucosa—valuable in all forms of schistosomiasis, (3) Immunological techniques, particularly complement-fixation test and enzyme-linked immunosorbent assay (ELISA). (4) Cystoscopy. (5) Sigmoidoscopy.

Prophylaxis of Schistosomiasis
Education. Propaganda against bathing, washing, or drinking in canals, ponds and rivers.
Hygiene. Provision of piped, safe water supply and adequate latrine facilities.
Destruction of snails. Cleansing of weeds from waterways; destruction of snails by 5,2-dichloro-4-nitro-salicylic anilide (Bayluside), sodium pentachlorophenate, acrolein, dinitrophenol compounds, or copper sulphate; periodic drying of canals.
Treatment of infected persons
    Note: In Egypt, where canals are a special difficulty, degree of infection is only falling slowly with methods in force, but the incidence of severe complications is being reduced by treatment.

Treatment of Schistosomiasis
Praziquantel (Biltricide). Effective against all varieties. Given orally 20 mg/kg t.d.s for one day. Few side effects.
Oxamniquine (Vansil). A quinoline derivative. Effective against *S. mansoni* only. Sensitivity of strains varies. Dosage 15–20 mg/kg body weight orally, daily for 1–5 days. Few side effects.
Metriphonate (Bilharcil). An organophosphorus anticholinesterase. Given orally, 7·5 mg/kg body weight once every 2–4 weeks for 2–3 doses. Acts against *S. haematobium* only. Avoid suxamethonium in anaesthesia for 48 h after giving metriphonate because of anticholinergic action of both.
Hycanthone (Entrenol). A lucanthone derivative. Effective against *S. haematobium* and *S. mansoni*. Administered i.m. as a single dose of 0·75–3 mg/kg body weight. Significant cure rate but hepatoxicity may occur with higher dosage.
Niridazole (Ambilhar). Largely replaced by praziquantel but effective against all types. Given orally in doses of 20–25 mg/kg body weight daily for 7–10 days. Vomiting, abdominal pain, psychoses, convulsions and aspermogenesis reported in adults, especially if liver damaged or venous anastomoses permit portal blood containing absorbed drug to bypass the liver where conjugation and detoxification occur. Children tolerate it well.
Sodium antimony tartrates. Still used, especially in Middle East; i.v. injections only (solution causes necrosis of tissue).
    Solution: 1 or 2% in normal saline or 5% glucose (30–60 mg in 10 ml), inject very slowly. *Dosage*: commence with 30 mg, increasing to 120 mg. Maximum individual dose, 2 mg/kg body weight; injections daily or on alternate days according to tolerance to total for course of 1·2–1·8 g. Kills adult parasites. Results checked by examinations for ova. *Toxic effects* of all antimony compounds: coughing, spasmodic and transient; vomiting, flushing. More severe reaction: headache, arthritic pains in shoulder joint, constriction of chest. Rarely cardiac collapse. Causes electrocardiographic changes, reduction in amplitude or inversion of T wave and upward sloping of S–T segment sometimes with prolongation of Q–T interval. ECG tracings should be taken before treatment and at intervals of 3–4 days during treatment, which should be suspended if changes marked.
Antimony dimercaptosuccinate (TWSB, Astiban). Probably the most effective of the antimonials which may be given i.m. Usual dosage 8 mg/kg body weight, maximum 0·5 g daily or on alternate days for 5 doses.

Fouadin, Neoantimosan. Therapeutic activity poor but toxicity low. I.m. injections of 6·3% solution. *Dosage*: 5 ml, 10–15 injections in 3–4 weeks. (First dose 1·5 ml.) May be spasms of coughing. Relapse rate 50% or more.

Anthiomaline (Lithium salt of Antimony thiomalate). In 6% solution, *I.v. injection*: adult 1·5 ml alternate days up to 4 ml. Also i.m. Toxic effects slight. Results poor and relapse rate 50% or more.

   Note: Pentavalent antimony compounds, e.g. neostibosan, have little effect.

Chapter 56   # DISEASES CAUSED BY CESTODES
                    (Taeniasis)

---

1. Intestinal Tapeworms

Tapeworms are flat worms of various types and size. Structure is in general a minute head and narrow neck forming the scolex, from which develop a series of flat segments or proglottides: these become larger and more mature distally. There is no alimentary canal: nutriment is absorbed direct from the intestine. Most tapeworms require an intermediate host. *Hymenolepis nana* is an exception.

Cycle in Man
Definitive host. Infected by ingesting animal meat (or fish) infected with larval cysticercoid form. Cysticerci develop in man into mature tapeworms and inhabit small intestine. Ova and segments escape in faeces.

Cycle in Animal
Intermediate host. Ingests ova: larval forms develop, enter bloodstream and are deposited in muscle and solid organs where larval cysts form.

Important Varieties in Man
1. *Taenia solium*, pork tapeworm.
2. *Taenia saginata*, beef tapeworm.
3. *Hymenolepis nana*, dwarf tapeworm. Host: predominantly man and man-to-man transmission under unhygienic conditions is the usual mode of infection but infection from faeces of infected rats, mice and hamsters is well known. Some of these infections are from pet animals. Length 5–45 mm: about 200 segments. In warm climates only. Large numbers may be present. No intermediate host required, as ova hatch in intestine.
4. *Diphyllobothrium latum* (syn.: *Dibothriocephalus latus*): Especially in Baltic countries and Switzerland; parts of Central Asia and Far East; rare elsewhere; imported to USA. Host: man, dog. Intermediate host: pike and other fish. Can produce blood changes identical with pernicious anaemia, but curable on discharge of worm.

   The principal characteristics are given in the table overleaf.

INTESTINAL TAPEWORMS

Characteristics		T. solium	T. saginata	T. echinococcus	Dibothriocephalus latus
Distribution		India; parts of Africa, Latin America. Rare in Britain, USA and Canada	Widespread; commonest type	Middle East, East Africa, Sudan, sheep-rearing areas almost anywhere. Australia and New Zealand.	Around Great Lakes in North America and Scandinavian lakes. Was common in Finland but control measures have much reduced its incidence. Rare elsewhere
Host (adult worms; in intestines)		Man only	Man only	Dog, also wolf and jackal (never in man)	Man, dog
Intermediate host (larval forms; in muscles and solid organs)		Pig, man	Cattle, never in man	Hog, sheep, cattle and man	Pike and other freshwater fish
Length		2–4 m	5–6 m	5 mm (including head)	8–10 m
Head		Small pin's-head; 4 suckers; rostellum with hooklets	Larger than T. solium; 2 mm 4 suckers; no hooklets	4 suckers; double row hooklets (hooklets barbed)	2 lateral grooves; no hooklets
Proglottides	Number	Many hundreds	Many hundreds	4 including head (rarely 3 or 5)	Many hundreds
	Size	10 × 7 mm	17 × 8 mm	Elongated	10 × 2 mm
	Shape	Elongated	Elongated	—	Broad and short
Sexual pore		Lateral	Lateral	Only terminal segment mature	Central
Uterus		Usually 8–12 branches, always less than 15	15 or more lateral branches	—	Rosette: in centre of proglottis
Ova		Nearly spherical; thick shell; contains embryo (rarely visible hooklets)	As T. solium (differences slight); no hooklets		Segmentation marked

Cysticercoid Forms

Two larval cystic forms occur in man with serious results: (1) *Cysticercus cellulosae*: larval form of *T. solium*; (2) *Echinococcus granulosus*: adult of which infects dogs, wolves, jackals.

Taenia Solium

Life cycle: the uterus contains numerous ova; if ova are ingested into stomach of pig, embryo becomes free, penetrates wall, reaches muscles (also brain and liver), develops into larval form or *Cysticercus cellulosae*, constituting 'measly pork'. Cysticerci are known as measles or bladder-worms. Frequent sites: tongue, muscles of mastication, shoulders, neck, diaphragm. In man, eating such pork, larvae develop into adult worms. Larval forms also occur in man (*see* Cysticercus Cellulosae, p. 258) *with serious results*.

Taenia Saginata

Life cycle resembles *T. solium*, but cattle form intermediate host. Cysticerci most common in muscles of jaw. Larval forms never occur in man.

Symptoms

May be none. Usual complaint is passage of segments. May be vague gastrointestinal disturbances, e.g. anorexia, with wasting, especially in children. Occasionally urticaria and other allergic symptoms occur.
Blood. Eosinophilia very rarely present except in hydatid disease. IgE may be increased.

Diagnosis

Proglottides are pathognomonic. Ova in stools may be distinctive but are absent unless segments have disintegrated in intestine.

Prophylaxis

(1) Inspection of meat. Cysticerci in beef die in 3 weeks, but in pork live longer. (2) Sufficient cooking of meat. (3) Destruction by burning of all tapeworm segments passed in stools. At all sewage farms precautions should be taken to ensure the tapeworm segments from faeces are not consumed by birds, rats, or other animals. Cysticercoid disease in cattle has been attributed to scattering of ova by the faeces of these animals. Those infected with *T. solium* or *H. nana* should guard against auto-reinfection or cysticerci may develop.

Treatment

Object is to ensure that the head of the worm releases its hold on the intestinal mucosa; unless it does so the worm will again become fully grown in approximately 3 months. Administer anthelmintic in a form in which it is able to act directly on the head of the worm; capsules and other containers for drugs may not rupture and so liberate their contents until they have passed the head of the worm.

Treatment of Taenia Saginata and Diphyllobothrium Latum Infections

Niclosamide (Yomesan, FBA). Now the most used remedy. No solid food is given for 12 h before treatment which is normally taken in the morning. The dose for children over 8 years and for adults is 1 g (2 tablets) followed in an hour by a further gramme. For those between 2 and 8 years one-half these amounts and for those under 2 years one-quarter of these amounts are administered. Food may be taken 2 h after the last tablet has been swallowed. The treatment is probably not as effective as that with male fern and as the worm may be disintegrated evidence of a cure is not usually obtained.

Niclosamide and dichlorophen may give rise to liberation of tapeworm eggs in the gut of the treated patient and if the worm is *T. solium*, cysticercosis is known to have followed. For this reason it is inadvisable to use these drugs for infections with that worm and as a corollary to this point species identification of the worm before treatment is essential.

Praziquantel. No special preparation needed. A single oral dose of 25 mg/kg is given. Mild side effects, headache, dizziness, drowsiness, nausea, abdominal pain, pruritus, urticaria, arthralgia and myalgia are common.

Paromomycin (Humatin). Effective in dosage of 30–50 mg/kg body weight on one day only. Total dose divided into four individual doses given orally at 15-min intervals.

Dichlorophen (Antiphen, M & B). The makers consider no preparatory treatment necessary and to adults a dose of 5 g is given usually in the morning. The worm is disintegrated. Side-effects include abdominal discomfort, diarrhoea and urticaria. Should not be used for *T. solium* infections.

Treatment of Taenia Solium Infections

Aspidium oleoresin, extract of male fern. On day before treatment give food containing no significant residue, and 15–30 g of sodium or magnesium sulphate, to clear intestine, facilitate access of the anthelmintic to the worm and to render the head of the worm more easily identifiable if passed. On the day of treatment three doses each of 2 ml male fern extract (B.P.) are given at 30-min intervals to adults followed by another 15 g sodium or magnesium sulphate. A child of 2 years may be given up to 2 ml extract in divided doses. The male fern is best made into a draught with flavouring agent. After administration all stools are saved and searched until the head of the worm is recovered or until 24 h following treatment have elapsed.

The treatment may be repeated after a week's interval. Toxic effects are very rare.

Treatment of Hymenolepis Nana Infections

Praziquantel the drug of choice or if not available aspidium oleoresin, 2 or 3 courses at weekly intervals to kill worms emerging from cysticerci in intestinal mucosa. Avoid drugs which cause rapid liberation of ova in intestine as these are infective to man.

2. Cysticercosis (Cysticercus Cellulosae)

This is the presence in man of the larval form of *T. solium* (pork tapeworm). The pig is the usual intermediate host for cysticerci; man acts as such if ova enter the stomach or upper small intestine where their shells are digested.

Cysticercus Cellulosae

Elliptical shape, about 8 mm by 6 mm: semi-transparent (hence called 'bladder-worms'). Where pressure is slight, e.g. in ventricles of brain, may be larger.

Mode of Infection
(1) Proglottides reach stomach or upper small intestine by own movement or ova liberated from them may be taken there by reversed peristalsis accompanying nausea or vomiting; (2) Ova are ingested from presence on fingers (auto-reinfection); (3) Contaminated food, e.g. salads. Flies are known transmitters.

Distribution
Any tissue in body but commonest sites are: (1) Subcutaneous and in muscle, usual site; (2) Central nervous system.

Symptoms
Depend on site and number of cysticerci. While cysticerci are alive they provoke little or no inflammatory reaction. Symptoms including epilepsy usually only occur when cysts die.
Subcutaneous and muscular. Patient complains of lumps beneath skin or in tongue. Often no symptoms. If numerous, rarely severe pains. Cysticerci palpable as small, subcutaneous, often tender nodules.
Central nervous system. In brain, may produce train of various cerebral symptoms over many years, e.g. epilepsy; also pressure symptoms especially with cysts in fourth ventricle and in basal meninges: headache, various paralyses, latter may sometimes be due to cysts in spinal cord; altered personality and psychotic states may also develop. Many cases in British soldiers who served in India. Symptoms may not occur for many years after exposure.
Eye. May be present in vitreous humour and affect sight.

Diagnosis
By removal of subcutaneous nodules, or very rarely by presence in eye.
Casoni skin test. May be positive from cross-reacting antibodies.
Cysticercal complement-fixation test. Available and useful in conjunction with clinical features but cross-reacts with hydatid and other larval tapeworms.
Radiographs. Cysticerci calcify in 4–5 years and are then (but not previously) opaque to X-rays.
Cerebrospinal fluid. May contain eosinophils and increased protein—mostly IgG.

Treatment
Symptomatic for epilepsy. Surgical if internal hydrocephalus caused by cysts in 4th ventricle.
Praziquantel. Has been given in doses of 15 mg/kg t.d.s. orally for 10–14 days. Kills cysticerci but may thereby provoke epilepsy—sometimes in those not known to have cerebral cysts. Coincident steroid therapy therefore needed to minimize surrounding inflammatory reaction and anticonvulsants if epilepsy develops.

3. Hydatid Disease: (Larval Taenia Echinococcus or Echinococcus Granulosus)

Infection in man by larval forms of *E. granulosus*, the adult of which lives in the intestine of dogs and certain related species.

Echinococcus Granulosus
For characteristics, *see* Table (p. 256).

Hydatid Cysts

Development. Terminal segment of the adult worm is discharged in dog faeces, and ova swallowed by intermediate host. From ovum, six-hooked embryo ('oncosphere') escapes, penetrates upper intestine and reaches blood vessels, whence carried to liver and in many cases beyond liver to lungs and other tissues where cyst forms.

Histology of cyst wall. Two layers: (1) External, laminated, chitinous layer—'ectocyst'; (2) Internal, parenchymatous layer or germinal epithelium—'endocyst'. Surrounding layer of fibrous tissue forms from host.

Development in cyst. From the 'endocyst' outgrowths form which develop:

1. *Secondary cysts*: Exactly resembling primary cyst. These may become free. Also tertiary cysts may similarly develop, the whole sometimes growing 25 cm in diameter.

2. *Scolices*: Immature heads of *T. echinococcus*, characterized by 4 suckers and hooklets. May be 60 000–70 000 scolices inside one cyst. In intestine of dog a scolex develops into adult tapeworm.

'Daughter cysts' may be: (1) Endogenous: occur in man, developing within primary cyst as above. (2) Exogenous: usually in animals, buds penetrate cyst wall and develop externally; never very large.

Contents of hydatid cysts. Clear fluid: no albumin (unless repeatedly tapped); specific gravity 1005–1010; contains chlorides. *Characteristics*: (1) Daughter cysts; (2) Scolices, as above; (3) Barbed 'hooklets'. Cysts are often sterile, and many contain neither scolices nor hooklets.

Fate of cysts. (1) Death of parasites, followed by inspissation and calcification. Characteristic wall and hooklets may be present. Not uncommon; (2) Rupture; (3) Suppuration. The last two are serious.

Principal Situations in Human Body

(1) Liver most frequent; (2) Lungs and pleura; (3) Less commonly bone, kidneys, nervous system, omentum. No site is immune.

Hydatid Cyst of Liver

Symptoms

None when small. When large, may be dragging pain, or tumour in abdomen; or cough, depending on direction of enlargement. Until cyst dies its walls are relatively impervious to its fluid content. After death of cyst absorption of fluid occurs and allergic symptoms may follow—asthma, urticarial weals. Cysts in spine may cause paraplegia or other symptoms due to compression of spinal cord. General health usually unaffected unless *complications* occur, viz.:

Rupture of cyst. Spontaneous or result of trauma. Patient often conscious of 'something giving way'. Urticaria and oedema common. May be massive and cause oedema glottidis. Directions: (1) Peritoneum; may be fatal peritonitis, unless operated on and fluid removed early; (2) Lungs; fragments of cysts coughed up. Often fatal from suppuration, haemorrhage, gangrene of lung, suffocation. May rupture into pleural cavity; (3) Stomach and intestines; may discharge for weeks, recovery, or death from suppuration; (4) Other directions may be: bile ducts, extreme jaundice; pericardium; vena cava.

Suppuration. With or without rupture. Symptoms of sepsis: rigors, sweats, pyrexia.

Physical Signs
Depend on position of cyst. Most common in right lobe. Great enlargement of liver; (1) Downwards, resembling tumour of liver and appearing in epigastrium or hypochondrium: especially if cyst on anterior surface or in left lobe. (2) Upwards: by compressing lung, resembles pleural effusion: heart may be displaced: especially with cysts on posterior surface and in right lobe. In spine cyst may destroy vertebra causing paraplegia and/or dislocation.
Palpation. Elastic sensation if cyst is large and superficial, occasionally with fluctuation. *'Hydatid thrill'*: on sharp pressure with fingers a thrill may be momentarily felt, like 'quivering jelly', ascribed to impact of daughter cysts: rarely obtained. More probably caused by tension and elasticity of cyst wall.

Diagnosis
1. *Clinical.* Great enlargement of liver, persistent, but associated with *good health.* Physical signs: elasticity, fluctuation, thrill and painlessness.
2. *Cyst fluid.* After aspiration: (1) Scolices; (2) Barbed hooklets. Either distinctive, but both may be absent if cyst sterile. Urticaria and toxic symptoms may follow aspiration which should only be carried out with surgical exposure of cyst. Needle aspiration of unexposed cysts is dangerous and should be avoided.
3. *Radiograph.* Cyst has definite outline which, however, may not be seen if cyst is in relatively radiopaque organ such as liver. Even calcified outline may then require care to detect.
4. *Blood.* Eosinophilia.
5. *Immunological tests.* The Casoni intradermal test may be helpful in clinically suspicious cases but needs care in interpretation as it cross-reacts with other larval cestodes. Complement-fixation tests are performed in some laboratories. Reagents are commercially available for the complement-fixation, latex agglutination, indirect haemagglutination and immunoelectrophoresis tests. Indirect haemagglutination and latex tests are useful for initial screening and immunoelectrophoresis for confirmation. Detection, by immunoelectrophoresis, of the genus-specific antigen 'Arc-5' is almost diagnostic.
6. *Scintillography.* Scanning over liver after administering radioactive material may reveal filling defect.
7. *Ultrasound.* Capable of localizing cysts very accurately.

Differential Diagnosis
Carcinoma of liver. Often difficult. Absence of wasting and good general condition.
Amoebic abscess of liver. May be impossible to distinguish clinically from infected hydatid cyst.
Pleural effusion. May be impossible clinically: differentiated by puncture fluid.
Hydronephrosis. Catheterization of ureter may be necessary.
Dilated gallbladder. Usually mobile and the shape distinctive.
Syphilitic liver. No fluctuation.
Pancreatic and similar cysts

Hydatid Cyst of Lung
Most frequent site next to liver. Symptoms result from effect on the lung tissue, pressure on bronchi, etc., which may produce: (1) Bronchitis; occasionally foetid bronchitis, bronchiectasis, gangrene; (2) Compression of lung with signs of

consolidation; (3) Haemoptysis; (4) Cavitation; (5) Pleurisy and empyema. Condition may suggest phthisis. Prognosis serious. Hooklets may be present in sputum. Radiograph of thorax often decisive; shadow of cyst has sharp, regular, curved outline.

Hydatid Cyst in Pleura

Less common. Simulates pleural effusion. General health good until complications occur—viz. (1) rupture—into lung or occasionally external; (2) suppuration—when prognosis is serious.

Hydatid Cyst of Kidney

Not common. May resemble hydronephrosis. Rupture into pelvis and passage of contents in urine, or into peritoneum and tissues.

Hydatid Cyst of Brain

Rare. Symptoms of tumour, usually cerebral.

Hydatid Cyst in Bone

May cause pathological fracture. In vertebral bodies pain and neurological complications. Prognosis serious. Remove surgically, if possible.

Treatment of Hydatid Cyst

Many, particularly those of liver, best left alone and symptomatic treatment given when required for allergic reactions. Cysts of lung usually relatively easy to remove surgically. Elsewhere, if producing symptoms usually best to swab the operation site with cetrimide 0·1% as a scolicide, aspirate cyst contents without leakage and replace with 0·1% cetrimide. If cyst is dissected out the fibrous wall should be left behind to reduce bleeding. If suppurating, treatment as for abscess.

Chemotherapy. Mebendazole in large doses, enough to produce plasma levels of 100 mg/ml has been given orally for approximately 20–200 days. No consistent results have been obtained.

Albendazole recently tried and appears to be more effective. Given orally 10 mg/kg daily for 6 weeks. It is best reserved: (1) for patients with numerous and/or inoperable cysts; (2) as treatment preliminary to surgical removal of operable cysts; or (3) following surgery, to prevent recurrence or to kill cysts not removed. Over the 3–4 months following treatment, cysts may become dead and flaccid. Cysts in bone and those of *E. multilocularis* appear to be resistant. To date experience in man with the drug has been limited and most work has been done in animals.

Chapter 57   # DISEASES CAUSED BY NEMATODES

Ascaris Lumbricoides (Roundworm)

Parasite

General resemblance to the earthworm. Cylindrical; pointed both ends; yellowish colour; transverse striations; four longitudinal bands. Male: length 15–30 cm.

Female: length 20–35 cm.
Ova. Oval: very thick mammillated capsule. Capsule of some (decorticated) eggs may be missing: no sign of embryo: numerous in faeces, stained brown by bile. Size: 80–95 μm by 40–60 μm.
Life cycle. No intermediate host. After ingestion of ova, embryos hatch in upper portion of small intestine, penetrate mucous membrane, enter lymphatics and reach bloodstream via thoracic duct or portal capillaries, and reach liver. After a few days latter embryos enter hepatic veins, pass through right heart to lungs, escape into bronchi, pass up trachea, and down oesophagus to stomach and intestines, where they reach maturity one month after ingestion; cf. Ancylostomiasis (p. 270).
Mode of infection. By water or uncooked vegetables contaminated with mature ova from infected faeces.
Number. Vary from 1 or 2 to many hundreds.

Symptoms

During migration of embryos may be urticaria, cough and pneumonitis. These probably result from death and absorption of some invading larvae. Masses of tangled worms can cause intestinal obstruction, particularly in children. Intestinal colic not uncommon. Diarrhoea and some blood in stools occasionally. Heavy infections in persons on poor diet may aggravate or cause malnutrition. Worm's products impair protein digestion.

Wanderings of adult worms relatively uncommon: into bile ducts, producing jaundice (rare); into appendix; into stomach, subsequently being vomited or withdrawn by subject from pharynx. Rarer situations: perforation of intestine and peritonitis; pancreatic duct and fatal pancreatitis.

Eosinophilia may occur during invasive stage due to death and absorption of larvae.

Diagnosis

By demonstration of ova in faeces.

Treatment

1. Piperazine salts (adipate, hydrate, phosphate and citrate) among most successful and least toxic remedies. Dose for persons of all ages 4 g. A saline purge 2 h after taking the anthelmintic helps to expel worms. Piperazine hydrate or citrate, prepared in an elixir, particularly suitable for treatment of children. Occasionally incoordination and confusional states have followed its use but it remains one of the safest anthelmintics.
2. Bephenium hydroxynaphthoate (Alcopar) also effective in doses of 2·5 g for adults, half that amount for those under 2 years of age.
3. Tetrachlorethylene given emulsified in mucilage, in adult doses of 4 ml, still much used in many parts of tropics.
4. Thiabendazole. Has a broad spectrum of anthelmintic activity. Dosage 25 mg/kg twice daily for 2–3 days. Maximum single dose not to exceed 1·5 g and total daily dose not more than 3·0 g. Course may be repeated after 1 week's interval. Side effects include anorexia, nausea and vomiting.
5. Pyrantel embonate (Combantrin). Another broad-spectrum anthelmintic. Dosage 10 mg/kg orally. Single dose often given but may be repeated after 24–48 h. Very safe but may occasionally produce nausea.

6. *Levamisole.* Effective against *Ascaris* and has very mild side-effects. Not active against hookworms or in strongyloidiasis. Dosage 2·5 mg/kg orally as a single dose or repeated in 24 h. Many now regard it as the drug of choice for ascariasis.
7. *Mebendazole.* May be given orally in doses of 100 mg b.d. for 3 days to all over 2 years of age.

Toxocariasis

Aetiology
Infection in man with larval forms of *Toxocara canis* and rarely *T. cati*. Definitive hosts of these worms are respectively dogs and cats in whose intestines the worms develop, reach a length of 7·5–12·5 cm (look like small earthworms or *Ascaris lumbricoides*), and produce ova which are passed in animal's faeces. Mature ova, on being swallowed by man, develop into larvae in intestine, invade intestinal wall, and via blood or lymph, are carried to all tissues of body but do not develop beyond larval stage. Damage in human tissues is produced by larvae in burrowing and by granulomas that develop around dead larvae.

Ova of *T. canis* measure 80 µm by 60–70 µm. Their surface is pitted, not covered in nodular projections as are ova of *A. lumbricoides*, but otherwise the two types of ova have a rough similarity.

Epidemiology
Prevalence of infection in dogs. Even 5–10% of best cared-for dogs such as those at top dog shows are infected and in some tropical regions infection rate is over 80%.
Soil reservoir of infection. Investigation has revealed that only about half of humans infected have had a dog or cat in their household. This led to investigation of the prevalence of toxocaral ova in soil of public parks, children's playing grounds and similar areas and between 5 and 25% of soil samples have been found to be infective. In the original study (Borg and Woodruff) infectivity of ova recovered from soil was proved by feeding them to mice. Contamination of soil with ova has now been demonstrated worldwide.
Predilection for children. Although many new infections are of adults, majority are of children. This led to the belief that children with pica were those affected. This, however, is not so, all children to an extent much greater than adults, put unwashed fingers in their mouth, or while in playgrounds handle sweets with contaminated fingers. In many parks children and dogs play together and the dogs contaminate the play area.
Role of cats. T. cati poses less of a hazard than *T. canis*. This was demonstrated by examining sera of Icelandic blood donors among whom no toxocaral antibodies were found although cats are numerous in Iceland; dogs have, however, been forbidden for over 40 years as part of the programme to eliminate hydatid disease. Cats, moreover, do not roam in children's playgrounds and parks to same extent as do dogs, being more peridomestic in their habits.

Pathology
Distribution of larvae. Larvae in blood are eventually halted by capillaries in which they become lodged. Their diameter is 16–20 µm i.e. approximately half that of *A. lumbricoides* larvae and this facilitates their passage, unlike those of *A. lumbricoides*, through the capillary plexuses in liver and lungs and thus enables them to reach systemic circulation and be carried to any organ in the body.

Tissue damage. Burrowing larvae cause tissue damage, leaving tracks which become filled with inflammatory cells, especially eosinophils. Dead larvae become surrounded by granuloma in which eosinophils are prominent. Later, fibrosis supervenes.

Humoral response to infection. Serum globulins, principally IgG and to a lesser extent IgM and IgE are increased. In blood some degree of eosinophilia is common.

Symptoms

Symptoms depend on: (1) number of ova ingested and consequent number of larvae in tissues; (2) site to which larvae are carried. Most persons swallow only very small number of ova at a time and unless larvae enter vital structures, infection is asymptomatic. Even lightest infections are, however, potentially dangerous.

Systemic symptoms. If many ova are swallowed together there may be fever, malaise, cough and eosinophilia.

Ophthalmic lesions. Sudden loss of sight in an eye is commonest mode of presentation. Children are particularly affected and usually begin to squint as a result of visual impairment. Tumour-like lesion may be present in fundus or there may be a small, slightly raised, pale retinal spot. These appearances overlie the toxocaral granuloma. Haemorrhage may surround affected area and there may be vitreous haze.

Toxocaral larvae have no predilection for the eye but their presence there is readily noted as they damage sight. In many other organs their presence may pass unnoticed.

Hepatic lesions. Larval invasion may produce enlargement and tenderness with eosinophilia.

Lung lesions. There may be bronchitis and allergic response to infection may cause asthma.

Cerebral lesions. Larvae have been demonstrated in brain and there is evidence that they may cause encephalitis and occasionally epilepsy.

Diagnosis

Immunological tests. Enzyme linked immunoabsorbent assay (ELISA) using antigen from cultured larvae is highly specific.

Fluorescent antibody test using second stage *T. canis* larvae treated with acid-pepsin and albumin is sensitive and specific if patient's serum is first adsorbed with ascaris antigen.

Differential Diagnosis

Retinoblastoma. This is simulated clinically but if serological tests for toxocariasis are positive and particularly if eosinophilia is also present toxocariasis is suggested.

Toxoplasmosis. Toxoplasmal lesions are usually multiple; often they affect both eyes and are flat. Those of toxocariasis are usually unilateral, single and raised.

Uveitis and enophthalmitis from non-toxocaral causes is unlikely to be associated with positive toxocaral serology.

Hepatic capillariasis. Causes hepatomegaly and eosinophilia but serology differentiates and liver biopsy may reveal ova of *Capillaria* species.

Treatment

Diethylcarbamazine in doses of 3 mg/kg t.d.s. for 21 days kills the larvae. Initial doses should be of 1 mg/kg, increased to 3 mg/kg over 3–4 days. Thiabendazole in doses as for strongyloidiasis (p. 274) is less effective.

In ophthalmic toxocariasis coincident administration of corticosteroids is advisable to reduce reaction around killed larvae.

Prognosis

Active infection is readily brought to an end but damage already done to sight is usually permanent but slight improvement may occur.

Prevention

1. Limit or prevent contamination of soil in public parks and especially in children's playgrounds.
2. Dog owners to have their dogs wormed at least annually and to remove their animal's excreta when deposited in public places.
3. In developed countries, stricter licencing of dogs and certificate of worming to be produced as condition of licencing.

Enterobius (Oxyuris) Vermicularis (Threadworm)

Parasite

Male: length 2–5 mm, tail coiled in spiral. Female: 8–13 mm, tail long and pointed. In faeces often in large numbers: resemble short pieces of thread, moving slowly.

Modes of Infection

By swallowing eggs which are relatively resistant to drying. Vehicles include food contaminated by infected persons, vegetables and occasionally water. Airborne spread is possible. After ingestion of ova, worms mature in small intestine, copulate and male dies. Females migrate to caecum and rectum, pass through anus, especially during warmth in bed, to lay ova on perineum and cause great irritation. Resultant scratching leaves ova on fingers and reinfection follows. Ova also may mature in perineal region and larvae return through anus to mature in rectum ('retro-infection'). Attention recently drawn to nail biting as an aetiological factor.

Symptoms

Mainly in children, but also in adults, causing pruritus ani. Sleep may be disturbed by this. Symptoms ascribed to infection but with inadequate supporting evidence: irritability, picking nose; nervousness.

Eosinophilia occasionally present to slight degree.

Diagnosis

Eggs on perianal skin may be collected and identified by applying adhesive transparent tape to the skin and then sticking it to a microscope slide. Eggs may also be recovered by swabbing or scraping skin of the area. Eggs should be searched for immediately on waking and before those deposited during sleep have been washed away. Eggs rarely present in stool.

Treatment

If reinfection can be prevented, worms present will die and patient therefore be cured in approximately 4–6 weeks. Reinfection usually occurs as a result of scratching anal region, contaminating fingers and nails with eggs and thus transmitting eggs to mouth or to food. The most useful hygienic measures for preventing reinfection are:

1. A morning bath, to rid perianal region of eggs deposited there during the night.

2. Scrubbing fingers with nail brush before every meal and after each visit to toilet.

3. Closely fitting underpants may be worn at night to prevent contamination with eggs, of fingers and bedclothing.

Drug treatment. Piperazine salts (citrate, adipate, or phosphate), for children an elixir or syrup most suitable, e.g. piperazine citrate (Antepar), dose up to 2 years 50–75 mg/kg; 2–4 years 750 mg; 5–12 years 1·5 g; children over 12 years and adults 2 g. Each dose repeated daily for 7 days.

Pyrvinium pamoate. Dosage 5 mg (base)/kg; single dose reported effective but dosage best repeated after 48 h.

Thiabendazole (Mintezol) in dosage 25 mg/kg b.d. and repeated after 7 and 14 days is effective but may cause gastrointestinal upsets.

Pyrantel embonate administered as for ascariasis is effective.

Mebendazole (Vermox) in single oral dose of 100 mg to persons of all ages also recently found satisfactory.

Trichiniasis*

Infection of human being by *Trichinella spiralis* results in a stage of gastric irritation during development of adult worm in intestine, and a more characteristic stage of myositis due to migration of embryos to voluntary muscles.

Parasite

1. Adult form. Both sexes are cylindrical, the oral end being pointed. Male: length about 1·5 mm: two projections from posterior end resembling the jaws of a pair of pincers hold the female in coitus. Female: length 3–4 mm. Characteristic: the oesophagus is lined by a *single layer of large cells*, readily recognized at the anterior portion of the parasite, and known as the '*cell body*'.

2. Embryos. Newborn larvae are 100 μm by 6 μm.

3. Larval form, or muscle trichinellae. Oval laminated capsule, length about 0·6–1 mm: contains a distinct coiled worm with pointed head and rounded end. In early stages capsule translucent; subsequently impregnation with lime salts occurs, and then easily visible with a hand lens. May be two, and rarely three or four, worms in single capsule.

Mode of Infection

In man by eating trichinous pork or occasionally wild hog or bear meat. No

---

*The terminology has become confused. The original name, *Trichina spiralis*, given to the parasite was not admissible, as *Trichina* was previously in use, hence it was altered to *Trichinella spiralis*. The clinical condition is often referred to as 'Trichinosis', but more correctly is 'Trichiniasis', or most correctly 'Trichinelliasis'.

intermediate host is necessary, and thus among hogs in large herds probably spreads by feeding on offal of other infected animals. In hog, symptoms are slight even with large infections; also calcification of capsule is less common and cyst more difficult to recognize. Rats may be true host.

Muscle trichinellae are resistant to heat below boiling-point, thus thorough cooking of pork renders it safe, but at centre of a cooked joint temperature may be less than 100 °C.

Geographical distribution is universal, but human infection is rare except in Eastern Europe and S.E. Asia, where raw pork is consumed.

Tends to occur in small outbreaks, but isolated cases are not infrequent. The disease has become increasingly important in recent years in Africa as a result of transmission from meat of wild pig and warthogs and in Northern Canada and Russia from meat of bears. There is evidence that the strain or subspecies of the parasite differs in these regions from that responsible for infection in domestic pigs.

Cycle in Human Body and Mode of Spread

1. On ingestion of muscle trichinellae, capsule is digested and larval trichinellae enter duodenum and jejunum.

2. By third day, adult worm is fully grown and sexually mature. The male dies after copulation.

3. By sixth to seventh day, embryos are fully developed. The adult female is ovo-viviparous, penetrates intestinal wall, and discharges free embryos in large numbers from uterus into lymph spaces; dies after discharging many hundreds of embryos during 5 or 6 weeks.

4. *Spread of embryos*. From the lymph spaces, embryos enter veins, reach intermuscular connective tissue, and finally enter *voluntary muscle-fibres*. Embryos have been found in blood between the 7th and 25th day; also numbers have been found in peritoneal and other serous sacs.

5. *Embryos in muscle*. The embryo coils, becomes less active, and in 2 weeks from ingestion of meat definite 'muscle trichinellae' are present. Local myositis results and an oval capsule forms in about 6 weeks. If fresh muscle be teased on a warm slide, embryo may be seen to move; can remain alive for many years, but undergoes no further development.

Calcification of capsule: in man occurs in a minimum of 4–5 months; may, though rarely, render capsule visible on radiography.

6. *Muscles affected*. Most frequent are diaphragm, intercostals, muscles of neck and eyes, and larger voluntary muscles, especially near tendinous insertions of voluntary muscles; in man biceps and gastrocnemius especially liable.

Note: Life cycle is similar in pigs.

Symptoms

Cardinal features: (1) Fever; (2) Oedema of eyelids—most constant and often earliest pathognomonic sign; (3) Eosinophilia; (4) Muscular pains. Manifestations very variable. Severity of symptoms depends on number of larvae per gram of tissue which may vary from 3 or 4 in subclinical infections to 1000 or more in life-threatening disease. May be very slight, or merely *vague rheumatic pains*. The following stages are rarely distinct.

Stage of gastro-intestinal irritation. Corresponds to growth of adult worms in small intestine, sexual activity, and possibly penetration of gut by females. *Onset*: may be within 24 h, usually 2–3 days after ingestion. *Abdominal pain, vomiting*, often diarrhoea.

This stage is frequently absent, but may be of *choleraic severity* with muscular cramps: intensity is no guide to subsequent stage, as vomiting and diarrhoea may discharge many adult worms before embryos are free.

Stage of myositis. Corresponds to migration of embryos and encapsulation in muscles. *Onset*: 7th to 14th day, usually 9th or 10th. (1) *Fever*: 38·9–40 °C (102–104 °F) remittent or intermittent; (2) *Myositis* (may be absent): Muscles swell, become hard, very tender, and all movements painful. Position in bed: limbs semiflexed to relax muscles, most typical being *flexed forearm* owing to great *infection of biceps*. Other special muscles commonly affected are: (*a*) Diaphragm (cough and respiratory troubles, may be extreme dyspnoea); (*b*) Muscles of mastication and larynx (aphonia); (*c*) Muscles of the eye; (*d*) Gastrocnemius; (*e*) Myocardial invasion may lead to arrhythmias and sudden death or to tachycardia and various degrees of myocardial insufficiency; (3) *Oedema of eyelids* (allergic), most characteristic and often initial sign: frequently extreme. May be oedema in other sites (genitals usually escape). Subsides gradually. Urticaria and sweating. Albuminuria is rare; (4) *Eosinophilia*: Leucocytes 20 000–30 000/mm^3 and eosinophils may be 50%; rise commences after onset of symptoms; (5) May be drowsiness and lethargy. May suggest typhoid. Involvement of nervous system in some epidemics, resembling meningitis. In severe infections, pulmonary symptoms, rapid emaciation and toxaemic state may develop.

Duration
Mild cases recover in 2 weeks. *Severe cases* convalescent in 6–8 weeks. Many months of weakness follow.

Prognosis
Best in children, and with much early diarrhoea resulting in excretion of adult worms.

Mortality has varied greatly in different outbreaks: depends on degree of infection of flesh at fault; varies from 1 to 30%, but often about 5%. *Death* usually occurs in 4th to 5th week while myositis severe. From: (1) Weakness of myocardium, diaphragm and intercostals, and extreme dyspnoea; (2) Pneumonia; (3) Typhoid state.

Diagnosis
In epidemic, diagnosis often simple. Diagnostic methods are:

Suspected food. Tease on slide and examine by hand lens or microscope for larval forms or feed to laboratory rats and examine their muscles for larvae.

Parasites in human faeces. Dilute faeces in conical glass: examine sediment against black background for minute parasites; under microscope identify by 'cell-body'.

Biopsy. Excise small slips of biceps or deltoid and examine.

Immunology. Several tests carried out in different laboratories. Bentonite flocculation and enzyme-linked immunosorbent assay (ELISA) most reliable.

Eosinophilia. Examine for.

Radiographs. Calcified cysts are small and rarely recognizable.

Differential Diagnosis

Typhoid: In trichiniasis: no headache, no splenic enlargement, no spots, but pain and swelling of muscles and oedema. Also eosinophilia.

Pleurisy: Myositis of intercostal muscles may simulate pleurisy but does not produce pleural rub.

Rheumatic fever: Distinguish by gastrointestinal stage.

Nephritis: Albuminuria rare, but may be abundant.

Dermatomyositis: Clinically may resemble trichiniasis but the various investigations for the parasite negative.

Treatment

(1) Thiabendazole in doses of 25 mg/kg body weight b.d. for 5 days may remove some adults from intestine. Mebendazole 100 mg b.d. for 3–4 days or pyrantel embonate 10 mg/kg daily for the same period may act similarly. (2) Thiabendazole has also been used to kill larvae in tissues but may provoke severe allergy in doing so. Mebendazole in doses of 5 mg/kg/day may be more successful but care is needed in using it. (3) Corticosteroids may be life-saving in severe cases by controlling allergy and oedema. In emergencies 5–10 mg dexamethasone may be injected i.m. or i.v. Usually 40–60 mg prednisone orally daily suffice.

Analgesics required for muscle pain.

Prophylaxis

Thorough cooking of all pork is best, and is efficient prophylactic measure, with rare exceptions.

In herds of hogs, measures advised are: (1) Destruction of rats; (2) Uncooked offal of hogs not to be used as food; (3) Examination of flesh in the abattoirs. (4) Heating of food given to pigs; (5) Wild pig and bear meat to be avoided or thoroughly cooked before eating. Camp fire cooking or barbecueing is often inadequate.

Ancylostomiasis (Hookworm Disease)

Geographical Distribution

In tropical and subtropical countries: widespread, particularly in hot moist regions. Mines and long tunnels, hot, damp, and with defective latrines, liable to infection in any climate.

Parasite

Two principal subgroups: (1) *Ancylostoma duodenale*, in Old World; (2) *Necator americanus* in New World. Not confined to this distribution. Both are small, cylindrical nematodes.

1. Ancylostoma duodenale. Mouth is large orifice with two pairs of hooked-shape ventral teeth. Male: length 10 mm; at posterior end is an expansion, the 'caudal bursa'. Female: length 10–18 mm.

2. Necator americanus. Differs from last in having 4 sharp lancets external to mouth on dorsal aspect, also single tooth and pair of semilunar plates in place of hook-shaped teeth. Other slight differences.

Ova. Characterized by segmentation within capsule: usually 4 or 8 cells when examined from fresh faeces. Often in enormous numbers. Size 60–75 μm by 35 μm.

Larvae. Embryos may emerge 1–2 days after ova leave body, depending on warmth and moisture. Embryos then moult twice, after which they are infective. Can occur within 4–5 days. May live for months subsequently. Development most favourable in faeces mixed with earth.

Mode of Infection (Domestic animals are not infected)
1. Through the skin. Larva penetrates skin, enters veins, passes through heart to lungs, escapes into bronchi, passes up trachea and down oesophagus to stomach and intestines, course occupying 7–10 days. (*See Ascaris lumbricoides*, p. 263.) In the intestine, larva moults again, and then matures. Ova are present in faeces in about 7 weeks from entry.
2. Through the alimentary canal. By infected drinking water and uncooked vegetables. Larvae may enter through buccal mucous membrane.

Pathology
The adult worm lives in the jejunum, scanty in duodenum; by its teeth it attaches itself to mucosa and draws blood thereby predisposing to iron-deficiency anaemia and hypoproteinaemia. In mucosa of jejunum, ecchymoses and erosions present. Fatty change of heart and other organs if anaemia advanced.

Degree of Infection in Relation to Symptoms
Infection with few worms is of little importance. Degree of anaemia depends on iron intake and nutritional value of diet as well as on number of worms present. From experience in dealing with infections in large populations, the Rockefeller Institute and other workers have arrived at the following conclusions:
Relation of ova to worms harboured. It is estimated that 44 ova per 1 g formed stool corresponds to one female worm.
Severity of infections. Cases are grouped according to number of worms thus estimated to be harboured:
   1. *Infection very light*: 1–25 worms; or *Light*: 26–100. Harbourers usually have no obvious symptoms but infection may contribute to iron and protein depletion.
   2. *Infection moderate*: 100–500 worms. Patients usually physically below normal, lethargic and apathetic.
   3. *Infection heavy*: 500–1000; or *Very heavy*: 1000–3000 worms. Serious symptoms as below. Constitute only a small percentage of total affected.

Mode of Production of Symptoms
Entry of larvae through skin. Causes 'ground itch' and local eruption.
Passage of larvae through bronchi and lungs. Cough, pneumonitis.
Parasites in jejunum. Anaemia caused by loss of blood. Work with isotopes has shown that in *N. americanus* infections 0·05 ml blood may be lost per worm per day and that this figure may be trebled for *A. duodenale*.

Symptoms
'Ground itch' occurs at site of entry of larvae. Vesicular eruption, becoming pustular ('bunches'). Commonly under toes. In miners on arms and hands. Heals in 1–2 weeks. May be bronchial symptoms as larvae pass through lungs.
Symptoms in well developed case. (1) *Hypochromic anaemia*, with *palpitation, oedema* and *lethargy*; (2) *Gastrointestinal disturbances*: Pain, vomiting. In severe forms, anorexia; (3) *Wasting* not common; (4) *Fever*: Variable; (5) *Mental*

inertia: Listless expression, apathy; (6) *In children*: Underdevelopment; small stature; puberty delayed; growth may continue until 25 years.

No enlargement of spleen, or liver.

Blood Changes

Classically those of iron deficiency.

Erythrocytes and haemoglobin. Haemoglobin often about 5–6 g/100 ml blood, but lower values occur. Mean corpuscular haemoglobin concentration low; normally 30–35% reduced sometimes to 20–24%. Red cells rarely under 2 000 000. Anisocytosis common.

Leucocytes. Eosinophilia, if numerous larvae migrating at same time.

Reticulocytes. Normal: may rise to 10% on treatment.

Plasma proteins. May be much reduced, especially albumin fraction.

Blood volume. Increased.

Faeces

Occult blood, but obvious haemorrhage rare.

Examination of stools for ova. Flotation method: Ova float in saline of sp. gr. 1130 while other faecal matter sinks; ova removed from surface on glass slide.

Count of ova in stools. Stoll's method: measured amount of stool diluted quantitatively and ova counted in measured quantity.

Prognosis

Life of *A. duodenale* 4–6 yr, *N. americanus* 10–15 yr. Eradication of worms and treatment of anaemia not difficult. Repeated infections common. Prognosis also influenced by: (1) Dietary deficiencies; (2) Mixed infections, amoebae and schistosomiasis; (3) Intercurrent infections.

Diagnosis

In infected areas, usually simple: microcytic anaemia, eosinophilia and ova in stools (not always present).

Treatment

Two essential objects: (1) *Eradication of worms*: Many effective drugs. Ova should be absent from stools 3 weeks afterwards. Reinfection common: treatment usually simple. (2) *Treatment of anaemia*: Ordinary methods with iron effective. To restore iron reserves, continue iron therapy for few weeks after haemoglobin restored to normal. If anaemia moderate and clinical condition fair, commence with eradication of worms. If anaemia severe, treat first with iron until haemoglobin reaches 7 or 8 g/dl blood. Diet important, especially protein, both during treatment and convalescence.

The following anthelmintic drugs have been extensively and successfully used:

Tetrachlorethylene. Probably still the most widely used for hookworms and is cheap. Dosage by mouth: 0·2 ml for each year of age up to 15 years, for adults 3 ml. Suspend in mucilage and flavouring agent. Avoid capsule as may not rupture till past the worms. Dose of magnesium sulphate 3 h later. Two treatments usually suffice. Cheap and effective.

Bephenium hydroxynaphthoate (*Alcopar*, Wellcome Ltd). Non-toxic and very effective. Dose 5 g, children under 12 years 3 g. Taken with water and followed in

2 h by saline purge. Repeat in 1–2 days. More effective against *A. duodenale* than *N. americanus*.

Bitoscanate. Acts on adult and larval hookworms. Dosage for adults 100 mg thrice at 12-hour intervals. Children 10–14 years two doses and aged 5–9 years two doses of 50 mg; capsules not to be chewed or buccal injection results. Drug slowly eliminated so treatment not to be repeated with this drug for 8 weeks.

Pyrantel embonate. Also active against *Ascaris lumbricoides* and *Trichuris trichiura* so useful in those with these concomitant infections. Dosage 10–20 mg/kg as a single dose. Few side-effects.

Levamisole. Oral dosage 2·5 mg/kg daily for 1–2 days.

Mebendazole. Effective against *A. duodenale* and *N. americanus*. Dose 100 mg orally b.d. for 3 days to persons over 2 years of age.

Thiabendazole. Has action against the hookworms less than the above but may be used if other drugs not available. Dosage as for ascariasis.

Prophylaxis
Infection is spread by faeces, especially in hot damp soil. Important measures are: (1) Disposal of faeces. Cleanliness of latrines. Special care in mines; (2) Pure water-supply. In absence of this, water to be boiled; (3) Wearing of shoes.

Strongyloidiasis

Aetiology and Epidemiology
An infection of man with *Strongyloides stercoralis* endemic in the Far East and tropics generally.

The life cycle is complicated. Only filariform larvae can infect man. Adult females measure approximately $2 \text{ mm} \times 50 \mu\text{m}$ and usually live in mucosa and submucosa of small intestine. Eggs produced contain rhabditiform larvae which hatch in intestine, are passed in faeces, and in soil develop either into free-living forms which give rise to further progeny, some of which become filariform and capable of infecting man by penetrating skin or mucous membranes. Alternatively, rhabditiform larvae in soil may transform directly into filariform larvae without maturing into free-living adults. After penetration larvae are taken in blood to lungs, may mature there or migrate to epiglottis, and be taken with food to intestine where they burrow into submucosa. Occasionally rhabditiform larvae in intestine become filariform and penetrate intestinal mucosa to migrate to mesenteric lymph nodes and other tissues or they may emerge from the anus and penetrate perianal skin.

Pathology
Worms in intestinal mucosa produce granulomatous reaction; in lungs produce pneumonitis. Larvae migrating from intestine may disseminate bowel microorganisms.

Symptoms
Most infections asymptomatic. Encysted worms in intestinal mucosa may cause gastrointestinal irritation, colic, and, in heavy infections, diarrhoea. Cause malabsorption in massive infections.

Invasion of perianal skin by filariform larvae causes irritable lesions similar to cutaneous larva migrans. Such invasion responsible for perpetuation of infection which may continue many years.

Encysted worms in lungs produce cough, sputum and pneumonitis.

Diagnosis
By demonstration of larvae in stools, duodenal juice or rarely in sputum. In duodenal juice, the larvae are most easily recovered by getting the patient to swallow a gelatine capsule to which a brushed nylon string is attached. This is later withdrawn and the juice it has absorbed is examined microscopically. The filarial complement-fixation test is usually positive in low dilution in strongyloidiasis. When positive, diagnoses of filariasis and strongyloidiasis have to be considered and the final diagnosis decided on clinical grounds. Concomitant eosinophilia usual.

Treatment
Thiabendazole. Drug of choice. Dosage 25 mg/kg for 3–5 days.
Mebendazole. Dosage 100 mg b.d. for 4 days. Drug of second choice.
Levamisole or *pyrantel embonate*. May be used if other drugs not available. Dosage as for ascariasis, *see* p. 264.

Trichuris Trichiura (Whipworm; Trichocephalus dispar)

Inhabits caecum and large intestine of man. Distribution probably universal and occurrence frequent.

Worm
Length: male 4 cm; female 5 cm. Shape resembles a whip: anterior portion very thin and posterior portion thick, being in female straight and in male coiled.

Ova
Oval: dark brown. Characteristic light-coloured protruding 'knob' at each end.

Mode of Infection
Direct by contamination of food or drink by ova which have matured and become infective. No intermediate host.

Symptoms
Usually none but in heavy infections and especially in young children may cause diarrhoea, sometimes with rectal prolapse.

Treatment
Difficult to eradicate.
Mebendazole. Dosage for all ages 100 mg b.d. for 3–4 days. Little drug absorbed.
   Recently reported effective:
Flubendazole. Dose 200 mg daily for 3 days.
Albendazole. Single dose of 400 mg.

Capillariasis

Aetiology
The nematode whipworm *Capillaria philippinensis* infects the human small

intestine in the Philippines and Southern Thailand. Certain small fish and crustaceans are thought to be the intermediate hosts and man is infected by eating these raw or only lightly cooked. In man the adult males measure 1·5–3·9 mm and the females 2·3–5·3 mm.

Clinical Features
The capillaria invade jejunal crypts and cause malabsorption with protein-losing enteropathy.

Diagnosis
Ova of *C. philippinensis* are found in the stools and are similar to those of *Trichuris trichiura* but have a more rectangular shape, a pitted, not smooth, shell and bipolar plugs which do not protrude beyond the egg's contour as do the plugs of *T. trichiura*.

Treatment
Mebendazole 400 mg orally daily for 10–30 days. A less satisfactory alternative is thiabendazole 25 mg/kg daily for 30 days and then on alternate days for up to 6 months.

Gnathostomiasis

Aetiology
Adult worms are nematodes of dogs and cats and produce eggs which are passed in faeces and develop further in freshwater cyclops and then in fish, frogs, snakes or birds which have consumed the cyclops. Man is infected by contact with or by eating raw infected intermediate hosts.

Clinical Features
In man the larval worm does not develop further but migrates to subcutaneous tissue where it causes swelling and pruritus. In the Far East the larval worms have invaded the brain and caused eosinophilic meningitis.

Treatment
Surgical where possible, otherwise symptomatic relief only is possible and for this corticosteroids and antihistamines are used.

Other Animal Nematodes

The herringworm *Anisakis marina* may infect man when herrings are eaten raw. Eosinophilic granulomas of the bowel result.

Angiostrongylus cantonensis is a rodent nematode of which the larval stage develops in freshwater shrimps and molluscs. Consumption of these may lead to eosinophilic meningitis in man.

Treatment is symptomatic and the disease is usually self-limiting. Removal of 10 ml amounts of spinal fluid, corticosteroids and analgesics are of benefit.

Ancylostoma braziliense, the hookworm of dogs and cats, produces eggs which are passed in the animal's stools and which develop into larvae in soil and sand. Man is infected when the larvae penetrate exposed skin and produce an irritable migrating linear eruption (cutaneous larva migrans). Treatment with thiabenda-zole in dosage as for strongyloidiasis (p. 274) is curative. Topical thiabendazole can also be used but with little advantage—500 mg/5 ml with 0·1% dexamethasone cream covered with an occlusive film.

Filariasis

Three main types: (1) Bancroftian filariasis or infection with *Wuchereria bancrofti*; (2) Loiasis or infection with *Loa loa*; (3) Onchocerciasis or infection with *Onchocerca volvulus*. Guinea worm *Dracunculus medinensis* also member of filarial family.

Wuchereria Bancrofti Infection

Geographical Distribution
Widespread in tropics and subtropics.

Parasite
Adult parasite. Hair-like worm, length: female 5–10 cm, male 3–5 cm; in many coils.

Site in body: in lymphatic channels, especially of testis region and lymph nodes, most frequently those of inguinal, axillary and para-aortic groups. Lives many years.

Embryo (Microfilaria). About 300 μm × 10 μm. Contained in a 'sheath', which *it does not fill* at the ends, and in which it moves back and forwards. Present in peripheral blood.

Life Cycle
1. *Mosquitoes*. Are intermediate host. Main vectors of periodic *W. bancrofti* in India, Asia and around the Indian Ocean are *Culex pipiens quinquefasciatus* and *C. pipiens fatigans*. In Africa *Anopheles* spp. *A. gambiae*, *A. funestus* and others are responsible and in Melanesia *A. punctulatus* and others. The vectors of the non-periodic *W. bancrofti* var. *pacifica* are *Aedes polynesiensis* and *Aedes vigilax*. Withdraw embryos from definitive host when feeding. In stomach of mosquito, embryo ruptures sheath, reaches thoracic muscles and there develops for 12–20 days. Thence it passes to base of proboscis. When mosquito feeds, larva bursts from base of proboscis (not through salivary glands), escapes onto skin, and penetrates it near, but not necessarily at, puncture.
2. *In man*, these larvae reach lymphatics, mature and produce embryos, which pass through lymphatics to veins and into peripheral circulation.

Periodicity
Embryos are present in blood especially at night, about 10 p.m. to 2 a.m. During day, in lungs and blood vessels of thorax. Cause of periodicity uncertain. May be connected with nocturnal habit of usual intermediate host, viz. the mosquito *C. fatigans*. Recently introduced blood-filtration techniques have shown that in all but lightest infections some microfilariae present in blood even during day. Such techniques particularly important for surveys as nocturnal collection of blood is often difficult.

Non-periodic filariae. In Fiji and islands near, embryos are present also during day. Parasite is identical, but intermediate host are day-feeding *Aedes* spp.

Pathology

Embryos, being breadth of red cells, can pass through capillaries without difficulty; often present in man without symptoms, and in animals. Symptoms produced by inflammation of and blockage of lymphatics by larvae and adult worms, and by obliterative lymphangitis.

1. Lymphatics distal to blockages greatly dilated. Those especially affected are in pelvis, paravertebral, renal and thoracic regions. May form varicose masses containing chyle. Thoracic duct may be stenosed. Groin nodes often enlarged. Rupture of varices into urinary system causes chyluria. Parasite may be dead and no embryos in blood.

2. *Elephantiasis.* Blockage of lymph vessels alone does not produce this (confirmed experimentally by ligature in animals), inflammation also necessary. This occurs in recurring elephantoid fever with lymphangitis. Protein in extracellular fluid of affected limb increased and probably assists by raising osmotic pressure of the fluid.

Relationship of elephantiasis to filariasis. Embryos are not usually present in blood: probably owing to previous blockage of lymphatics. Relationship is inferred from: (1) Geographical distribution identical; (2) Both are lymphatic diseases with recurrent lymphangitis; (3) Elephantiasis is common sequel of, or coexists with, filarial lymph scrotum. Much elephantiasis latterly found in non-filarial regions and attributed to accumulation of silicaceous material in lymph nodes (Price). The material is thought to originate in soil and enter through abrasions in skin of feet of those who use no, or inadequate, footwear.

Symptoms

Incubation period. Variable: probably 6 months to 2 years after infection before clinical symptoms appear. *Lymphangitis* usually first complaint; often retrograde, i.e. develops proximally and extends distally. Associated with fever and malaise.

1. *Lymphatic swelling.* 'Lymph scrotum': lymphatics dilated and varicose over scrotum: subsequent elephantiasis common. 'Varicose groin glands': chronic, bilateral: frequently with lymph scrotum. *Lymphangitis.*

2. *Chyluria.* Passage of milky urine, usually bloodstained. No symptoms, or may be pain in back and pelvis. Occurs intermittently, at intervals of weeks or months, over many years: but if frequent it may aggravate malnutrition or iron-deficiency anaemia in those who are already so predisposed from other causes. *Urine* sometimes clots on standing. The pink coagulum contracts and expresses milky fluid. Later a layer of fat globules may form on surface—clears with ether. Embryos often present in blood and urine.

3. *Elephantiasis. Legs* most commonly affected, especially below knee. Scrotum not infrequently. Enlargements sometimes enormous. Mammae and arms less frequently. Fluid is lymph, not chyle.

Elephantoid fever. Recurrent attacks of fever, pain and swelling in limb, and lymphangitis. After attack, limb remains larger. Embryos seldom present in blood.

Diagnosis

Mainly on clinical and epidemiological features and demonstration of microfilariae in night blood. Occasionally adult worms are found in biopsy material, especially that from epididymis or scrotum.

Complement-fixation and other immunological tests may be positive.

Treatment
Specific therapy. Diethylcarbamazine (*Banocide, Hetrazan*) kills microfilariae in day or two and adult worms in few days. Cures in early and intermediate stages of infection. Does not improve elephantiasis but may prevent further damage to lymphatics of elephantoid tissues. Dose 2–3 mg/kg body weight t.d.s. for 21 days. Begin with 1 mg/kg body weight and increase according to tolerance. Herxheimer type reactions common in first few days' treatment; include headache, vomiting, allergic skin rashes and pyrexia.

Chyluria. Rest, limit fluids, avoid fats. Disappearance of chyle does not prove rupture is healed: can be tested by drinking glass of milk and watching for reappearance of chyle.

Elephantiasis. Carefully protect from injury and sepsis. Elevate limb and wear elastic stocking during waking hours.

Elephantoid fever. Rest, cooling lotion to sites. Bandage firmly subsequently. Give course of diethylcarbamazine if patient not already had one. Antibiotics if evidence of bacterial infection.

Elephantiasis of scrotum. May be removed by operation.

'*Groin glands*' and '*Lymph scrotum*'. Operation inadvisable. In latter, elephantiasis of leg may follow.

Brugia Malayi Infection

Geographical distribution. Rural South-East Asia.

Parasite
Compared with *W. bancrofti* the adult is about half as big and the microfilaria are smaller being 170–260 μm × 4–7 μm, have two discrete nuclei at tip of tail and in stained preparations their curves are less smooth. There are nocturnal periodic forms transmitted by anophelines and by mosquitoes of the *Mansonia uniformis* group. Subperiodic forms are mostly transmitted by *M. bonneae* and *M. dives*.

Symptoms
Similar to bancroftian filariasis but following exposure, symptoms develop more rapidly. Elephantiasis is milder and less common and seldom involves the genitalia.

Treatment
As for bancroftian filariasis.

Loiasis

Geographical Distribution
Confined to tropical Africa, particularly the region around eastern part of Gulf of Guinea.

Parasite and its Vectors
Adult females measure 5–7 cm by 0·5 mm and males 3–3·4 cm by 0·35–0·43 mm; live in subcutaneous tissue and move freely. Produce microfilariae measuring 250–300 μm, are sheathed, and have diurnal periodicity. Transmitted by various species of *Chrysops*, flies normally inhabit foliage of high rain-forest trees.

Pathology
Adult worms wander in subcutaneous tissue and cause the Calabar swellings which are typical of the condition. Injection of worm protein produces swelling similar to Calabar swelling which therefore has been considered to be localized allergic response to worm protein.

   Encephalitis: has been reported in patients whose CSF contained microfilariae of *Loa loa*.
Immunological changes. Infection leads to production of complement-fixing antibody, mostly IgG and IgM, in serum but this exerts little protective action against worms.

   Eosinophilia is characteristic of this and many other helminthic infections.

Clinical Features
Calabar swellings (classic): affect principally regions of medium-sized joints, face and orbit; are diffuse, usually 7·5–10 cm in diameter; usually last 2–3 days; frequency varies. Develop not less than 3 months after exposure to infection, may ache, seldom really painful. Sometimes associated with pyrexia, often with malaise. Ulnar and medial nerves have been injured by swellings and worms.
Adult worms: may appear beneath skin or conjunctiva and visibly migrate for minutes or hours.

Diagnosis
Definitive diagnosis: depends on identification of microfilariae of *L. loa* or adults.

Serological Diagnosis
The complement-fixation, indirect fluorescent antibody and enzyme-linked immunosorbent assay (ELISA) tests are done in specialized laboratories and if positive indicate present or past filarial infection. They do not differentiate between filarial species.

Blood Changes
Eosinophilia usual and forms useful general guide to helminthic, including filarial, infections.

Treatment
Diethylcarbamazine (*Banocide, Hetrazan*) very effective. Given in doses as described under Bancroftian filariasis. Kills adults as well as microfilariae. Allergic reaction during early stage of treatment sometimes severe. May be controlled by promethazine (Phenergan) 10–25 mg once or twice daily or other antihistamine or, failing this, small doses of corticosteroids. These, however, are very seldom required. During treatment adult worms occasionally die beneath

the skin where their outline is visible. Allergic skin rash is not uncommon during treatment. High eosinophilia also common during and for 3 or 4 months following treatment.

Mansonella Perstans (*Acanthocheilonema Perstans*)

Geographical Distribution
Tropical Africa, particularly rain forest areas, also parts of Central and S. America; in Africa often found along with *L. loa*.

Parasite and its Vectors
Adults in serous cavities, mesentery, and connective tissue, commonly retroperitoneal. Females measure 7 cm by 130 µm, males 4 cm by 70 µm. Microfilariae aperiodic, measure 100 µm by 5 µm, are unsheathed and found in blood. Transmitted by *Culicoides* species.

Pathogenicity
Pathogenicity doubtful, causes eosinophilia.

Treatment
Difficult to eradicate but responds slowly to full courses of treatment with diethylcarbamazine as for *W. bancrofti, see* p. 278.

Onchocerciasis

Infection by filariae *Onchocerca volvulus*.

Geographical Distribution
O. volvulus: West, Central and East Africa; Sudan, Yemen, Guatemala, Venezuela, Colombia, Mexico and Brazil.

Parasite and its Vectors
Female, length 35–55 cm; male shorter. Inhabits subcutaneous and connective tissues of man. *Simulium damnosum* and *S. naevi* convey infection in Africa; ingest embryos from skin in which microfilariae live. *S. ochraceum, S. metallicum* and *S. amazonicum* are the main vectors in Central and S. America.

Pathology
Adult worms. When they die, stimulate production of fibrous tissue and nodules. Little reaction around living worms.
Microfilariae. In skin produce, when they die, small foci of inflammatory cells and eosinophils; death in cornea produces small area of punctate keratitis approximately 1 mm diameter. Heavy infection over many years may produce permanent interstitial keratitis. Similar process in iris produces iritis.
Elastic tissue. Appears to be damaged by the parasites and in chronic cases subcutaneous nodules may loosen skin surrounding them and come to hang in folds especially in groin where appearance of inguinal hernia develops although no hernia present. Chronic dermatitis with super-added bacterial infection common. Patchy depigmentation results from scratching and removal of superficial melanophore-bearing layers.

Cell-mediated immunity is usually marked in those with much skin disease and is weak in those with many microfilariae in skin but little dermatological pathology. IgE is usually increased in those with active skin disease, and by adhering to mast cells enables them to combine with antigen and to release heparin, histamine, serotonin and other vasoactive substances promoting skin reactions.

Symptoms

1. Skin. Pruritus: usually with maculopapular eruption is earliest complaint: limbs or trunk may be affected; symptoms worse when patient hot, e.g. after hot bath or when in bed. Scratching leads to scarring and depigmentation. In longstanding cases elastic tissue damage causes premature wrinkling. Some degree of oedema is common.

Nodules seldom develop until patient has been infected for several years—commonest site is around iliac crest, greater femoral trochanters, and along lower ribs. In Guatemala, commonly on scalp. May be painful when over pressure points.

Erysipela de la Costa. Especially in Guatemala a dermatitis known as 'erysipela de la costa' may occur; is painful and irritable. Thought to result from secondary infection of onchodermatitis.

Mal morado also occurs in Central American foci. Is a raised plaque-like, purplish lesion found in areas of skin subject to friction.

Leonine facies like 'hanging groin' results from atrophy of elastic tissue and stretching of skin affected by longstanding infection.

2. Ocular manifestations. Earliest is punctate keratitis usually associated with a conjunctivitis and if treated in early stages recovery is complete. Later iritis occurs and in neglected cases pin-point pupil bound down to lens and sometimes occluded by organized exudate may develop and cause blindness. Thus in longstanding cases cornea may become opaque from much keratitis. Choroidoretinitis develops in some with heavy prolonged infection.

3. Other manifestations. Lymphadenopathy and/or elephantiasis may develop. 'Hanging groin' in longstanding heavy infections results from atrophic lax skin developing around nodules in groin.

Diagnosis

A definitive diagnosis depends upon recovery of microfilariae from skin shavings or snips of skin, or identification of adults in excised nodules. In lightly infected patients, serological methods as for *W. bancrofti* are valuable, *see* p. 278. On giving a dose of diethylcarbamazine the skin symptoms are aggravated and temporary erythema develops. This has been used as a diagnostic test (Mazzotti reaction) but is not recommended as by destroying microfilariae it makes definitive diagnosis difficult or impossible. Eosinophilia usually present and is a general guide to helminthic infection.

Treatment

Diethylcarbamazine. Microfilariae in skin destroyed by standard course of diethylcarbamazine. After temporary exacerbation of symptoms patient usually completely freed from symptoms for variable period, in heavy infections a few weeks or months, in light infections perhaps several years or may be permanently cured. In view of exacerbation of symptoms during early phase of treatment, treatment must be commenced with very small dosage, usually ¼ mg/kg body weight once or twice daily and successive doses doubled until 3 mg/kg body weight is given 3 or 4 times daily and maintained at maximum for 21 days. Close supervision necessary particularly in early phase of treatment. Allergic manifestation may be controlled by antihistamines or, if severe, by small doses of corticosteroids.

Adult worms killed only slowly by diethylcarbamazine but in light infections may be killed by this drug.

Antrypol (Suramin) may be used for its action on adult worms, 1 g dissolved in 10 ml sterile distilled water injected intravenously at weekly intervals for 5–7 weeks. Give preliminary test dose of 0·2 g to ensure patient does not have severe reactions to the drug. Is nephrotoxic and important to ensure urine is free from albumin and casts before each injection.

Invermectin (Merck, Sharp, Dohme). Single oral doses of 200 µg/kg appears to have good microfilaricidal and macrofilaricidal action and is currently undergoing trial.

Mebendazole. In large doses such as 25–50 mg/kg orally daily for 3–4 weeks reduces microfilarial production by adult worms and causes reduction of microfilariae in skin for about a year without causing allergic skin reactions. Simultaneous administration of levamisole in doses of 7·5 mg/kg once weekly for the same period has a synergistic effect.

Streptocerciasis

Geographical Distribution
Western and central Africa, especially in rain forests.

Parasite and its Vectors
Mansonella streptocerca (formerly *Dipetalonema streptocerca*) are approximately 27 mm by 75 µm (female) and 17 mm by 50 µm (male). The microfilariae are 180–240 µm by 2·5–5·0 µm and have a characteristic 'shepherd's crook' shaped posterior extremity. Adults and microfilariae are found in the skin and are transmitted by *Culicoides grahami*.

Symptoms
Usualy none but may cause pruritus with papules and sometimes dermal thickening with hypopigmented macules which have been confused with leprosy.

Diagnosis
By identifying microfilariae in skin snips.

Treatment
Responds well to diethylcarbamazine as given for onchocerciasis *see* p. 281.

Dracontiasis (Guinea-worm Disease)

Infection by *Dracunculus medinensis*.

Geographical Distribution
Parts of India and Africa, especially West Africa and Southern Sudan. Distribution limited by prevalence of intermediate host. Not endemic in America, but has been reported from Caribbean.

Parasite

Female guinea-worm is about 80 cm long by 1·5 mm in breadth: shape, cylindrical. On tail is a minute hook. Uterus occupies almost entire body, is packed with up to 3 million embryos, which are discharged by prolapse of the uterus through the mouth. The male measures only 2·5 cm and dies shortly after fertilizing the female.

Life-cycle. Two phases: (1) Man—definitive host; (2) *Cyclops*, minute water crustacean—intermediate host. Several features are related to the host's habitat, thus the guinea-worm develops in parts of the human body where it can discharge embryos into water.

1. *Cycle in man*: infection occurs by drinking water containing cyclops. Larva freed by digestive juices. Female penetrates intestine after impregnation: reaches subcutaneous connective tissue usually of leg and there develops over ensuing year. A toxin is secreted which produces penetration of the skin, a small vesicle forms and bursts; through this erosion the tip protrudes and embryos are discharged when site is cooled. Occasionally worm becomes calcified under skin.

2. *Cycle in cyclops*: embryo after entry moults twice and reaches the infective third stage in approximately 14 days.

Symptoms

Generalized urticaria of allergic origin, with aching pain where vesicle forms, and worm palpable or visible under skin: may be vomiting, diarrhoea and collapse. Itching before surface penetrated, then for 2–3 weeks milky fluid containing embryos is discharged whenever the area is cooled as by exposure to water. Eosinophilia. Constitutional symptoms rapidly subside when vesicle over tip of worm ruptures, secondary infection of track common and important: tetanus may result.

Treatment

1. Douche site with water daily or spray track of worm with ethyl chloride to cool, stimulates uterine contraction, and expulsion of embryos; worm then easily extracted. May then, but not before, be rolled on sterile stick; keep moist with saline or eusol dressing or it will break.

2. Treat secondary infection. Immunize against tetanus.

3. Niridazole in doses of 25 mg/kg body weight daily for 10 days the first drug shown to reduce period of disability and make worm easier to extract. Side-effects of drug, nausea, dizziness and occasionally psychological disturbances make many consider the drug unsuitable for guinea-worm treatment but it may be valuable in endemic areas where many are affected, incapacity considerable and dressing of lesions difficult to supervise.

The following all have a similar effect and have been used since niridazole was first employed in this infection.

> 3.1. Metronidazole in adult doses of 400 mg orally daily for 10–20 days.
>
> 3.2. Thiabendazole, 50 mg/kg orally daily for 3 days.
>
> 3.3. Mebendazole 400–800 mg for adults, orally daily for 6 days.
>
> None of these drugs affect the pre-emergent worm nor do they abolish infectivity of the larvae.

Prevention
Prevent contamination of drinking water by excretion from guinea-worm ulcers or
if contaminated filter the water.

8

Chapter 58   *NUTRITIONAL DISEASES*

Kwashiorkor (Protein-calorie Malnutrition; Malignant Malnutrition)

Geographical Distribution
Most of tropics, particularly common in W. Africa.

Aetiology
Main cause. Imbalanced diet mainly consisting of carbohydrate and low in protein. Cassava with its very low protein content is the vegetable staple most prone to be associated with kwashiorkor. Psychosocial factors are important, e.g. child's misery and neglect resulting from being semi-abandoned to the 'extended family' as parents go away for work or other purposes. Infections such as diarrhoea, malaria or measles often then act as precipitating factors.

In absence of adequate quantities of protein-containing lipotrophic substances, liver cannot metabolize carbohydrate adequately, and carbohydrate then becomes converted into fat and is stored in the liver, hence fatty liver develops.
Age. Most patients aged 1–3 years, but some are older and some features of kwashiorkor may be seen in persons of older age groups. Demand for protein created by rapid growth important. Peak incidence probably results from child's diet being changed from breast milk to 'starchy paps' low in protein. Under such circumstances subcutaneous fat may first be utilized for metabolism and then protein may be similarly utilized so that cytoplasm of cells becomes impoverished.

Sex incidence equal in infants and children. Pregnant women sometimes present some manifestations of kwashiorkor probably due to increased demand for protein created by growth of fetus.

Pathology
Morbid anatomy. Tissues generally wasted. Much muscle wasting but some oedematous subcutaneous fat persists.

Liver: Moderately enlarged and yellowish in colour as result of fatty change within it. Microscopically, fat commences in periphery of liver lobule as fine droplets; in later cases involves whole lobule and droplets large. In severe cases liver may resemble adipose tissue. This condition considered by some authorities to predispose to reticulin hypertrophy and later fibrosis but this disputed. Probable that protein-calorie malnutrition plus chronic malaria or viral hepatitis leads to fibrosis in cases in which neither alone would cause fibrosis. Such fibrosis most marked in portal triads and extends to become perilobular.

Pancreas: Macroscopically, size reduced and microscopically, cytoplasm of acinar cells diminished. This results in nuclei of cells becoming crowded together with loss of glandular structure. Zymogen secretory granules lost and pancreatic secretion and enzymes reduced. Later fibrosis may occur and possibly calcification. Considerable increase in incidence of pancreatic calcification in tropics thought possibly to be a result of protein malnutrition in childhood.

Small intestines: Atrophic and mucosal villi small, may become almost flat. Malabsorption may occur and steatorrhoea has been reported.

Blood: Plasma proteins often normal in total amount but albumin much reduced, sometimes to levels less than 1 g% and globulin greatly increased. Gross reversal of albumin/globulin ratio occurs. Moderate anaemia usual even in absence of intercurrent hookworm or other infections. Anaemia usually normochromic and normocytic but occasionally megaloblastic, and in such cases folic acid deficiency has been demonstrated. In the absence of an over-riding deficiency of folic acid or iron, anaemia may result from protein deficiency alone. Blood urea, blood sugar, and serum cholesterol are also low. Distinctive amino acid patterns in plasma described

Muscles: Much wasted from metabolism of muscle as a reserve of protein.

Clinical Features
Basic symptoms are (Jelliffe): (1) Oedema; (2) Growth failure; (3) Psycho-motor change, i.e. lethargy, apathy, whining misery and withdrawal; (4) Wasting of muscles. This tetrad indicates a clinical diagnosis of kwashiorkor in areas where protein-calorie malnutrition is a public health problem. Pitting oedema is a cardinal feature. Growth failure recognized by failure to gain weight on serial measurement or by low weight for age. May be masked by oedema.

Hair. Normally crisp and dark, becomes straight and inelastic, and may lose colour. When treatment instituted, colour returns to new hair and contrast between new and old constitutes the 'flag-sign'.

Skin. Over oedematous areas has shiny appearance; superficial skin then peels leaving depigmented patches, so-called 'crazy-pavement dermatosis'; this is most common in flexures and portions of skin subject to friction, e.g. groins, patellar and cubital regions. Skin generally may become lighter in colour than normal. Ulcers and secondary infection common. Cancrum oris is a mutilating and often fatal complication.

Gastrointestinal features. Diarrhoea common and stools may be fatty. Anorexia usual and/or buccal ulcers frequent. Liver often slightly enlarged. Ascites may be present.

Cardiovascular system. Heart small, myocardium atrophied, output low and pulse thin, tachycardia usual. Electrocardiogram of low-voltage type, ST segment deep, T wave depressed and prolongation of Q–T interval common.

Prognosis
Always serious and mortality considerable even in relatively mild cases, but with prompt and efficient treatment may be reduced to very low levels. Now generally considered that liver cirrhosis is not a sequel of uncomplicated kwashiorkor. Immediate prognosis made worse by intercurrent infection. Bronchopneumonia a common terminal event.

Diagnosis
Made on clinical grounds—the cardinal clinical features already described, plus a history of low intake of protein and calories. Supporting features are low plasma albumin and fatty change in liver. Liver biopsy of great value in establishing diagnosis.

Distinguished from beri-beri by absence of neurological lesions and from pellagra by oedema and by skin lesions being particularly found in flexures rather than on extensor surfaces and areas exposed to sunlight.

Treatment
Twin principles are to clear up intercurrent infections and provide an easily digested diet rich in protein. Malaria, bronchopneumonia, enteritis and skin infections are commonest secondary conditions to be given immediate attention.
Dietary treatment. The diet in initial stages of severe kwashiorkor should be liquid or semi-solid. It should be as full and varied as possible with frequent small meals. Supplement with 1–2 pints milk daily. Add eggs and meat as child able to take these.

For severely ill patients a gruel was devised by Medical Research Council's Infantile Malnutrition Group, Kampala. Aim is to give approximately 4 g protein per kg body weight per day with adequate potassium and magnesium. Daily ration consists of 50 g calcium caseinate, 50 g dried skimmed milk, 20 g sugar, and 30 ml cotton-seed oil. Dried skimmed milk made into paste with cold water, hot water then added, and mixture boiled. Sugar and oil are added and mixture put in high-speed electric blender. Total made up to 1 litre with water. May be given by intragastric tube in child too ill to take food normally.

Potassium deficiency common, orally administered supplement of 1 g daily valuable.

Folic acid if megaloblastic or macrocytic anaemia present. Iron if indicated by low mean corpuscular haemoglobin concentration.

Marasmus

Syndrome of severe protein-calorie malnutrition characterized: (1) by growth failure with a body weight 60% or less than expected for age, (2) by very wasted muscles and subcutaneous fat.

Aetiology
In first year of life usually from failure of lactation and resulting contaminated bottle feeds—a combination of malnutrition and diarrhoea. Lactation failure may result from taking oral contraceptives. Late marasmus—the result of low protein, low calorie diet—common in famines.

Clinical Features
Extreme growth retardation and severe wasting of muscle and fat. Associated diarrhoea is usual. Other signs of malnutrition common, e.g. anaemia, vitamin deficiencies, especially keratomalacia and ariboflavinosis.

Treatment
As for kwashiorkor.

Pellagra

Chronic, relapsing disease characterized by: (1) symmetrical dermal lesions especially on exposed parts of the body—a photosensitive rash; (2) diarrhoea and glossitis; (3) psychic disturbances.

Aetiology
Due to dietetic deficiency especially of niacin, but also riboflavine and pyridoxine (vitamin B_2 complex). Occurs where maize is the staple food. Other factors are protein deficiency, especially of that providing tryptophan; chronic alcoholism; chronic infective and wasting diseases; cirrhosis of the liver; chronic diarrhoea; pregnancy and lactation. It is more common in adults than in children. Worldwide in distribution but mainly in maize-eating areas: southern European countries, Egypt, parts of Africa, India, the Far East, and the West Indies. Formerly in southern USA. Sporadic cases occasionally in mental hospitals.

Niacin is an essential component of nicotinamide adenine dinucleotide and nicotinamide adenine dinucleotide phosphate which are concerned with oxida-tion-reduction systems.

Pathology
Marked general wasting with atrophy of wall of alimentary tract and of heart, liver and spleen. Skin shows erythema, pigmentation and exfoliation. Nervous-system lesions are variable: oedema of brain and degenerative changes in the cord.

Clinical
Skin. Affected areas: those exposed to light, especially brow and cheeks ('butterfly' rash), neck and upper chest ('Casal's necklace'), backs of hands and wrists, and dorsal surfaces of feet. Initially like sunburn with erythema followed by brown pigmentation. Later roughening and desquamation and sometimes secondarily infected fissures.
Alimentary tract. Glossitis ('beet tongue'), cheilosis and angular stomatitis. Proctitis sometimes present. Anorexia, abdominal pains and severe weight loss occur. Diarrhoea is always present.
Nervous system. Headache, muscular cramps, sleeplessness are common. Coarse tremors of tongue and hands occur. Depression leads on to psychosis, most often melancholia, rarely mania. Delirium, confusion common.

Diagnosis
In patient eating maize as staple article of diet, combination of symmetrical dermatitis on exposed parts, glossitis, diarrhoea and mental abnormality, especially depression, points to pellagra. In children kwashiorkor must be considered, and in adults tinea, chronic eczema, syphilis, chronic discoid lupus erythematosus, alcoholism and chronic mercury poisoning must be excluded.

Treatment
Nicotinic acid, or nicotinamide, 25–50 mg t.d.s. The latter substance does not cause the burning and vasodilatation often brought about by nicotinic acid. If the mouth is very sore i.v. fluids to which nicotinamide is added must be given initially.

Pyridoxine in doses of 20–50 mg orally or parenterally a valuable adjuvant, improving oral and neurological lesions. Riboflavine in doses of 5–10 mg is also often necessary for full recovery from oral lesions.

Diet to include fresh meat, liver, eggs, fresh vegetables and yeast.

Prognosis
Good, if dietetic alterations are maintained. Relapse very likely if the diet is poor in protein and vitamin-B complex.

Beri-beri

Nutritional deficiency disease due to insufficiency of thiamine (vitamin B_1, aneurin), occurring where polished rice is the staple article of diet and characterized by variable symptomatology including congestive cardiac failure with oedema (wet beri-beri) or symmetrical polyneuritis particularly affecting the feet and legs (dry beri-beri). Wernicke's encephalopathy is a manifestation.

Aetiology and Epidemiology
Thiamine is found in whole cereals, yeast, peas and beans, nuts, pork, liver and eggs. Cooking, if it is not prolonged and the medium is alkaline, causes relatively small losses. The husk and germ of rice contain much thiamine which is removed by polishing to obtain white rice. Beri-beri occurs in rice-eating populations, especially Far East, parts of India, S. America and southern USA. Additional causal factors may be alcoholism, fevers, especially malaria, digestive and other alimentary diseases, pregnancy, increased physical exertion on poor diet.

Pathology
Heart. Dilated, especially right side. Macroscopically appears to be fatty degeneration, but microscopically separation of muscle cells and bundles by oedema. Hydropericardium common. Hyperkinetic circulatory state occurs with low peripheral vascular resistance and consequent retention of sodium and water by kidneys. There is an increase in blood volume and venous pressure.
Lungs. Pulmonary oedema, serous effusions in pleura.

Passive congestion of liver, spleen and kidneys. Subserosal and submucosal petechiae may be seen.
Peripheral nerves. Wallerian degeneration with cellular infiltration. Patches of degeneration may be found in posterior columns of spinal cord.
Wernicke's encephalopathy. Capillary damage and haemorrhage in the tegmentum of the medulla, the region of the vagus nucleus and mammillary bodies.

Clinical
Wet or cardiac beri-beri. Usually gradual onset: pain and tenderness in calves on walking and shortness of breath on mild exertion. Muscular wasting of legs masked by oedema. Heart sounds, particularly the pulmonary second, are loud. Pulse rapid and full. Sudden cardiac failure with death may occur.
Dry beri-beri. Usually gradual onset with numbness, paraesthesiae and burning sensations of extremities as longest nerves are affected first. There are anorexia, weight loss, weakness and tenderness of leg muscles. Patient has difficulty in getting up from squatting position. Tendon reflexes first exaggerated, later lost. Wrist-drop and especially foot-drop with high-stepping gait result.

Wernicke's encephalopathy: only in very deprived, e.g. prisoners of war, or those with complicating vomiting, diarrhoea or alcoholism. Paralysis of cranial nerves, especially IIIrd, ptosis, nystagmus, papilloedema, confusion and delirium may occur and be followed by Korsakoff's syndrome.

Infantile beri-beri. Usually acute onset in breast-fed babies where mother's diet is deficient in thiamine. Vomiting, refusal to feed and weight loss are early symptoms. Abdominal cramps and tender muscles in the legs occur. The knee jerks are diminished. Convulsions or sudden cardiac failure may result in death.

Diagnosis

In a predominantly rice-eating population an adult presenting with high output cardiac failure in regular rhythm must be considered likely to have cardiac beri-beri. Evidence of peripheral neuritis in a person who has taken a deficient diet, and especially if alcoholism is present, should raise the question of beri-beri neuritis. Infantile beri-beri is difficult to diagnose and may be confused with cerebral malaria, tetanus, or virus encephalitis. Urinary thiamine absent. Blood pyruvic acid elevated.

Treatment

Infantile beri-beri and Wernicke's encephalopathy are medical emergencies and require i.v. thiamine hydrochloride, 50–100 mg. This may be repeated i.m. daily for some days. Treat mother with thiamine and improve her diet.

Thiamine propyl disulphide found to be the most effective form of the vitamin where rapid and sustained response is needed.

Cardiac beri-beri may require similar urgent treatment. Usually i.m. injections of thiamine 20–50 mg daily for 2 weeks are needed. Absolute rest in bed with careful nursing is essential. The dramatic therapeutic response helps to confirm this diagnosis.

Dry beri-beri. Usually 5–10 mg of thiamine orally daily will be adequate. Where there is muscular weakness bed cradles, splints and physiotherapy are required.

General. In all cases the diet should be revised. Fulminating beri-beri responds rapidly to thiamine administration, but the polyneuritic patients often improve slowly and may be left with persisting ataxia.

Deficiency Anaemias in the Tropics *(see also Chapter 60)*

Iron-deficiency Anaemia

Seldom results from dietary deficiency of iron; more commonly caused by hookworm infection. Sweat and particularly cell-rich sweat may contain significant amounts of iron. Under conditions of maximal termperature and humidity 1 mg iron may be lost in cell-rich sweat per day. Normally considered that 1·5 mg iron needs to be absorbed per day for maintenance of normal haemoglobin levels and approximately 10% dietary iron is absorbed.

In determining cause of anaemia full investigation for parasites necessary.

Treatment is with iron; orally administered iron satisfactory. Parasitic infections present must be treated.

Megaloblastic Anaemia

Sometimes results from deficiency of vitamin B_{12} in food, particularly of vegetarians. More commonly, megaloblastic anaemia results from deficiency of, or disturbance in, metabolism of folic acid. Such deficiency may be conditioned by malabsorption as in sprue.

Megaloblastic anaemias may be severe, with low haemoglobin values, a megaloblastic marrow and mean corpuscular volume raised above the normal range (82–95 fl). Conditioned folate deficiency also results from longstanding haemolytic states as in haemoglobinopathies.

Administration of 5–20 mg folic acid orally daily or 1000 µg vitamin B_{12} parenterally usually an effective cure.

| Chapter 59 | ALIMENTARY DISORDERS OF PARTI-CULAR IMPORTANCE IN THE TROPICS |

Tropical Sprue (Steatorrhoea or Malabsorption Syndrome of Tropics; Sprue)

Definition
Disease characterized by diarrhoea with pale stools, and weight loss in milder cases and also glossitis and megaloblastic anaemia in more chronic cases.

Epidemiology
Although it often affects Caucasians of middle age or over residing in parts of the tropics, it was during the Second World War shown to be common among young adults. Sprue-like syndromes have been described among indigenous inhabitants of the Caribbean and of India, especially in the South. It occurs particularly in coastal districts of India and the Far East but is uncommon in Africa. In S. India it has been reported to have reached epidemic proportions in certain villages.

Aetiology
Still not certainly known. Epidemiological evidence suggests both nutritional and infective causes. Considerable outbreaks have occurred in particular localities suggesting an infective cause, and although not uncommon among ill-nourished persons it is also frequently encountered among those on a good diet. An abnormal jejunal flora comprising enterobacteria has been found in Indian and white patients who acquired sprue in India. Slowed small bowel transit may be a factor which allows this microflora to persist. Broad-spectrum antibiotics are beneficial and may eradicate this microflora. In the Second World War sprue commonly occurred at same time as outbreaks of intestinal infection.

Folic acid shown to have very considerable effects on well-being of patients with sprue and although its administration has no immediate effect upon fat absorption there is considerable need for it for maintenance of proper rate of replacement of intestinal cells. Folic acid concerned with synthesis of deoxyribosenucleic acid (DNA) of cell nuclei; deficiency results in foamy nuclei and enlarged nucleoli. Rate of turnover of cells lining intestinal tract and the bone marrow great. Probable that some deficiency of folic acid plays a part in causation of both the megaloblastic anaemia and malabsorption of sprue. Folic acid absorption may be impaired and body stores last only 3 months.

Pathology and Biochemistry
General picture is of wasting subcutaneous tissue and of atrophy of small intestines and other internal organs. Liver, spleen and kidneys 20–35% below normal weight.

Intestinal villi atrophied and flattened. These are normally long, finger-like processes, but in tropical sprue become shortened and thickened, though not so markedly as is seen in coeliac disease. Cellular infiltration occurs between crypts.

Absorptive capacity of bowel reduced; fat, carbohydrate and vitamin B_{12} absorption most readily measured. Plasma protein and serum calcium values reduced in longstanding cases. Folate depletion (low red cell folate) in more prolonged cases.

Clinical Features
First symptom usually diarrhoea, soon becoming most marked in early morning, stools pallid and often frothy and obviously fatty. Stool may float in water because of gaseous content but does not contain blood, unless complications such as haemorrhoids also present. Malabsorption of intestinal contents associated with abdominal distension, most marked in latter part of day.

Glossitis and angular stomatitis develop in longstanding cases. Mucosal inflammation may extend to pharynx and oesophagus causing dysphagia. Flatulence and flatus toublesome. Lethargy prominent, weight loss almost invariable, much of latter due to fluid loss consequent upon sodium depletion; occasionally tetany results from hypocalcaemia or hypomagnesaemia in longstanding cases. Skin becomes dry and flaky and occasionally malar and frontal hyperpigmentation develop. Follicular hyperkeratosis described as a result of vitamin A deficiency. Nocturnal diuresis may result from delayed absorption of water ingested during day. Oedema occurs in advanced cases secondary to hypo-albuminaemia.

In fully developed cases clinical picture highly characteristic with pallid faeces, glossitis, general wasting and protuberant abdomen.

Low blood pressure usual and consequent upon sodium depletion.

Haemoglobin seldom much reduced in early cases but more marked anaemia may develop in advanced cases with megaloblastic erythropoiesis.

Diagnosis
Radiological. Mucosal pattern in the jejunum lost as valvulae which formed 'herring-bone' pattern disappear. Loops of small bowel become dilated and barium in them becomes pooled. These changes are non-specific.

Determination of fat absorptive defect. Estimation of total fat content of 24-h output of faeces more reliable, though still a crude index. In health 95% ingested fat is absorbed and diets containing more than 100 g fat/24 h very rarely consumed. Therefore in health 24-h stool sample should not contain more than 6 g fat. Amounts in excess of this indicate malabsorption.

Absorption of sugars. In sprue blood-sugar curves following oral administration of 50 g glucose are usually flat in advanced cases, i.e. rise by less than 30 mg/dl.

Xylose absorption and excretion test: xylose not utilized by body, and its metabolism therefore does not interfere with the test; 25 g in 500 ml water given orally, and normally 5–6 g excreted in urine in first 5 h, i.e. 20–25%. In sprue less than normal excreted in first 5h and more between 5 and 24h after administration, i.e. absorption and therefore excretion have been delayed.

Folic acid. In severe sprue red cell folate well below normal range.

FIGLU test: Histidine normally metabolized to glutamic acid, but if folic-acid-deficient, formiminoglutamic acid, an intermediate product of metabolism, accumulates and is excreted in urine in which in patients with sprue and folic-acid deficiency it may be detected after an oral dose of 15 g histidine.

Vitamin B_{12}. Impaired absorption usually present and revealed by Schilling test done with intrinsic factor.

Serum calcium. Normally 9–11 mg/dl (4·5–5·7 mEq/l) usually reduced.

Bone marrow. In cases in which anaemia is marked, marrow may be megaloblastic.

Intestinal biopsy. Portion of jejunal mucosa may be obtained by biopsy. In sprue absence of villi, deep crypts and cellular infiltration will be found. *Note*: racial variation in villous pattern, even in health, well recognized.

Differential Diagnosis

Sprue in or from tropics must be distinguished from steatorrhoea following gastrectomy or removal of part of small intestine, and from steatorrhoea associated with gluten enteropathy, regional enteritis, strictures of small intestine, blind loops, pancreatitis, giardiasis, strongyloidiasis, capillariasis, intestinal TB, jejunal diverticulosis.

Intestinal atrophy and steatorrhoea may also follow severe malnutrition, radiation, and prolonged use of neomycin.

Prognosis

Formerly poor, but with modern treatment good. Recovery usual in 1–2 months and relapses infrequent.

Treatment

Basis of treatment is an adequate diet and on this alone 30% of patients very rapidly improve. Infusions of saline may be needed by those who are severely dehydrated.

Broad-spectrum antibiotics, such as tetracycline in doses of 2 g daily, bring about rapid improvement in two-thirds of cases and this supports view that bacterial upset often plays a part in causation of sprue.

Folic acid improves general condition; valuable particularly if anaemia present; 10–12 mg daily orally and, in severe cases, 50 mg may be given i.m. daily. During convalescence 5 mg folic acid daily for 6–8 weeks usually recommended.

If anaemia severe, transfusion of packed red cells valuable along with injection of 1000 μg hydroxocobalamin or cyanocobalamin.

Attend to plasma electrolytes. Replace sodium and potassium deficiencies. Of potassium give not more than 1·5 g of chloride i.v. in 4h and repeat if hypokalaemia persists. Control by laboratory estimation of electrolytes and ECG valuable.

Veno-occlusive Disease

Definition

Disease of the liver associated with ascites occurring most often in poor children in the W. Indies.

Aetiology

Pyrrolizidines are alkaloids present in various plants especially *Senecio* and *Crotalaria* species which are used as 'bush teas' in the W. Indies, especially Jamaica and Barbados. Bread made from wheat contaminated with these plants has also been incriminated. The disease has been reported from Ecuador, India and S. Africa. A similar disease has occurred in cattle and horses fed on ragwort, which contains these alkaloids.

Children 2–5 years of age are most affected, but adults occasionally.

Pathology

Liver enlarged, congested and of nutmeg appearance in acute cases. Diffuse fine cirrhosis in subacute cases. Histological changes in acute cases result from subendothelial swelling of intima of medium- and small-sized veins in the liver. Swelling at first seems due to oedema, later to collagen deposition. There is centrilobular block with distension of the sinusoids and sublobular hepatic vein obstruction. In the subacute cases the thickened intima is seen with centrilobular fibrosis. In chronic cases there is cirrhosis which is not portal in distribution, but later, portal hypertension, ascites and oesophageal varices occur.

Clinical

Gradual painless abdominal distension with low fever, loss of appetite and sometimes diarrhoea. Liver may be enlarged to level of umbilicus. Spleen is usually palpable. Occasionally mild jaundice. Ascites develops slowly except in very acute cases.

Diagnosis

This is mainly from other causes of painless hepatomegaly.

Treatment

Rest in bed. High-protein diet. Appropriate general treatments for ascites may be needed. General improvement in the whole diet, with more protein, and avoidance of all 'bush teas' are needed to prevent further liver damage. Often great improvement when consumption of 'bush teas' discontinued.

Vomiting Sickness of Jamaica *(Ackee Poisoning)*

Acute disease in undernourished children characterized by hypoglycaemia, drowsiness, vomiting and sometimes convulsions preceding death, and associated with eating Ackee fruits.

Aetiology

Ackee fruit (*Blighia sapida*) contains polypeptides which can produce hypoglycaemia in laboratory animals. Occurs in Jamaica, especially in months of December to March. If Ackee is eaten by a family, children aged 1–10 years may suffer, while breast-fed babies and adults usually escape the disease.

Pathology

Extreme hypoglycaemia; may be as low as 22 mg%. Liver shows almost complete absence of glycogen.

Clinical Features
Early morning vomiting with profound prostration. Very acute cases develop froth in the mouth, twitching, unconsciousness, convulsions and death. Others show temporary remission, sometimes with recovery and sometimes with further vomiting, drowsiness and death.

Diagnosis
Vomiting sickness is most often seen in children over 1 year of age who have eaten Ackee, and usually in the first quarter of the year. Malaria, food poisoning, epilepsy and tetany may all be considered in differential diagnosis.

Treatment
I.v. drip infusion of dextrose solution. Intramuscular injection of aneurin, 25–50 mg, should also be given. In severe cases gastric lavage may help. There is need for general improvement in child care and feeding in the affected area.

Bantu Siderosis

Generally thought to result from high iron intake. Bantu reported to cook food in unenamelled iron pots with consequent very high iron content of diet and overloading of liver with iron. Malnutrition probably also a factor by interfering with iron-handling enzymes in liver cells. Kaffir beer may contain much iron. Liver frequently cirrhosed and cells show heavy iron deposits.

Infantile Cirrhosis

A condition occurring in Indian, especially Hindu, infants and marked by severe cirrhosis of liver. Cause uncertain. High levels of copper in liver. Corneal changes do not occur, cf. Wilson's disease.

Chapter 60   # ANAEMIAS OF THE TROPICS

Anaemias form one of the commonest medical problems in the tropics, in some places overshadowing all others, and as the great infective disorders in the tropics are increasingly brought under control, anaemia emerges in many regions as the condition most deserving attention on a public health scale. It is commonly secondary to helminthic infection but may also be a deficiency disorder or result from a genetic abnormality. The main anaemias of the tropics may be classified as follows; several causes may be present in any one case:

Deficiency Anaemias
Iron
   Primary dietary deficiency.
   Conditioned deficiency (most commonly by hookworm infection).
Vitamin B$_{12}$
   Primary dietary deficiency.
   Conditioned (as by *Dibothriocephalus latus* infection).

Folic acid
   Primary dietary deficiency.
   Conditioned (usually by malabsorption from intestine or by increased demand caused by chronic haemolysis).
Vitamin C
Pyridoxine deficiency (vitamin B₆)
Protein

Haemolytic
Infective
   1. By invasion of erythrocyte with parasite, e.g. malaria and Bartonella infection.
   2. By production of complement deviating immune complexes, e.g. kala-azar, trypanosomiasis and other infections.
Genetic
Haemoglobinopathies.
Glucose-6-phosphate dehydrogenase deficiency.
Toxic (e.g. snake venom poisoning).

Anaemias associated with Chronic Infections
(Overlap with infective haemolytic anaemia (2, *above*).)
Tuberculosis
Sepsis (often urinary)
Fungal infections

Anaemias Secondary to Special Diseases
Nephrosis (especially secondary to quartan malaria).
Neoplasms

Iron-deficiency Anaemias of the Tropics

Aetiology
May be primary, i.e. due to deficiency of iron in diet or secondary to iron loss from body.
Primary or dietary deficiency of iron. Comparatively uncommon in tropics, many diets relatively rich in iron but in some regions iron content low, particularly if both meat and green leafy vegetables scarce.
Secondary deficiency, i.e. loss of iron from body
   1. Hookworm commonest cause of chronic blood loss leading to iron-deficiency anaemia in tropics. *Ancylostoma duodenale* can cause loss of up to 0·1 ml blood per day and *Necator americanus* about one-fifth of this amount. Infections with up to 100 worms or more not uncommon, so blood loss may be considerable.
   2. Schistosomiasis, especially infection with *Schistosoma haematobium*, may also cause chronic blood loss.
   Daily blood loss of 10 ml will represent iron loss of up to 5 mg, depending on the haemoglobin concentration in the blood lost.
   3. Sweat and particularly sweat containing many skin cells responsible for some iron loss from body. Maximal sweating causes loss of approx. 0·5 mg iron daily.
   These figures should be considered in conjunction with knowledge that average diets contain approximately 12–15 mg iron daily and that 10% of this is absorbed.

Excretion in all forms by adult males and non-menstruating females averages 0·6 mg, so that normally a person is in positive iron balance to extent of approximately 0·5 mg. Menstruation, pregnancy, and in childhood bodily growth, approximately double demands for iron.

Epidemiology

Hot moist regions in tropics without adequate disposal of night soil are usually those with most hookworm infection and anaemia therefore most prevalent there. Coastal regions especially affected.

Clinical Features

Minor degrees of anaemia difficult to detect clinically, more severe degrees cause increasing lassitude, weakness, dyspnoea on exertion, palpitations, glossitis, and pallor of mucous membranes. Capacity to work impaired and therefore economic repercussions of widespread anaemia need consideration.

Clinical picture usually complicated by coincident helminthic infection and/or protein malnutrition.

Diagnosis

Clinical appearance unreliable especially in persons with pigmented skin. Skin folds on palms of hands, tarsal conjunctiva, and lips may be guide.

Haemoglobin estimation by standard method necessary. Tallquist method unreliable except as very rough guide.

Mean corpuscular haemoglobin concentration (MCHC) reduced in iron deficiency and is very valuable guide. Normal value 32–36%. Values below this indicate iron deficiency.

Plasma iron normally 80–140 µg/dl is reduced.

Mean cell volume (MCV) normally 82–92 fl reduced; microcytosis and poikilocytosis present.

Treatment

Iron either as sulphate, gluconate, or ferric ammonium citrate most commonly used. The sulphate in doses of 100–200 mg in tablets twice daily usually sufficient, larger doses commonly cause nausea. Ferrous gluconate in doses of 300 mg in tablets twice daily.

Continue treatment till 1 month after haemoglobin reaches normal to replace iron reserves, which are usually exhausted before anaemia develops.

Coincident treatment of malnutrition and of hookworm infection or other cause of blood loss important. *N.B.* Treatment of hookworm infection alone will not immediately benefit anaemia; it will merely stop abnormal iron loss.

The parenteral administration of iron. Iron dextran, e.g. Imferon (Fisons) may be given intramuscularly or intravenously and iron-sorbitol-citric acid complex stabilized with dextrin, e.g. Jectofer (Astra), may be injected intramuscularly. Usual daily dosage 100 mg iron, i.e. 2 ml Imferon or Jectofer or 1·5 mg/kg body weight. One dose daily till haemoglobin normal. Considerable amount of intramuscularly injected iron remains in tissues and is slowly absorbed over months; may stain skin.

Total iron replacement therapy. In 70-kg person deficiency of 1 g haemoglobin per 100 ml blood needs approximately 300 mg iron for replacement of haemoglobin and iron stores. Amount of iron required for treatment may be very approximately calculated from this information. The calculated amount of iron needed may be given intravenously at rate of 200 mg/day. Care needed and admission to hospital advisable during treatment. Patients with large spleens may have considerable expansion of plasma volume and anaemia may be less marked than appears from haemoglobin value.

Anaemia due to Deficiency of Folic Acid or Vitamin B₁₂

Aetiology
Primary dietary deficiency. Dietary deficiency of vitamin B_{12} has been reported in vegans who eat nothing of animal origin, i.e. exclude from diet not only meat but eggs, milk, butter, etc. Such dietary deficiency may occur among those who by choice or necessity are vegetarians in tropics, especially those of poor means.

Dietary deficiency of folic acid less common in view of folic-acid content of green leaves which in many regions form substantial part of diet.
Conditioned or secondary deficiency

1. *In malabsorption syndromes.* Folic acid and vitamin B_{12} may not be absorbed and deficiency, especially of folic acid, may result.

2. *In infection with* Dibothriocephalus latus. If the worm is situated high up in the intestine, the human host may be deprived of vitamin B_{12} as a result of the worm absorbing it from the intestinal contents before host has opportunity to do so.

3. *In chronic haemolytic states.* Increased demand for folic acid created by increased haemopoiesis may lead to insufficiency. Sicklaemic states, thalassaemia, and chronic malaria most likely to be those responsible.

4. *In pregnancy.* Folic-acid and vitamin-B_{12} deficiency may occur possibly partly as a result of increased nutritional demands imposed by foetus, but also as a result of altered metabolism of these vitamins.

Epidemiology
Occurs throughout tropics and especially reported from India. Strict Hindus particularly vulnerable. Causes considerable problems, but not as important to the public health as iron-deficiency anaemia.

Clinical Features
Those of anaemia in general (*see* Iron-deficiency Anaemia, p. 297) with, in addition, greater tendency to glossitis, oesophagitis and gastro-intestinal upset, especially diarrhoea. In chronic vitamin-B_{12} deficiency signs of central nervous system involvement may occur though they have only been rarely reported.

Marrow in well-developed cases megaloblastic; in less severe degrees of deficiency some degree of arrest of nuclear development present and erythrocytic series of cells slightly larger than normal—macronormoblastic reaction. Mean cell volume usually increased above normal range of 82–92 fl. Erythrocyte diameters increased. MCHC normal unless coincident iron deficiency present.

Treatment
In cases of folic-acid deficiency usually best to start with intramuscular injection 50 mg folic acid, followed by folic acid tablets given orally, dose 5 mg once or twice daily till blood-picture completely restored.

If vitamin B_{12} deficient, usually give 1 mega unit (1000 µg) vitamin B_{12} parenterally and 100 µg weekly till blood picture normal.

Important to treat any coincident iron or protein deficiency.

Anaemia Secondary to Vitamin-C Deficiency

In severe vitamin-C deficiency states and when scurvy is present, a megaloblastic anaemia may result and respond to treatment with vitamin C. It is considered to result from interference in the metabolism of folic acid in which vitamin C plays a part.

Anaemia Secondary to Pyridoxine Vitamin-B₆ Deficiency

This is microcytic and similar to iron-deficiency anaemia but responds to pyridoxine—100–200 mg daily.

Anaemia associated with Protein Malnutrition

Anaemia has been recognized as an accompaniment of kwashiorkor and other syndromes caused by protein malnutrition since these syndromes were first described. The anaemia was first considered to result from the protein deficiency, then iron, folic acid, and other coexisting deficiencies were thought to be responsible, but evidence has accumulated indicating that protein deficiency is in considerable measure responsible. It is often complicated by other deficiencies.

Blood Picture
In these cases erythrocytes tend to be broad but thin, giving the appearance of poorly filled macrocytes, and hence some cases have been confused with anaemia due to coincident deficiency of iron and a specific haemopoietic factor such as folic acid or vitamin B_{12}.

Haemoglobin values commonly around 8 g% and MCHC normal, i.e. $34\% \pm 2\%$. Serum albumin low.

Marrow usually normoblastic, but may exhibit slight maturation arrest of erythrocytic series of cells.

Treatment
High-protein diet and attention to any other coincident deficency or infection.

It has been shown that high-protein diet may cause expansion of plasma volume with consequent haemodilution which masks improvements in blood picture. Dietary treatment must be continued for several weeks.

Haemolytic Anaemias

Haemolytic Anaemia in Infection
1. May result from direct invasion of erythrocyte by infecting agent, e.g. malaria or bartonella.
2. Recently shown that haemolytic anaemia occurs independently of erythrocyte invasion in malaria and some other protozoal infections, e.g. kala-azar and African trypanosomiasis.

Pathogenesis

An immune reaction involving complement deposition on erythrocyte surface. Erythrophagocytosis in such anaemia underlies much of the splenomegaly in these infections and is likely to be the basis of some of the 'big spleen' syndromes associated with malaria and other parasitic infections.

Haemoglobinopathies

Sickle-cell Anaemia and Sickle-cell Trait

Aetiology

Structure of haemoglobin genetically determined according to classical Mendelian principles. Haemoglobin molecule is composed of 4 chains of amino acid residues, two of the chains designated α have 141 amino acids and two designated β have 146 amino acids. A single substitution changes normal to abnormal haemoglobin and in sickle-cell haemoglobin (HbS) this is of valine for glutamic acid in the 6th position of the β chain. This abnormal haemoglobin may be designated $\alpha_2\beta_2^s$, or $\alpha_2^A\beta_2^s$ in contrast to the designation for haemoglobin A which is $\alpha_2\beta_2$ or $\alpha_2^A\beta_2^A$. The letter 'S' right superscript to the letter β indicates that the abnormality is on the β chain.

Each of the paired chromosomes in man has on it approximately 3000 genes situated at fixed points (loci); two genes determine each character, one on each chromosome. Thus synthesis of haemoglobin A controlled by pair of genes for α chains and pair for β chains. Genes for the different haemoglobin chains are alleles, i.e. can only occupy their own exclusive position. If paired genes are identical for a character, e.g. HbS, the person is said to be homozygous for that character; if they differ he is heterozygous. A person homozygous for HbS will have no HbA in his blood and will be said to have sickle-cell anaemia; a person heterozygous for it will have approximately 50% of his haemoglobin in the A form and 50% in the S form and will be said to have the sickle-cell trait.

Epidemiology

Gene found only among those of the Negro race or Negroid extraction and particularly prevalent in areas where incidence of *Plasmodium falciparum* malaria is high. Sicklaemia affords partial protection against malaria and enables proportionately more children with sicklaemia than normal children to survive the first year or two of life in which malarial mortality is highest. After this period, acquired partial immunity exceeds in effect resistance conferred by sicklaemia and no difference in malarial morbidity or mortality discernible between sicklers and non-sicklers.

Up to 20–25% of indigenous inhabitants of coastal regions of West Africa possess the sickling gene, and among Baamba in East Africa sickling rates of up to 45% have been reported.

In regions of low malarial endemicity the gene tends to be eliminated as it is there a disadvantage rather than an advantage to the possessor.

Pathology

Basic pathological processes. Two basic processes are haemolysis and infarction. Both result from formation, when HbS is deoxygenated, of intracellular tactoids, semicrystalline structures of elongated form that distort the erythrocyte causing it to assume at first a demi-lunar and later a crescentic shape. The distortion ruptures erythrocytes, hence causing haemolytic anaemia, and the distorted cells may also form tangled masses instead of sliding over one another intravascularly and hence intravascular thrombi form and produce infarcts.

Bone marrow. Marrow hyperplastic unless an aplastic crisis develops, sometimes from folic-acid insufficiency. Hyperplastic red marrow of skull and long bones erodes cortex leaving behind islets of unabsorbed bone causing 'hair-on-end' appearance radiologically.

Erythrocytes. Erythrocytes when unsickled are thin and target cells may be present. Osmotic fragility decreased.

Spleen. Spleen enlarged in childhood; later becomes fibrotic from repeated infarction and shrinks. Enlarged spleens are congested and sinuses and Malpighian corpuscles compressed. Infarcts commonly form in it.

Liver. Liver large, sinusoids congested, and Kupffer cells enlarged due to erythrophagocytosis. Plasma bilirubin usually increased.

Infarction. Intravascular thrombi affect particularly spleen, liver, lung, kidney and long bones, especially head of femur, and the choroid and retina of the eye.

Foetal haemoglobins. At birth 80% haemoglobin of normal persons is foetal or haemoglobin F, consisting of two α chains and two γ chains, the latter taking the place of the β chains in haemoglobin A (haemoglobin F therefore is $\alpha_2\gamma_2$). Ability to produce haemoglobin F rapidly declines with age in normal persons; at 6 months only 5% haemoglobin normally is F and in adult life less than 3%. In sicklers who cannot produce normal β chains, production of γ chains continues into adult life and haemoglobin F may then constitute up to 50% of the haemoglobin possessed. Haemoglobin F resists action of alkalis better than haemoglobin A and its presence may be detected by this characteristic. *N.B.* (1) The presence of alkali-resistant haemoglobin suggests the presence of foetal haemoglobin—it is not proof of its presence. (2) Foetal haemoglobin may be increased in thalassaemia and other haemoglobinopathies.

Clinical Features

The sickle-cell trait. Usually persons so affected are symptom-free and live normal lives, the haemoglobin value being within the normal range but erythrocytes sickle when oxygen tension reduced, e.g. when patient is at high altitudes or when blood flow is impeded. Flying with recognized airlines very seldom subjects persons to sufficient anoxaemia to cause erythrocytes of trait carrier to sickle.

Small thrombi may form in kidneys, lung and brain of persons with sickle-cell trait. In kidneys thrombi may cause haematuria. Loss of tubular function leads to impairment in power of concentrating urine.

Infants and young children with sickle-cell trait are more resistant to *Plasmodium falciparum* infections than normal children and this may help them to survive years when mortality from malaria is greatest. Later acquired immunity to malaria usually overshadows resistance conferred by sickling trait.

Sickle-cell anaemia. Child develops normally until end of first year of life, by which time foetal haemoglobin dropped to level at which it fails to protect against effects of sickling. Anaemia and painful limbs develop.

Painful limbs often confused with rheumatism. Are usually due to infarction of bone and may be accompanied by swelling over affected bone; in young children phalanges often affected, long bones in older children. Infarcts near joints may cause effusion.

Haemolytic crises occur especially after fever. Haemoglobin falls to especially low level; jaundice develops, spleen and liver enlarge, may reach umbilicus or below. Infarcts of either not uncommon.

Between crises blood picture of slightly microcytic normochromic anaemia. In blood film many target cells and usually a few sickled cells. Prolonged haemolysis causes drain on folic acid for haemoglobin production and megaloblastic change in marrow may occur.

'Milestones' delayed, child underdeveloped.

Cardiac enlargement usual and exercise tolerance diminished.

Occlusion of branches of retinal artery causes retinal damage and bleeding into eye. Leg ulcers common and in males priapism.

Aggravation of symptoms or complications may be brought on by fever from any cause or by dehydration, acidosis, hypoxia or large alcohol consumption.

Diagnosis
Suspect sickle-cell anaemia in Negro children with anaemia, 'rheumatism', hepatosplenomegaly, and especially if history of recurrent abdominal pains.

Tests. Seal drop of blood under cover-slip using petroleum jelly. As cells use up oxygen sickling occurs. Process accelerated by adding a drop of 2% solution sodium metabisulphite. The Sickledex test (Ortho) is a convenient rapid method. It utilizes the principle that deoxygenated sickle haemoglobin is relatively insoluble.

Haemoglobin electrophoresis on paper or starch gel. Haemoglobin S moves more slowly than haemoglobin A, more rapidly than haemoglobin C.

If haemoglobins S and A present, patient has sickle-cell trait. If S and no A present, either patient has sickle-cell anaemia or sickle-cell thalassaemia.

In most haemoglobinopathies percentage of foetal haemoglobin increased and especially so in sickle-cell anaemia and sickle-cell thalassaemia. Detected by alkali-denaturation.

Prognosis
In sickle-cell anaemia 5–30% survive into adult life. Prognosis improved by prevention of fever producing infections. Longer child survives, usually the milder the disease becomes.

Treatment
Maintain good nutrition and hygiene. Prevent infections wherever possible as by malaria prophylaxis. Treat infections promptly. Beware especially of upper respiratory infection. Patient may be immunologically compromised by fibrosed, almost non-functioning, spleen.

Folic acid, 5–10 mg daily, if signs of megaloblastic change in marrow present.

Blood transfusion may be needed in crises and before surgical operations or parturition.

During anaesthesia ensure good oxygenation.

Sickle-cell Haemoglobin C Disease

Aetiology
Results from inheritance of S gene from one parent and C gene from the other.

Epidemiology
Found especially among West Africans in Ghana and Nigeria. Gene for haemoglobin C occurs with greatest frequency in Northern Ghana.

Pathology
Seldom any marked anaemia, haemoglobin usually 11 g% or more, yet erythrocytes sickle at oxygen tension very little lower than they do in sickle-cell anaemia. Hence tendency to form intravascular thrombi greater than in sickle-cell anaemia in which there are usually fewer erythrocytes available to sickle. Thrombosis of, or haemorrhage from retinal vessel relatively common. Red blood cells usually microcytic and thin; many target cells.

Clinical Features
Similar to those of sickle-cell trait, but tendency to develop infarctive lesions is greater.

Diagnosis
Often not recognized till patient has an operation when sickling complications develop. Early recognition of the disease therefore important.
    Sickling test as in sickle-cell anaemia.
    Haemoglobin electrophoresis—haemoglobin C moves very slowly, more so than haemoglobins S and E. Examine parents and relatives to complete genetic study.

Prognosis
Good; life seldom jeopardized.

Treatment and Management
As for sickle-cell anaemia and trait.

Other Aberrant Haemoglobins
Haemoglobin D is found principally in Sikhs and Gujaratis and causes no clinical abnormality, but sickle-cell haemoglobin D disease confers a greater tendency to morbidity than the sickle-cell trait alone.
    Haemoglobin E occurs principally in India and Far East. Homozygous inheritance may cause syndrome with splenomegaly, hepatomegaly, joint pains and icterus due to mild anaemia. Many target cells present.
    Possession of other haemoglobins usually confers no clinical abnormality. Is detected by haemoglobin electrophoresis.
    Haemoglobins C, E, S, D, L, G and F move more slowly than haemoglobin A at pH 8·6, though haemoglobins G and F have a mobility so close to haemoglobin A that special expertise is needed to detect the difference. Haemoglobins K, J, I and H move more rapidly than haemoglobin A.

Thalassaemia

Aetiology
Caused by inheritance of gene which suppresses formation of the ordinary but not the variant α or β haemoglobin chains. It is not allelomorphic to that for haemoglobin S and other haemoglobin variants, thus the thalassaemia gene can

be inherited as well as those for two haemoglobins, e.g. A and S; in the latter case formation of most haemoglobin A would be suppressed and the patient might be thought to have sickle-cell anaemia.

Epidemiology
β-Thalassaemia is commonest in Mediterranean countries and a synonym is 'Mediterranean anaemia'.

α-Thalassaemia is commonest in China and Far East. Cases have been reported from India and Burma.

Pathology
The α-thalassaemia gene suppresses the formation of the α chains of haemoglobin and the β-thalassaemia gene the β haemoglobin chains. Inheritance homozygously of α-thalassaemia is incompatible with life and leads to stillbirth or death a few minutes after birth. Infant exhibits features similar to hydrops foetalis due to Rh or ABO blood group incompatability. Formation of all the normally present haemoglobins is suppressed thus:

$$\text{Haemoglobin A} = \cancel{(\alpha/_2)}\ \beta_2.$$
$$\text{Haemoglobin A}_2 = \cancel{(\alpha/_2)}\ \delta_2.$$
$$\text{Haemoglobin F} = \cancel{(\alpha/_2)}\ \gamma_2.$$
$$\cancel{(/)} = \text{suppression.}$$

The β and γ chains continue to be formed and may combine into molecules known as tetramers, consisting either of four β or four γ chains; thus β_4 = haemoglobin H and γ_4 = haemoglobin Bart's.

Heterozygous inheritance of the α-thalassaemia gene leads to partial suppression of formation of haemoglobins A, A_2, and F with an excess of β chains, which form so-called haemoglobin H and particularly in early life an excess of γ chains forming haemoglobin Bart's.

Homozygous inheritance β-thalassaemia gene causes complete suppression only of the formation of haemoglobin A thus:

$$\text{Haemoglobin A} = \alpha_2\ \cancel{(\beta/_2)}$$
$$\text{Haemoglobin A}_2 = \alpha_2\ \delta_2.$$
$$\text{Haemoglobin F} = \alpha_2\ \gamma_2.$$
$$\cancel{(/)} = \text{suppression.}$$

Haemoglobins A_2 and F continue to be formed in amounts greater than normal.

Heterozygous inheritance of β-thalassaemia gene causes mild pathological states with partial suppression of haemoglobin A formation.

Erythrocytes thin and misshapen with many target cells. They have a shortened life span and haemolytic anaemia present.

Clinical Features
Those of chronic haemolytic anaemia, degree of severity depending on the pathological state present—*vide supra*. MCV and MCH diminished. Splenomegaly, tendency to leg ulcers.

Bone changes as in sickle-cell anaemia except that infarction of tissues other than spleen is uncommon. Chronic haemolytic anaemia increases demand for folic acid.

Diagnosis
By microcytosis, target cells, family study where possible, and haemoglobin electrophoresis. Haemoglobin A_2 increased in β thalassaemia; moves very slowly in electrophoretic studies; mobility similar to haemoglobin C. Osmotic fragility of erythrocytes diminished.

Radiological appearances of bone similar to sickle-cell anaemia.

Treatment
Blood transfusion may enable survival till inevitable deposition of iron in myocardium usually leads to cardiac failure and death in second or third decade. Treatment with desferrioxamine may postpone the fatal outcome.

Folic acid valuable.

Anaemia in Glucose-6-phosphate Dehydrogenase Deficiency

Aetiology
Deficiency of this enzyme results from a gene inherited on the X chromosome. There are two main varieties, the Mediterranean and, in Negroes, the A minus, but over 150 less common variants occur. As the gene is carried on the X chromosome the disease, like haemophilia, does not usually affect women unless they inherit, homozygously, genes on both of their X chromosomes. Haemolytic anaemia occurs when the defective erythrocytes are exposed to various compounds, especially drugs such as 8-aminoquinolines.

Epidemiology
Negro or A minus type commonest and may affect up to 20% of inhabitants in West and Central Africa. The Mediterranean variant is less common but usually causes more severe disease.

Full expression occurs in heterozygous males with no normal allele to exert its effect or in homozygous females, both of whose X chromosomes carry the gene.

Pathology
Older erythrocytes deficient of the A minus enzyme and all erythrocytes deficient of the Mediterranean variety disintegrate when exposed to certain drugs. These include 8-aminoquinolines, sulphonamides, some antipyretics and analgesics, sulphones, nitrofurans, phenylhydrazines, chloramphenicol, quinidine and the essential constituents of fava beans.

Haemolysis may be severe and cause haemoglobinuria or methaemoglobinaemia with marked icterus. Reticulocytosis follows haemolysis.

Clinical Features
Those of haemolytic anaemia with haemolytic jaundice and, in severe cases, haemoglobinuria. Renal complications, however, rare. Coexistent bacterial or viral infection aggravates haemolysis. Haemolysis following ingestion of fava beans develops particularly in the Mediterranean variety. Haemolysis tempor-

arily ceases when older erythrocytes haemolysed in A minus variety but continues as long as drugs and fava beans are taken in Mediterranean type.

Diagnosis
Heinz bodies found in erythrocytes during first few days of drug administration; they are denatured protein or methaemoglobin. Stain cells supravitally with crystal violet.

Most useful test is based on a colorimetric estimation of the enzyme (Berger, L. (1961), *Tentative Technical Bulletin*, No. 400, St. Louis, Mo., Sigma Chemical Company—this company produces a kit for performing the test).

Treatment
Avoid drug or beans to which sensitive. Blood transfusion, if anaemia warrants it.

9

Chapter 61

TROPICAL ULCER. TROPICAL SLOUGHING PHAGEDENA (Ulcus Tropicum; Naga Sore; Vincent's Ulcer)

Chronic sloughing ulcers usually on the legs occurring in hot moist climates.

Aetiology
Uncertain. Many organisms present, usually including *Treponema vincenti* and *Bacillus fusiformis*. Has not been transmitted. Nutritional factor possible.

Symptoms
Ulcer commences at an abrasion, often an insect bite: usually on ankle or leg. Painful papule or bulla: rapidly ruptures leaving ulcer with moist sloughing base. Edges inflamed and extended. Foul-smelling discharge. Usually superficial but may be deep. Glands enlarge. Constitutional symptoms vary. Heals after months with scarring and contractions. Rarely septicaemia and death.

Treatment
Difficult. Penicillin, locally and intramuscularly gives best results. Improvement in nutritional status.
Locally. Many systems advocated by enthusiasts. General principles: (1) remove infection chemically or mechanically; (2) allow healing by avoiding interference: hence occlusive dressings. Rest the part; (3) encourage epithelization, e.g. by skin grafts.
   Surgical excision later followed by grafting often shortens the duration of stay in hospital.

Prevention
Adequate early first-aid measures for every abrasion. Wearing protective clothing on legs.

Chapter 62

VENOMOUS ANIMALS

Venomous Fish

Many fish cause injury but three families are known to have caused death in humans: stingrays; weaver fish; and scorpion fish.

Stingrays

Stingrays (*Myliobatoidea*) are found in tropical and subtropical seas, especially in estuaries. They range in size from 25 cm to 4 m in length. they lie buried in sand, and most injuries result from stepping on them.

Venom. On the tail is a serrated spine enclosed in a sheath of skin and venom-secreting glands lie in ventrolateral grooves of the spine. When the barbed spine enters the victim, the sheath is torn and venom released.

Weaver Fish

Weaver fish (*Trachinidae*) are found in flat coastal areas of the Atlantic and Mediterranean. They are less than 45 cm long. They lie buried in mud or sand.

Venom. There are several dorsal spines with associated venom glands.

Scorpion Fish

Scorpion fish (*Scorpionidae*) are found in tropical and temperate seas. They have dorsal, anal and pelvic spines similar to weaver fish.

Clinical

Wound usually on foot or ankle. Severe instant pain radiating up the limb. Morphine often insufficient to relieve. The edges of the wound are pale, later cyanotic, and then red. Oedema develops. General symptoms are those of severe shock, nausea, sometimes diarrhoea, hypotension, dyspnoea and sometimes fever, convulsions, respiratory suppression.

Treatment

Careful wound toilet to remove pieces of spines or sheath. Hot fomentations or soaking in hot magnesium sulphate solution. Local injection of procaine hydrochloride, 2% will help to relieve pain. Tetanus toxoid and antibiotic should be given. Vigorous resuscitation with plasma expanders may be needed for shock. If the laceration is extensive it may be sutured if drainage is provided.

Jelly Fish (Coelenterates)

Coelenterates include hydroids, jelly fish, corals and sea anemones. For paralysing their prey, all have tentacles with special organs named nematocysts.

Colonial Hydroids

Colonial hydroids (*Siphonophora*) include Portuguese men-of-war. May produce painful weals on the skin.

Box Jellies or Sea Wasps

Box jellies or sea wasps (*Cubomedusae*) are found in all the warmer oceans, especially in sheltered bays. Most fatalities are due to them, and death may occur within 3 hours of contact with them.

Clinical

Initial pain like that of nettle, but sometimes much more severe. Contact with the tentacles shows as linear weals which may fade and disappear in a few hours or may vesicate. In severe cases there is vomiting, muscular pain and spasm, dyspnoea, and there may be pulmonary oedema with eventual paralysis of the centres in the brain stem.

Treatment
Any adherent tentacles should be removed. Application of alcohol or oil will prevent further discharge from nematocysts. Local and systemic antihistamines are useful, and in severe cases cortisone should be used. Treatment of shock, and ventilatory support where necessary. If muscle spasm is severe intravenous injection of 10 ml 10% calcium gluconate.

Molluscs (Conus)

About 400 species of *Conus* found in the Pacific and Indian oceans under rocks, on coral, or moving on sandy beaches. The shells are attractive, and so injury usually occurs on the hands.

Venom. Normally a neurotoxic venom is produced to capture fish, worms, etc. for food. There is a sheath containing teeth to which a duct comes from a venom-secreting gland.

Clinical
Either excruciating pain or localized numbness, with some ischaemia and cyanosis of the injured part. Numbness may spread over the whole body, especially around lips. Dysphagia, aphonia and salivation may occur. Sometimes pruritus occurs. Some fatalities recorded in which muscular paralysis followed by cardiac arrest occurred.

Treatment
Remove as much venom as possible by suction and promoting bleeding. Soaking the limb in hot water (120 °F) containing magnesium salt for 30–60 min may help.

Poisonous Insects

Centipedes
Centipedes (*Chilopoda*) are segmented insects having a pair of legs attached to each segment, but the appendages of the first segment form poison claws through which venom is injected. Larger ones may cause very painful bite, but is not fatal.

Millipedes
Millipedes (*Diplopoda*) resemble centipedes, but have two pairs of legs attached to each segment of the body. From pores in the sides of the body they produce an irritant fluid which may cause a vesicular dermatitis.

Treatment
The part should be washed and dressed with a local antihistamine cream. In the case of centipede bites infiltration with local anaesthetic will relieve pain.

Scorpions
These insects which vary in length from 1·2 cm up to 10–12·5 cm belong to several families. The most dangerous belong to a family called Buthidae, found in the warmer areas of the world, from southern USA to S. America, and from southern Europe to Australia. All are nocturnal in activity and most live in dry desert areas, but some are found in damp rain forests.

Venom. Produced by a gland in the terminal segments of the creature. A sting is present in its up-curved tail. Venom produces severe local pain. In some cases it is neurotoxic or haemolytic in effect. Fatalities may occur, especially in children.

Treatment
Local pain sometimes relieved by injecting procaine hydrochloride 2%, but in others a local injection of emetine hydrochloride, 65 mg, proves very effective. Rest, immobilization of the limb and application of a tourniquet may help to delay absorption of toxins.

Where systemic effects show themselves it is useful to try corticosteroids. Antiscorpion serum is prepared in some countries, and may prove useful.

Spiders
About 8 out of 2000 genera of spiders are probably poisonous to man. The bite of large non-venomous spiders may be secondarily infected, however. Fatalities are known to have occurred after bites with spiders of the following species: *Latrodectus, Loxosceles, Phoneutria* and *Atrax*.

Venom. Produced in paired venom glands, from which it is conducted to paired chelicerae which end in sharp fangs. Venom duct passes through each chelicera and opens on convex side near tip of fang.

Latrodectus or Black Widow Spider is widely distributed throughout the world, but is common in USA. Normally lives in holes in the ground, among stones, in long grass, or in outhouses or privies. In the male the venom-secreting glands diminish in size as maturity approaches, but in the female they increase and become more active.

Loxosceles is found in USA, Central and S. America. The female causes toxic bites. The spider may get into houses and hide under furniture or among clothing.

Phoneutria is found in S. America. *Phoneutria fera* is the species which has caused most fatalities, especially in children.

Atrax is found in Australia and Tasmania and it makes funnel-shaped webs. In this species the venom of the male is more toxic than that of the female.

Clinical
Black widow spider bite. Actual bite may be unnoticed, but severe, radiating pain develops. Muscular spasm both of the abdominal muscles and sometimes of the intercostals may occur, resulting in abdominal rigidity and in dyspnoea. The pain reaches a maximum in 3 h, but may persist for 2 days. There is nausea and profuse sweating. Abdominal pain may suggest an intra-abdominal perforation.

Loxosceles bite. Results in mild to severe pain lasting 2–8 h. Transient erythema occurs at the site. Venom may cause local oedema and necrosis. If much venom is absorbed, haemolytic changes, including haemoglobinuria and jaundice, can occur.

Phoneutria bite. Venom is neurotoxic, and respiratory, cardiac and visual disturbance may occur.

Atrax bite. No severe local pain or reaction but neurotoxic symptoms develop.

Treatment. Patient is kept at rest. Firm compression bandage helps reduce spread of toxin. Site is dressed with antiseptics. Chlorpromazine will help to relieve pain. If muscle spasm is marked intravenous injection of calcium gluconate 10% solution will help.

Local and systemic antihistamines may be used where there is rash or evidence of local necrotic change. Corticosteroids may prove useful, where serious neurotoxic symptoms develop.

Prevention
Danger of spider-bite is usually overemphasized. Where Black Widow spiders are known to occur field workers should wear gloves. General cleanliness of outhouses, and insecticide spraying of privies, etc., will help to discourage the insects.

Venomous Snakes

Of some 2400 species of snakes in the world about 300 species are known to be venomous to man. However, the danger of an infected lacerated or punctured wound from the bite of a non-venomous snake must be remembered.

Venom apparatus. Modified parotid gland produces venom which is carried by a duct to the upper jaw of the snake. Here certain maxillary teeth, known as fangs, are adapted for producing punctured wounds. In Colubrine snakes, fangs are situated posteriorly and the duct opens at base of fang. In Elapine snakes, fangs are fixed, situated in the front of the maxilla, and are grooved for conveying venom into the punctures. In Viperine snakes, fangs are situated in front of maxilla, but are attached to movable section which can be rotated forwards, so that fangs, normally enclosed in sheath of mucous membrane on roof of mouth, are erected and so more effective in puncturing. In addition, are cannulated so that venom is injected down fangs.

Colubrine snakes
These must obtain a wide bite on the part if fangs are to enter. Produce venom which is mainly neurotoxic in effect.

Hydrophinae
Hydrophinae or sea snakes have short, fixed and anteriorly placed fangs. Characterized by flattened paddle-like tail. These snakes are found in shallow coastal waters of Indian and Pacific Oceans. Venom is neurotoxic and myotoxic. Fortunately, these snakes are sluggish and though often caught by fisherman in nets off the Malayan coast, they rarely bite. Venom, however, very toxic.

Elapinae
Elapinae include cobras, kraits and mambas. Fangs are anteriorly placed, fixed and grooved. Snake is long with pointed tail, and small head with no distinct neck. Upper surface of head has several large scales. Venom is mainly neurotoxic in effect.

Viperinae
Viperinae or vipers are widely scattered in the world and are dangerous. Fangs are movable, cannulated and anteriorly placed. Venom is cytotoxic and usually haemolytic in effect. Vipers are short, stumpy snakes, head being triangular and with numerous small scales on its surface.

Crotalinae
Crotalinae or pit vipers include rattle-snakes, so-called because of several dry

rings on tail which produce a hissing noise when snake is irritated. The 'pit' is a small depression between eye and nostril on side of head of snake, known as a Loreal pit, which is a heat receptor assisting snake to find warm-blooded prey in darkness. Venom may be cytotoxic and haemolytic, but in some cases is neurotoxic.

Clinical

Estimated that there are about 40 000 deaths a year from snake bite throughout the world. Usually fear and shock-like symptoms after any snake bite whether or not venomous.

Colubrine envenomation. Little local effect. After several hours petechiae may appear and sometimes haemolytic effects. In some, however, centres in medulla and pons are affected, with ptosis, dysphonia and dysphagia, and then respiratory or cardiac arrest.

Elapine envenomation. Locally there may be tingling or numbness but in some cobra bites local necrosis may occur. Systemic changes occur rapidly with ptosis, unsteadiness, and dysarthria and dyspnoea. In some cases severe abdominal pain occurs. Pupils at first are small, but as bulbar signs develop pupils become dilated. If no systemic symptoms have developed within 24 h of a bite, fatal outcome is unlikely. However, minor systemic symptoms in first 24 h may be followed by latent period of 3–4 days after which death occurs.

Hydrophinae (sea snake) envenomation. Locally little evidence is found and there is not much pain in bitten area. However, within ½ h muscle stiffness and aching occur, and in 3–6 h after bite myoglobinuria is present. Leucocytosis over 20 000 cells/mm^3 occurs. Severe symptoms are those associated with medullary and pontine damage.

Viperine envenomation. Locally, marked changes with oozing of blood from punctures, early oedema of part, and much subcutaneous haemorrhage. Crops of blisters may develop and spreading local haemorrhagic necrosis of tissues may progress for several days. Systemically nausea and vomiting are frequent, and pulse is thready. There is pallor, dyspnoea and often dilated pupils. Sometimes haemorrhage from mucosal surfaces will result in haematemesis, melaena, haemoptysis and haematuria. Rarely, where fang punctures a vein and venom injected intravenously, almost instantaneous death may occur from intravascular clotting. Usually death occurs several days after bite from blood loss with heart failure, from gas gangrene, or from pneumonia.

Treatment

Immediate: Where bite is on limb a broad, firmly applied band which obstructs venous return may be of help in delaying absorption of venom. Arterial tourniquet may be applied following bites by neurotoxic elapids, sea snakes and Australasian snakes when delay in getting to medical care may be between 30 min and 2 h. Release tourniquet for 15 sec every 30 min. Do not keep on tourniquet more than total of 2 h.

Wash the surface of wound and apply an antiseptic dressing. Immobilize the part.

Hospital treatment: Admit to hospital. Observe for 24 h. Treat patient for shock. If haemorrhage has been considerable, carefully matched blood may be transfused. If there is dyspnoea or respiratory failure positive-pressure respiration and administration of oxygen may be needed. Occasionally tracheostomy will be required. A booster dose of tetanus toxoid will be needed. Large dose of antibiotic such as penicillin 1–2 megaunits should be given.

Antivenene should be administered if systemic effects appear, i.e. (1) hypotension or cardiovascular toxicity; (2) signs of myotoxicity or neurotoxicity; (3) impaired coagulation; or (4) impaired consciousness. Rapid spread of local swelling is indication for immediate administration of rattlesnake antivenom. Ideally, snake should be identified and monovalent antivenene given, but in most cases polyvalent antivenene against the commoner snakes of the district must be used. Up to 100 ml may be given by intravenous infusion in total volume of 500 ml with normal saline over 1 hour. Patient must be carefully observed during infusion, noting pulse, BP and respiratory rates. Anaphylactoid reactions are the most common during the infusion. Treat with subcutaneous adrenaline. Pyrogenic reactions may occur soon after infusion. Serum sickness reactions occur 5–10 days post-infusion. Give prednisolone 20 mg/day for 7 days also chlorpheniramine.

If patient is seen some time after bite, and no systemic effects are found, no antivenene should be given.

Prognosis
Depends on numerous factors: the larger the snake the more likely that large dose of venom was introduced, but if snake recently bit some creature, very little venom may have entered. Size of patient also makes a difference: children are at greater risk than adults. Finally, the speed with which effective treatment is given may make an important difference to the outcome.

Chapter 63   # HEAT-INDUCED DISORDERS

Heat Hyperpyrexia

Definition
Condition induced by exposure to high environmental temperature and characterized by high fever, clouding of consciousness, and, in late stages, by coma.

Aetiology
Predisposing factors. Age, very old or very young. Long-continued exposure to high temperature, continued physical exertion, unsuitable clothing, alcoholism and minor pyrexia induced by infection. Malignant hyperpyrexia precipitated by inhalation anaesthetics.

Precipitating factors. Exercise in hot, humid, relatively still air after body temperature already slightly raised is particularly potent cause. Sweat under such conditions not fully evaporated and therefore ineffective in reducing body temperature, and when this rises beyond critical level sweating may diminish, thus aggravating pyrexial stage. High environmental temperature and muscular work are the most important factors.

Symptoms

Sweating may cease, patient becomes restless and weak. Headache, lassitude, giddiness and tachycardia follow. Temperature rises to 40·5–43·5 °C (105–110 °F). Delirium, semiconsciousness and coma may ensue. Urine often contains trace of albumin.

Pathology

Almost all internal organs congested and many contain petechial haemorrhages. Cloudy swelling in myocardium, liver, kidneys. Spleen not enlarged and, if palpable, other causes of splenomegaly should be sought.

Complications

Include subarachnoid haemorrhage, respiratory and cardiac failure.

Prognosis

Always serious; mortality considerable. Greatest in alcoholics and those with intercurrent disease.

Treatment

Place stripped patient on bed covered with water-proof sheet; then either sprinkle tepid water on skin and direct fan on patient, or wrap in sheet which has been dipped in water of temperature 7 °C (45 °F) and rub patient with ice allowing only the sheet to intervene between the ice and patient's skin. Intermittently massage patient's skin vigorously to counter skin vasoconstriction which prevents heat loss.

While cooling patient, take rectal temperature at 10-min intervals and cease cooling when temperature drops to 39 °C (102 °F). Temperature will then usually continue to drop to normal. If it does not, cooling procedure to be recommenced.

Watch for and if necessary combat cardiac failure. Counter dehydration; i.v. chlorpromazine to counter agitation and shivering.

Important not to overlook malaria as a possible cause or coexisting infection in patients with hyperpyrexia. Antimalarial treatment may be given as soon as blood films have been taken.

Heat Exhaustion

Classic type of heat exhaustion is caused by salt deficiency, less commonly anhidrosis and water deficiency. Mixed syndromes may occur.

Salt-deficiency Heat Exhaustion *(Heat Exhaustion, Type I)*

Aetiology

Salt lost in sweat and if insufficiently replaced by diet of person sweating and drinking freely, depletion rapidly develops. Person of 70 kg weight has approximately 170 g sodium chloride in body and under conditions of maximal sweating may lose 35 g salt per day. Food eaten daily normally contains approximately 10–20 g salt and 5 g added as table salt, so considerable deficit possible, particularly if anorexia present. Considerable amounts of salt lost in vomit or diarrhoea if present.

Clinical Features

Symptoms. Lassitude develops early and is followed by muscular weakness, anorexia, nausea and vomiting, headache, giddiness, orthostatic fainting, muscular cramps, and, in very advanced cases, disorientation and hallucinations. Vomiting increases salt loss in early stages, large amounts of fluid excreted in urine to raise osmolarity of extracellular fluid; later oliguria or anuria.

Physical signs. Skin moist, inelastic, eyes become sunken in sockets. Pulse rapid, blood pressure low, systolic pressure less than 95 mmHg in moderately severe cases and may fall to 60–70 mmHg.

Laboratory findings. Urinary chlorides low (normal 5 g/L urine); plasma sodium low (normal 132–143 mEq/L), blood urea increased (normally not more than 40 mg/dl blood), plasma volume (normally 40–50 ml/kg body weight) diminished, and haemoconcentration marked.

Fantus test useful for recognition when full laboratory facilities not available. To 10 drops of urine add 1 drop 20% potassium chromate solution, then drop in 2·9% silver nitrate till fluid turns from clear yellow to opaque brown. Drops of silver nitrate used equivalent in number to grammes of chloride in a litre of the urine. Same pipette must be used throughout test to standardize size of drops and it must therefore be thoroughly washed in distilled water between each operation. Normally 5 g chloride per litre urine; in heat exhaustion this amount much reduced.

Prognosis

Good in early and moderate cases if treated by intravenous infusion. Poor in advanced cases and severe once oliguria and uraemia have developed.

Treatment

Intravenous infusion of isotonic saline essential once clear symptoms have developed. Oral administration of salt causes nausea and vomiting and may therefore aggravate depletion.

Slightly affected patients will complain of giddiness and fainting and require 1–4 L isotonic saline.

If moderately affected, will complain of lassitude, giddiness, fainting and anorexia. Will require 4–6 L isotonic saline. If severely depleted, will, in addition to above, be apathetic and perhaps stuporose, and systolic blood pressure will be less than 90 mmHg.

To infants, half-strength saline (i.e. containing 0·425% NaCl), brought up to isotonicity with glucose, should be used as it is easy to overcorrect saline deficiency in them.

During recovery, potassium may also be administered but should be given orally and sparingly, 1 g twice or three times daily for 2–3 days.

Control treatment by reference to clinical condition, blood pressure, and urinary chlorides.

Anhidrotic Heat Exhaustion (*Thermogenic Anhidrosis; Heat Exhaustion, Type II; and Anhidrotic Asthenia*)

Aetiology

Occurs in persons who have or have recently had 'prickly heat'; sweat glands may not secrete adequately and this predisposes to pyrexia. This, however, will not explain all cases and central control of sweating may also be affected.

Clinical Features
Patient complains of exhaustion and lassitude, headache, dizziness. Temperature usually does not rise above 39 °C (102 °F), skin exhibits mammillaria as sequelae of 'prickly heat'.

Treatment
Place patient in bed in cool room. Recovery almost invariably rapid.

Prickly Heat

Definition
Papular eruption affecting moist area of body and associated with pricking discomfort without constitutional disturbance.

Aetiology
Result of blockage of ducts of sweat glands by swollen stratum corneum.

Clinical Features
Marked pricking sensation and pruritus affecting particularly trunk and areas most endowed with sweat glands.
   Affected region exhibits roughness composed of numerous small papules— mammillaria. Later may be capped by vesicles.

Treatment
Remove to cool environment.

Other Heat Disorders

Circulatory Deficiency Heat Exhaustion
Results from vascular pooling in skeletal muscles of unacclimatized persons. Patient feels faint and has symptoms similar to those of salt deficiency heat exhaustion but salt deficiency not present.
   Recovery with rest and cooling.

Water Deficiency Heat Exhaustion
Caused by water deprivation and resultant cellular dehydration. Patient complains of thirst and lassitude but plasma volume little impaired and blood pressure maintained. Urinary output much reduced. No sodium deficiency and salt content of urine high.
   Recovery with administration of water. Absorption from intestine good in contrast to poor absorption in salt deficiency heat exhaustion with haemoconcentration and increased blood viscosity.

Chapter 64   # MISCELLANEOUS DISEASES

Endomyocardial Fibrosis (EMF)

Type of heart disease characterized pathologically by fibrosis of the endocardium, especially of ventricles.

Aetiology
Cause unknown. Filarial infection has long been suggested. Occurs most often between ages of 10 and 20 years. Found in hot damp areas, especially equatorial belt of Africa, in Brazil, Malaya and Sri Lanka.

Pathology
Either or both ventricles may be affected. Endocardium is thickened with fibrous tissue obliterating apex of ventricle, and embedding papillary muscles. Chordae tendineae become shortened and thus incompetence of mitral or tricuspid valve occurs. In severe cases right ventricular cavity is virtually obliterated and there is marked dilatation of right atrium.
Early stage: pericardial effusion. Foci of cytolysis are found in myocardium. Endocardium shows hyperaemia and there is inflammatory cellular infiltration. Later fibrosis occurs and even calcification.

Clinical
Probably a non-specific initial illness in children or adolescents with low fever, tachycardia, lasting some weeks. Later breathlessness, palpitation and pain over the liver develop. If left ventricle is most involved, there are signs of mitral incompetence often with pulmonary hypertension.

If right ventricle is most involved, there is tricuspid incompetence with chronic venous congestion. Jugular venous pulse shows a large systolic wave. More than half the patients develop atrial fibrillation. Clinical picture is usually confusing because of variability of most affected parts of heart.

Diagnosis
By cardiac angiography, echocardiography and endocardial biopsy which is now possible in properly equipped centres. Demonstration of much reduced ventricular capacity suggests diagnosis.

Treatment
Symptomatic and routine for heart failure. Surgical excision of endocardial fibrous tissue and prosthetic replacement of incompetent valves has been undertaken in UK. No specific treatment.

Ainhum

Localized chronic inflammatory disease affecting proximal phalanx or little or adjacent toes in adult men, and often resulting in spontaneous amputation.

Aetiology
Cause is not known. It has been suggested that it might be related to tertiary yaws.

Occurs in tropical areas, especially E. Indies, Central Africa and Central and S. America. Most often in adult males.

Pathology
Area of chronic inflammation around base of little toe with dense fibrous tissue in subcutaneous tissue producing ring-like constriction. Distal part enlarges and becomes spherical in shape. Eventually natural amputation occurs, or patient seeks treatment to remove the troublesome terminal part of toe. Rarely other toes affected, and very rarely it has affected little fingers.

Treatment
Local dressing. Some have tried incising the constricting band, without much success. Amputation under aseptic conditions is best.

Acute Infectious Lymphocytosis*

Aetiology
Usually in children, but adults not immune. Small epidemics occur.

Symptoms
Mild febrile symptoms. Upper respiratory tract symptoms or abdominal pain usual onset. *Cervical glands*: Moderate general enlargement.

Blood Changes
Simple absolute lymphocytosis. Mononuclear cells: *mature small lymphocytes throughout course*; no immature cells. *Leucocytosis*: 20 000–100 000/mm^3; in children often over 50 000.

Heterophil Agglutinins
Absent.

Rash
Present occasionally.

Course
Pyrexia may continue after general symptoms abate. Lymphocytosis persists for several weeks. No complication recorded. Recovery complete.

*Considered here for convenience.

Index